Brain Research in Language

LITERACY STUDIES

VOLUME 1

While language defines humanity, literacy defines civilization. Understandably, illiteracy or difficulties in acquiring literacy skills have become a major concern of our technological society. A conservative estimate of the prevalence of literacy problems would put the figure at more than a billion people in the world. Because of the seriousness of the problem, research in literacy acquisition and its breakdown is pursued with enormous vigor and persistence by experts from diverse backgrounds such as cognitive psychology, neuroscience, linguistics and education. This, of course, has resulted in a plethora of data, and consequently it has become difficult to integrate this abundance of information into a coherent body because of the artificial barriers that exist among different professional specialties. The purpose of the proposed series is to bring together the available research studies into a coherent body of knowledge. Publications in this series are intended for use by educators, clinicians and research scientists in the above-mentioned specialties. Some of the titles suitable for the Series are: fMRI, brain imaging techniques and reading skills, orthography and literacy; and research based techniques for improving decoding, vocabulary, spelling, and comprehension skills.

The titles published in this series are listed at the end of this volume.

Zvia Breznitz
(Editor)

Brain Research in Language

Springer

Zvia Breznitz
University of Haifa
Haifa 31905
Israel
zviab@construct.haifa.ac.il

Series Editor:
R. Malatesha Joshi
Texas A&M University
College Station, TX 77843
USA

Library of Congress Control Number: 2007935911

ISBN-13: 978-0-387-74979-2 e-ISBN-13: 978-0-387-74980-8

Printed on acid-free paper.

9 8 7 6 5 4 3 2 1

springer.com

CONTENTS

BRAIN RESEARCH IN LANGUAGE

Zvia Breznitz
Neurocognitive Research Laboratory, Faculty of Education, University of Haifa, Haifa 31905 Israel

The human brain has existed for approximately 60,000 years while the alphabetic code has been in use for only 5000 years. It can therefore be argued that the ability to read is not part of our evolutionary heritage, as no brain system was specifically developed for the purposes of reading. The reading process is a highly composite cognitive task, which relies on brain systems that were originally devoted to other functions. In most cases, the reading process is successful, but in some cases it is not. Reading involves the decoding and comprehension of printed materials. Word decoding implies the activation of different brain entities such as the visual and auditory modalities and the orthographic, phonological, and semantic systems. Each entity has a different function in the reading process, and each has a different biological structure. Each is activated in different brain areas, and each processes information in a different manner and at a different speed. In addition, as a cognitive process, reading is based on information processing mechanisms and requires highly complex information processing skills. As such, this cognitive activity varies along the different stages of the information processing system. During the input stage, attention, perception and discrimination of alphabetic symbols in the visual and acoustic modalities are required. In the processing stage, activation of these symbols in short term memory (STM) and working memory (WM) is necessary, as are interpretations and retrieval of alphabetic representations from long term memory (LTM) and the mental lexicon (ML). At this stage, the orthographic, phonological and semantic systems are activated. During the output stage, reading requires activation of various motor systems. This process ends with the reader's responses. The complex nature of this process poses a major challenge for the human brain, which proves too much for some readers.

The majority of studies in this area have implemented behavioral methodologies, which provide information concerning the entire cognitive sequence at the conclusion of processing only, in the reader's output. The reader arrives at this stage following the completion of sensory, cognitive and motor processes (Bentin, 1989). As such, behavioral measures cannot specify all of the covert component operations that contribute to reading, nor can they determine the relative processing times required by the individual stages. Furthermore, they cannot determine which processes occur serially, which occur in parallel and which overlap in time (Brandeis & Lehmann, 1994; Johnson, 1995). This makes it difficult to determine, on the basis of behavioral measures alone, the extent to which dysfunction or slowness at any particular stage of processing contributes to reading deficits.

However, recent advancements in the field of neuroscience and cognitive development have added a new dimension with regard to the research into the universal and domain specific aspects of reading with the advent of innovative neurophysiological measurement techniques. The most common are electroencephalography (EEG) and functional magnetic resonance imaging (fMRI). These two methods provide researchers with the opportunity to examine, in-depth, the neural correlates of the reading processing with precise temporal and spatial resolutions, respectively. EEG techniques assess on-line processing of the cognitive activity utilizing Event Related Potential (ERP) methodology. This method permits direct observation of information processing at different levels of analysis, and can provide crucial information by means of real-time imaging of the neural system's responses to sensory stimulation (Bentin, 1989). Thus, it enables us to trace on-line the speed at which information is processed during the various cognitive stages of the reading activity.

The fMRI method focuses on the source of brain activity with time resolution that is not sufficient to trace temporal brain activation during the reading process. Even though these two methodologies are complimentary, it is important to note that precise time measurement of temporal resolution is a critical factor in reading research, and as such, the advantage of EEG measurement is clear.

Tracing the source of brain activity during reading is crucial for understanding both the accurate and impaired process and led various researchers to focus on developing new approaches for estimating the source localization of brain activity from ongoing EEG measures during performance of cognitive tasks such as reading, i.e., Low Resolution Electromagnetic Tomography (LORETA). The extent to which this estimation is similar to fMRI results remains unclear.

The current book contains chapters based on a series of lectures given at the annual conference held by the Department of Learning Disabilities at the University of Haifa in June 2006 on "The Use of Brain Activity Measures in Reading Research." The lectures presented data obtained from various studies employing behavioral, electrophysiological and imaging methodologies in different languages focusing on the regular reading process and the dyslexic population.

The first two chapters review the use of imaging and electrophysiological techniques employing the Evoked Related Potential (ERP) methodology in reading research. Data from studies focusing on measuring the brain activity of regular and dyslexic readers is presented.

The first contribution by Breznitz and Lebovitz offers evidence from post-mortem, structural and functional imaging studies in which the brains of dyslexic individuals are compared to those of regular readers. As phonological processing is a key concept in our understanding of the regular and impaired reading process, the majority of studies in the field focus primarily on the nature of neural activity within the phonological system. Data concerning the effect of phonological intervention training on the brain activity of dyslexics are discussed. Moreover, based on the fact that reading is an act of perceiving printed materials from the printed page via the visual system, data from studies focusing on activation in the visual system are also presented.

The second chapter contributed by Shaul and Breznitz surveys the different ERP components characteristic of brain activity during the reading process as well as the compelling results stemming from studies implementing this technique. The aim of this review is to gain a better understanding of the underlying causes of reading as a temporal process among developmental dyslexics for the purpose of effective diagnosis and remediation.

The next three chapters deal with processing in the different sensory modalities (auditory and visual) in written language. In the third paper, Been et al, present a research study on the auditory processing of 5-month-old infants, as part of a national longitudinal research program in the Netherlands on developmental dyslexia. Using the ERP methodology, they examined infants using a speech stimulus, comparing infants from dyslexic families to those from non-dyslexic families, while awake, watching a silent video or asleep. The hypothesis was made based on a dynamic neuronal model which predicted that the P200 ERP component would be reduced in infants at risk for dyslexia. Indeed, amongst infants from dyslexic families, in both hemispheres a reduced P200 was found in the frontal-central-parietal regions. In particular, there was a greater reduction in P200 amplitude while sleeping. These findings support previous evidence regarding the elevated risk for dyslexia in children from families characterized by the disorder.

The fourth article by Pratt provides an overview of electro-physiological functional imaging results in dyslexic and regular readers, while processing different kinds of auditory stimuli. It is known that the auditory system is a basis for phonological processing and findings indicate that the brain is a parallel processor that copes simultaneously with numerous aspects of processed materials, adapting this processing with experience.

In the fifth chapter, Sommer and Hohlfeld focus on visual perception by reviewing a series of studies investigating the effects of additional visual tasks on the N400 ERP component during an overlapping task paradigm. These researchers suggest, on the basis of the findings discussed, that the dual-task methodology is a useful tool for investigating processes that support language perception as well as the retrieval of semantic knowledge. They suggest a model, which refers to the use of semantic knowledge as part of the central cognitive processes and its' bottleneck like nature, allowing only one piece of information to pass through it at a time.

In terms of higher order processing during the reading process, the next contribution by Kutas and Delong discusses the advantages of ERP research in general, and language processing in particular. In some instances, ERP measures are more sensitive than regular behavioral measures and therefore reveal differences that are otherwise not clear-cut. An additional strong point of the ERP measure is that it does not require an external response and allows careful monitoring of cognitive events due to high temporal resolution and temporal span. It is also a convenient and noninvasive tool, which is important when dealing with a wide range of subjects. The ERP measures revels how the brain can extract meaning from both auditory and visual linguistic stimuli. In particular, these measures are sensitive to linguistic processes such as comprehension and production, as well as those difficult to measure such as prediction.

The seventh chapter by Leiken reviews several ERP findings obtained from studies investigating the grammatical function of words among regular and dyslexic Hebrew-speaking adult readers. The findings suggest that while processing different aspects within sentences, all readers, both dyslexic and regular, are affected by the grammatical roles of target words. However, these two groups of readers demonstrated distinctly different strategies when identifying the grammatical functions of words in a sentence. These differences were apparent in ERP measures. Whereas regular Hebrew-speaking readers were more apt to use a predicate-oriented morphologically based strategy, dyslexic readers tended to use a word-order strategy, which was reflected in higher amplitudes and longer latencies of N100/P200, P300 and P600 components.

The chapter submitted by Goldstein, Arzouan, and Faust discusses the implementation of ERP components in the examination of figurative language, in particular metaphor comprehension. The ERP method is useful in recognizing the processing stages at which metaphorical meaning is reached, as well as the specific locations activated in the brain. In particular, it is claimed that ERPs elicited by novel metaphors differ from those evoked by conventional metaphors in terms of amplitude and scalp distribution. In terms of hemispheric differences in literal and figurative language comprehension, it was found that both hemispheres work in unison, creating a complex and dynamic pattern for language comprehension. Similarly, Zaidel, Hill, and Weems present a study in which behavioral and electrophysiological correlates of hemifield tachistoscopic presentations of single words and nonwords for lexical decision were compared in English and Hebrew. It was shown that EEG differentiates between the relevant dimensions of the task. In other words, all lexical variables had physiological correlates were usually not the same in both hemispheres. Thus, the EEG can detect early stages of processing, which are not part of conscious decisions and tap different stages of processing. In addition, hemispheric error monitoring in English was studied. Findings show that the left hemisphere is superior for lexical decision, whereas the right hemisphere monitored errors more efficiently by slowing down and becoming more accurate. Thus, effective monitoring requires interhemispheric cooperation.

The final chapter by Sinai focuses on the study of high frequency EEG activity with ERP components in language research by using an electrocorticographic (ECoG) technique in an attempt to study the dynamics of brain oscillations in a variety of language tasks. In particular, the synchronization in gamma brain waves. Findings suggest an interaction between gamma oscillations in macroscopic local field potentials (LFP) and the timing of the performance. The use of this method in clinical and neurophysiological research is discussed.

REFERENCES

Bentin, S. (1989). Electrophysiological studies of visual word perception, lexical organization, and semantic processing: A tutorial review. *Language and Speech, 32,* 205-220.

Brandeis, D., & Lehmann, D. (1994). ERP mapping: a tool for assessing language disorders. In: H. J. Heinze, T. F. Mante, & G. R. Mangun (Eds.), *Cognitive Electrophysiology* (pp. 242-250). Boston, MA: Birkhauser.

Johnson, R. (1995). Effects of color on children's naming of pictures. *Perceptual and Motor Skills, 80,* 1091-1101.

1

NEUROBIOLOGICAL CORRELATES OF DYSLEXIA

A Review

Zvia Breznitz and Lilach Lebovitz

Neurocognitive Research Laboratory, Faculty of Education, University of Haifa, Haifa 31905 Israel

Abstract: The selective impairment of reading skills that characterizes dyslexia is a source of difficulty for children and adults in literate societies worldwide. As part of the increasing effort to reveal the underlying causes of this disorder, post-mortem and imaging methodologies are being used to study the neural structures and mechanisms of dyslexics. The following review presents post-mortem, structural and functional imaging studies comparing the brains of dyslexic individuals to those of normal readers, focusing particularly on the nature of neural activity at the levels of phonological processing (awareness) and reading, on underlying deficits in the sensory-linguistic transfer of information at the phonological level, and on representational (processing) deficits in the visual pathways of dyslexics. Findings from the post-mortem and structural imaging studies presented attest to various configurational changes associated with dyslexia, particularly in terms of altered hemispheric asymmetry. Research employing functional imaging methods has added to these findings, revealing characteristic changes in neural activation patterns during performance of various sensory and phonological tasks related to reading processes. While a number of brain systems, incorporating frontal, temporal and posterior areas, are shown to be associated with dyslexia, no single mechanism is consistently implicated, such that agreement has yet to be reached regarding the neural basis of the disorder.

Key words: developmental dyslexia, neuroimaging studies, phonological processing

1. INTRODUCTION

Developmental dyslexia can be viewed as a selective impairment of reading skills, specifically of word recognition (Lovett, 1987; Stanovich, 1991), despite normal intelligence, visual acuity, motivation, and instruction (Galaburda & Livingstone, 1993). There is a high incidence of developmental dyslexia (5-10%) in most known languages. In literate societies, a considerable disability results as reading deficits persist into adulthood.

Poor readers are characterized by slow and inaccurate word recognition (BPS, 1999), and many researchers agreed that dyslexia is based on deficits in the phonological system (Adams, 1990). More recent data indicate that deficits can also be seen in orthographic (Terepocki, Kruk, & Willows, 2002) or fluency-related systems (Breznitz, 2001; Wolf & Katzir-Cohen, 2001).

Many researchers agree that dyslexia has a neuro-developmental basis (Hynd & Semrud-Clikeman, 1989). However, the exact nature of the neural deficit underlying this impairment remains the subject of considerable debate. In an attempt to explore the origins of the dyslexia phenomenon over the past 30 years, various research teams have employed post mortem and brain imaging techniques to investigate neural activity patterns in dyslexic individuals and to study the activity of different brain systems in developmental dyslexia. These studies have focused on three principal issues, all of which are of great relevance to understanding the pathophysiology of dyslexia:

1. The nature of the neural activity signature for dyslexia at the level of phonological processing (awareness) and reading.
2. The underlying neural activity deficits in the sensory-linguistic transfer of information at the phonological level.
3. The nature of the representational (processing) deficits in the visual pathways of adult dyslexics.

Within the context of these issues, a central question underlying much of the research on the neurobiology of dyslexia pertains to whether the neural routes utilized by dyslexics in the reading process are the same routes employed by normal readers, though not as efficiently, or whether different, alternative routes come into play. In the present review, relevant findings from post mortem and imaging studies on these three issues will be presented.

2. POST-MORTEM STUDIES

Galaburda and his colleagues have performed the only comprehensive post-mortem studies of diagnosed cases of developmental dyslexia (Galaburda, Sherman, Rosen, Aboitiz, & Geschwind, 1985; Galaburda & Livingstone, 1993; Galaburda, Menard, & Rosen, 1994; Humphreys, Kaufmann, & Galaburda, 1990; Jenner, Rosen, & Galaburda, 1999; Livingstone, Rosen, Drislane, & Galaburda, 1991). All five cases (one female and four males) showed evidence of small areas of cortical dysgenesis (called ***microdysgenesis***) including ectopias (small nests of abnormally placed neurons) and dysplasia (focally distorted cortical lamination). The microdysgeneses varied in number and location from brain to brain but tended to involve the language-relevant perisylvian cortex. Furthermore, the observed structural deviances in the male specimens tended to be lateralized, selectively affecting the left hemisphere (Galaburda et al., 1985), whereas in the female brain a fairly symmetric distribution was observed (Humphreys et al., 1990; NB: specimen ORT-20-87). Because ectopias and dysplasias are found only rarely in routine autopsy analyses (or in other developmental disorders), usually omit perisylvian regions, and are located more frequently in the right side of the brain than in the left, Galaburda (1988, 1989, 1993; Sherman & Galaburda, 1999) considered the malformations to be specifically associated with dyslexia. According to Galaburda, the microdysgenesis might reflect neuronal migration errors that occurred during fetal development.

Changes in the pattern of hemispheric asymmetry of the planum temporale were also seen in dyslexic brains. The *planum temporale* is a triangular landmark situated on the supratemporal surface, just posterior to the first Heschl's gyrus inside the sylvian fissure. The left *planum* coincides with part of Wernicke's speech comprehension area (e.g., Galaburda, 1993; Shapleske, Rossell, Woodruff, & David, 1999). Large-scale post-mortem studies (Geschwind & Levitsky, 1968; Wada, Clarke, & Hamm, 1975), each including 100 normal adult brains, found that the *planum* was symmetrically sized between the hemispheres in 16% of specimens, whereas 10.5% showed a rightward and 73.5% a leftward asymmetry. Corresponding figures reported on 307 normal fetal or neonatal specimens were 29%, 16%, and 54% (Chi et al., 1977; Wada et al., 1975). Consequently, the *planum temporale* is thought to be an important substrate of left-hemisphere language lateralization (Geschwind & Levitsky, 1968; Wada et al., 1975). Returning to the five dyslexic brains (Galaburda et al., 1985; Humphreys et al., 1990), none was reported to show the typical planar asymmetry favoring the left side. Instead, these specimens exhibited symmetry due to an enlarged right-hemisphere *planum.* Galaburda et al. (1987) propose that symmetry reflects reduced cell death in the right *planum temporale* during late fetal development, which leads to enhanced survival of neurons and the formation of improper connections, resulting in a redefinition of the cortical architecture.

Another set of post-mortem examinations was performed on thalamic structures, specifically the lateral geniculate nucleus (LGN) of the visual pathway and the medial geniculate nucleus (MGN) of the auditory pathway. The magnocellular layers of the LGN were found to be more disorganized in dyslexic than in non-dyslexic brains (Livingstone et al., 1991). Furthermore, magno cell bodies were on average 27% smaller and appeared more variable in size and shape in the brains of dyslexic individuals relative to those of controls. Neither the parvocellular lamination nor the parvo cell sizes of the LGN differed between the population specimens. With respect to the auditory system, Galaburda et al. (1994) reported significantly smaller MGN neurons on the left side, compared with the right, in the same dyslexic autopsy specimens. No hemispheric asymmetry in MGN neuronal size was observed in ordinary brains. In addition, the brains of the dyslexic individuals were said to exhibit a relative excess of small neurons and a relative paucity of large neurons on the left side as compared to control brains. According to Galaburda et al. (1994), the structural deviances found in the LGNs of dyslexic brains are likely to be associated with slowness in early segments of the magnocellular channels, whereas the MGN differences may be related to the auditory temporal processing abnormalities described in language-impaired children.

Autopsy data on neuronal tissue in the primary visual cortex (area 17) were presented in a recent work by Jenner et al. (1999). In contrast to the atypical organization found in the magnocellular layers of the LGN, the dyslexic brains did not show consistent changes in the size of cortical neurons receiving thalamic input. The researchers suggested that this inconsistency might be due in part to blending of magnocellular and parvocellular pathways or to functional effects of cortico-cortical top-down projections. On the other hand, another example of changes in hemispheric asymmetry similar to those found in the *planum temporale* was observed. Primary visual cortex in the brains of non-dyslexic individuals contained larger neurons in the left hemisphere than in the right, whereas dyslexic brains showed no such lateralization. According to Jenner et al. (1999), neuronal symmetry in primary visual cortex is associated with abnormality in circuits involved in reading.

To date, Galaburda's group has presented autopsy data on nine brains of individuals (six males and three females) with a history of developmental dyslexia. Three of the male and one of the female patients were reported to have histories of delayed language acquisition (Galaburda et al., 1985; Humphreys et al., 1990). All dyslexic brains have displayed evidence of symmetric *plana temporali* (Galaburda, 1988, 1989; Humphreys et al., 1990). Neuronal ectopias and architectonic dysplasias were observed in all male cases and in two of the females (Galaburda, 1993). Other cerebrocortical deviances in dyslexic autopsy specimens such as microgyria and cortical scars were less uniform than the pattern of microdysgenesis (Galaburda, 1993). Overall, dyslexic female brains showed fewer and differently located microcortical malformations when compared to male brains (Humphreys et al., 1990). Histological differences in thalamic structures and the primary visual cortex are hitherto limited to reports on five dyslexic brains versus five (Jenner et al., 1999; Livingstone et al., 1991) or seven control brains (Galaburda et al., 1994). In interpreting the study results, Galaburda (1988, 1989, 1993; Galaburda et al., 1994) has hypothesized that dyslexia is an outcome of anomalous neural development, which might derive from brain injury during the prenatal stage. In this proposition, the chemical environment and maturation rate of relevant brain areas are assumed to interact.

To complete the picture, two post-mortem findings in language-impaired children should be briefly mentioned. Landau, Hoien, Lundberg, and Odegaard (1960) observed bilateral perisylvian cystic lesions with surrounding dysplasias and severe retrograde degeneration in the MON in a single male brain. In a female autopsy specimen, Cohen, Campbell, and Yaghmai (1989) found a dysplastic microgyrus in the left insular cortex and decreased asymmetry of the *plana temporali.*

Despite the robustness of most of the findings provided by Galaburda and his colleagues, there are methodological issues complicating the interpretation of their results. For instance, many of the dyslexic subjects had a history of comorbid disorders or prior head injuries, which would have prevented their participation in neuro-imaging studies (Galaburda et al., 1985; Humphreys et al., 1990). Furthermore, the number of autopsy specimens examined is small.

In a recent neuroanatomical study, Finch, Nicolson, and Fawcett (2002) examined the differences between the olivo-cerebellar path-ways of adult dyslexics and regular readers. A significant difference in mean cell area in medial posterior cerebellar cortex was identified, with the cells from dyslexic brains having a larger mean area than corresponding cells from normal readers. Furthermore, analysis of cell size distributions not only confirmed the significant differences in the posterior lobe, with an increased proportion of large neurons and fewer small neurons for the dyslexics, but also revealed a similar pattern of significant differences in the anterior lobe. Although it was not a large sample, the neuroanatomical data established from this study provides converging evidence of cerebellar abnormality in dyslexia.

3. NEUROIMAGING STUDIES

Based on neurobiological and cognitive theories, structural as well as functional brain- imaging studies in dyslexic individuals have focused on the areas subserving language. Because findings of atypical cortical asymmetry in known language regions may be related to deviances in interhemispheric transfer of information, the morphology of the *corpus callosum* has been another point of interest.

3.1 Structural Neuroimaging

Magnetic Resonance Imaging (MRI) studies have shown that individuals with dyslexia have a higher incidence of reduced or reversed asymmetry of temporo-parietal language regions than exhi-bited in the normal population (Dalby, Elbro, & Stodkilde-Jorgensen, 1998; Duara et al., 1991; Hynd, Semrud-Clikeman, Lorys, Novey, & Eliopulos, 1990; Kushch et al., 1993; Larsen, Hoien, Lundberg, & Odegaard, 1990; Robichon, Levrier, Farnarier, & Habib, 2000; Rumsey et al., 1986). Similar to the post-mortem findings of Galaburda and his colleagues, MRI studies have demonstrated atypical asymmetry (i.e., right = left or right > left) of the ***planum temporale*** in dyslexic individuals (Hynd et al., 1990; Larsen et al., 1990; Flowers, 1993). Larsen et al. (1990) found that 13 out of 19 dyslexic adolescents displayed symmetric *plana* as compared to only 5 out of 17 normal readers. Among the dyslexic readers exhibiting "pure phonological dysfunction" (p.297), none showed the typical leftward asymmetry of the *planum.* This led the authors to hypothesize that symmetrical *plana temporali* are a possible neural substrate for phonological processing impairments in developmental dyslexia. It is noteworthy that the source of symmetry differed among the studies. Larsen et al. (1990) and Flowers (1993) attributed the atypical asymmetry of the *planum temporale* to an increase in size on the right side (consistent with Galaburda's post-mortem results), while Hynd et al. (1990) showed differences resulting from shorter left *planum* length.

More recent MRI research has challenged the view of altered planar asymmetry in dyslexia (Best & Demb, 1999; Heiervang et al., 2000; Leonard et al., 1993; Robichon et al., 2000; Rumsey et al., 1997b; Schultz et al., 1994). For instance, Leonard et al. (1993) reported an exaggerated leftward asymmetry in a small group of compensated dyslexics compared with unaffected relatives and controls. Best and Demb (1999) observed that dyslexic adults with a magnocellular pathway deficit did not depart from the left-lateralized *planum temporale* type. According to Best and Demb, planar asymmetry may be associated with a subgroup of dyslexia.

With respect to Broca's area, Robichon et al. (2000) obtained similar results in 16 adult male dyslexics. Other MRI studies, targeting primarily posterior language regions, revealed no changes in *planum* lateralization among dyslexic subjects (Heiervang et al., 2000; Preis, Jaencke, Schittler, Huang, & Steinmetz, 1998). Analyzing the vertical part of the *planum,* the posterior ascending ramus (PAR) or so-called ***planum parietale***, Heiervang et al. (2000) found that dyslexic boys were less likely to show the expected rightward asymmetry than normally reading controls.

Leonard et al. (1993) reported a higher incidence of added gyri between the postcentral sulcus and PAR in a group of compensated dyslexics. Recent findings (Leonard et al., 2001) have further specified the significance of the abnormal gyral morphology of the *planum* and adjacent gyral structures. MRI scans of 13 dyslexic college students revealed greater leftward asymmetry of the summed planum and PAR areas among phonological dyslexics but not among control subjects and subjects with other types of reading deficits.

These findings led to the conclusion that this greater planar and PAR asymmetry is one of four anatomical measures differentiating phonological dyslexia from other unspecified reading deficits (the other three are 1. marked rightward cerebral asymmetry, 2. marked leftward asymmetry of the anterior lobe of the cerebellum, and 3. large duplication of Heschl's gyrus on the left). When normalized and summed, these anatomical measures predict short and long term phonological capabilities. Another differentiating anatomical measure, low cerebral volume, predicted oral and written comprehension skills among phonological dyslexics.

In contrast, the results of studies by Hiemenz and Hynd (2000) and Robichon et al. (2000) failed to support a possible association between sulcal pattern morphology and diagnosis of developmental dyslexia.

In summary, various changes in perisylvian-language regions have been reported in dyslexia. A very small number of studies, including some on families affected by language-based learning impairments, suggest that certain perisylvian deviances might increase the risk of developing problems in learning language. However, there has been no brain structure for which MRI findings have been replicated consistently. The *planum temporale* has been the most prominent landmark investigated in dyslexia. While some studies have indicated reduced or absent left-right planar asymmetry in dyslexic individual, others have not. The inconsistency of the studies examining the *planum temporale* may be attributed to several factors, including:

1. Research groups disagree on how to define the boundaries of the *planum temporale*; its structural ambiguity has led to some imaging measurements of unidimensional lengths rather than surface area (see Shapleske et al., 1999 for a review).
2. Different measurement techniques used to acquire images and to measure anatomical regions are associated with considerable variability in planar surface areas across studies. For example, Best and Demb (1999) compared three measurement methods on the *planum temporale* in five dyslexic and five normally literate adults. The first two methods adopted from relevant MRI studies included the tissue between Heschl's sulcus and the terminal upswing of the posterior ascending sylvian ramus, though the second one took into account neither the shape of the *planum* nor the small sulci on its surface. The third method approximated

those used in Galaburda's post-mortem work, revealing solely the bidimensional area on the superior surface of the temporal lobe. The results showed that both participant groups became less left-lateralized using the second and third procedure, which exclude sulcul tissue to an increasing degree.

3. Variation in certain characteristics of the participants (e.g., handedness, gender, intellectual capacity, oral language skills, or socioeconomic background) across studies might obscure the relationship between planar asymmetry and dyslexia (Eckert, Lambardino, & Leonard, 2001; for reviews see Beaton, 1997; Eckert & Leonard, 2000; Lambe, 1999; Shapleske et al., 1999). For instance, given that non-right-handedness is related to reduced or reversed asymmetry of the *planum temporale* and given that most studies reported normal distributions of handedness within the dyslexic group, careful control for handedness is essential in imaging studies of dyslexia.
4. Finally, certain methodological flaws, such as small sample sizes, criteria used to define dyslexia, the heterogeneity of the disorder, and codiagnoses (e.g., attention-deficit/hyperactivity disorder) might also contribute to conflicting information regarding morphometric changes in the *planum temporale* (e.g., Shapleske et al., 1999; Eckert & Leonard, 2000).

Although still highly controversial, it has been proposed that reported findings of reduced cerebral asymmetry in dyslexia may be associated with anomalous interhemispheric pathways coursing through the ***corpus callosum*** to the perisylvian-language regions (Filipek, 1995). The *corpus callosum* subserves communication and integration between the hemispheres and has been shown to be topographically organized with projections from specific cortical areas to specific callosal regions (de LaCoste et al., 1985; Pandya & Seltzer, 1986). Based on animal models, Galaburda's group (Galaburda et al., 1990; Rosen et al., 1989) has hypothesized that the commissural connections between the hemispheres are inversely related to cerebral asymmetrics. Thus, more symmetric brains have a stronger inter-hemispheric connectivity, which may be reflected by larger *corpus callosum* size and *vice versa.* To date, there are five studies using MRI techniques to compare *corpus callosum* size between dyslexic individuals and non-dyslexic controls (Duara et al., 1991; Hynd et al., 1995; Larsen et al., 1992; Robichon & Habib, 1998; Rumsey et al.,

1996). Duara et al. (1991) observed that the most posterior segment of the *corpus callosum*, termed the *splenium*, was larger in a group of 21 dyslexic adults than in 29 controls. However, this effect was primarily accounted for by female participants in the dyslexic group. In addition, both the (most anterior) *genu* area and the *corpus callosum* in general were larger in female than in male dyslexic adults. Larsen et al. (1992) failed to find differences of the total callosal area or the *splenium* in a predominantly male sample of 19 dyslexic adolescents and 17 normal readers. They also reported no deviances in size of the *corpus callosum* in subgroups of dyslexia related to reading profile or symmetry/asymmetry of the *planum temporale*.

Studying children, Hynd et al. (1995) obtained completely different results, with the dyslexic group (n = 16) showing a smaller *genu* region than the equally sized control group. Furthermore, moderate positive correlations were found between overall reading achievement and the (region of interest) measurements for the *genu* ($r = .40$) and *splenium* ($r = .35$) in these children. Rumsey et al. (1996) reported an increase in the area of the posterior third of the *corpus callosum* – roughly corresponding to the *splenium* and its rostrally adjacent segment, the *isthmus* – in dyslexic men (n = 21). Likewise, in a group of 16 adult male dyslexics, Robichon and Habib (1998) showed a larger total callosal area, in particular in the *isthmus*, but found that this result was accounted for by right-handed participants.

Taken together, three of the five studies reviewed above showed an increase in size of the *corpus callosum* in dyslexic adults, especially in the *splenium* (Duara et al., 1991; Rumsey et al., 1996) and the *isthmus* (Robichon & Habib, 1998; Rumsey et al., 1996). The *isthmus* contains fibers from the superior temporal and posterior parietal regions. The *splenium* includes all of the fibers connecting occipital cortex, but also links the superior parietal lobules and the temporo-parieto-occipital junctional area, the region including the *planum temporale* (de LaCoste et al., 1985; Pandya & Seltzer, 1986). Thus, these callosal segments are associated with posterior language regions, in which atypical cerebral asymmetries and other cytoarchitectonic deviances have been reported in dyslexia (e.g., Dalby et al., 1998; Flowers, 1993; Hynd et al., 1990; Kushch et al., 1993; Larsen et al., 1990; Leonard et al., 1993).

The works of Larsen et al. (1992) and Hynd et al. (1995) on *corpus callosum* morphometry in dyslexia provide conflicting results, however. In explaining this conflict, differences in subject characteristics (e.g., age, gender, handedness, comorbidity, or intellectual ability) as well as procedural variations in the methods used to acquire the scans and to define and measure the callosal subregions of interest, may play an important role (Filipek, 1995; Beaton, 1997; Lambe, 1999).

One of the most consistent locations exhibiting structural differences between dyslexics and normal readers is the cerebellum. Rae et al. (2002) observed significant cerebellar asymmetry (right grey matter > left grey matter) in controls, which was absent among dyslexic subjects. In the dyslexic subjects, the degree of cerebellar symmetry was correlated with the severity of the phonological decoding deficit. Eckert et al. (2003) found that dyslexics exhibit significantly smaller right anterior cerebellar lobes, bilateral *pars triangularis*, and brain volumes. The cerebellar measures were highly associated with deficits in rapid automatic naming and with the double-deficit subtype of dyslexia, correctly classifying 72% of the dyslexic subjects (94% of whom had rapid automatic naming deficit).

As acknowledged above, it is apparent that no consistent structural correlates have been associated with developmental dyslexia using MRI techniques. Several factors possibly accounting for the inconsistent findings were outlined previously. Further insight has been expected from functional brain-imaging methods.

3.2 Functional Neuroimaging

Among the developmental disorders, functional measures of cerebral blood flow or metabolism such as Positron Emission Tomography (PET) and functional Magnetic Resonance Imaging (fMRI) have been applied most often in studies of adults with dyslexia (Filipek, 1999).

3.2.1 Brain Activation During Phonological Tasks

One of the first functional imaging studies examining phonological processing in dyslexia was that of Rumsey et al. (1992). PET scans were obtained from 14 adult male dyslexics and 14 normal literate controls while performing two tasks: a phonemic awareness task in which participants were asked to press a button if two auditorily presented words rhymed with each other, and a non-phonological attentional task in which they were required to push a key whenever a target tone in a series of (simple) tones was detected. In normal literate subjects, the left temporo-parietal cortex (angular/supramarginal gyrus) was activated during rhyme judgment but not during tone detection. Dyslexic individuals showed reduced blood flow in the left temporo-parietal regions activated in controls while performing the phonological task but did not differ from controls in these regions during rest or attentional testing. Thus, dyslexic individuals demonstrated left temporo-parietal dysfunction associated with the phonological demands of the rhyming task.

A subsequent PET study (Paulesu, Frith, Snowling, & Gallagher, 1996) employed two visually presented phonological tasks: a rhyming task ("*Does the letter rhyme with B?*") and a short-term memory task ("*Was 'K' among the last 6 letters you saw?*"). In normal literate men (n = 5; all right-handed), both tasks activated a number of perisylvian structures in the left hemisphere, including Broca's area, Wernicke's area, and the insula, whereas parietal operculum activation was specific to the phonological memory task. In dyslexic men (n = 5; all right-handed), only a subset of brain regions normally involved in phonological processing was activated, including Broca's area during rhyme judgment and left temporo-parietal cortex during short-term memory demands. The insula of the left hemisphere was never activated. Paulesu and his colleagues thought the left insular cortex to be crucial in the conversion of whole-word phonology (temporo-parietal regions) to segmented phonology (inferior-frontal regions). They speculated that phonological deficits in dyslexia might result from a weak connectivity between anterior and posterior language areas.

Paulesu et al. (1996) support the findings of Rumsey et al. (1992) founding their report of reduced activity in the left temporo-parietal regions in dyslexic adults during performance of simple rhyming tasks. They extend these findings by showing task-dependent activations of only a subset of left-hemispheric perisylvian-language areas. It deserves mention, however, that the two PET studies used different methodological approaches. While Rumsey et al. (1992) employed a region of interest method, which is governed by preconceived anatomical considerations; Paulesu et al. (1996) utilized whole-brain scanning and voxel-based image analysis, permitting a more detailed investigation of brain areas.

Using whole-head PET scanning, Rumsey et al. (1997a) compared 17 right-handed dyslexic men and 14 non-impaired controls who performed two kinds of print tasks with stress on phonological or orthographic features. The first type of task, referred to as 'pronunciation' included (phonological) decoding of pseudowords (e.g., *phalbap, chirl*) and (orthographic) reading of low frequency irregularly spelled words (e.g., *pharaoh, choir*). The second type of task involved lexical decision-making with a phonological instruction (*Which one sounds like a real word?*; e.g., *jope-joak*) or an orthographic one (*Which one is a real word?*; e.g., *thurd-third*). In comparison to normal literate controls, dyslexic subjects displayed reduced blood flow in temporal regions bilaterally and in inferior parietal cortex, mainly on the left, during both pronunciation and lexical decision-making. However, their activation of left inferior frontal cortex (Broca's area) during both phonological and orthographic decision-making did not differ from the control group. Thus, the Rumsey et al. (1997a) results contrast with the data from their earlier study (Rumsey et al., 1992) as well as with those of Paulesu et al. (1996). Rumsey et al. (1997a) comment on the absence of different activation loci in phonological versus orthographic tasks, which might result, they suggest, from more basic deficits in phonemic awareness. They further hypothesized that the dyslexic group may have approached unknown irregular words in a manner closely resembling the letter-by-letter reading of unfamiliar pseudowords.

In line with the latter interpretation by Rumsey and associates, Shaywitz (1998) designed a set of hierarchically organized print tasks thought to make progressively greater demands on phonological analysis. The tasks required same-different judgments concerning: line orientation (e.g., *[\\V]-[\\V]*), presumed to reflect visual-spatial processing; letter case (e.g., *[bbBb]-[bbBb]*), thought to predominantly explore orthographic processing; single-letter rhyme (e.g., *[T]-[V]*); as well as pseudoword rhyme (e.g., *[leat]-[jete]*), assumed to add increasingly more phonological processing demands; and semantic category (e.g., *[corn]-[rice]*), believed to make demands on transcoding from print to phonology, but also requiring activation of the mental lexicon to determine meaning. Brain activation patterns of 17 regions of interest per hemisphere were measured by means of fMRI in 29 right-handed dyslexic adults and 32 controls. On tasks making explicit demands on phonological processing (e.g., pseudoword rhyming), dyslexic individuals showed relative underengagement of left posterior perisylvian and occipital sites (Wernicke's area, angular gyrus, and striate cortex), coupled with a disproportionately elevated response in a left anterior region (inferior frontal gyrus) compared to non-impaired readers. According to Shaywitz and her colleagues, these findings suggest a functional disruption in those posterior cortical systems that are engaged by phonological decoding and, possibly, a compensatory reliance on Broca's area.

A more recent study by Shaywitz et al. (2001) compared the performances and brain activation patterns of 29 dyslexic readers (DYS) and 32 non-impaired readers (NI). Findings revealed significant differences in brain activation patterns between the two groups during tasks that made progressive demands on phonological analysis. During non-word rhyming, dyslexics exhibited a disruption in several critical posterior components involving the posterior superior temporal sulcus (Wernicke's area), BA 39 (angular gyrus), and BA 17 (striate cortex), and a concomitant increase in activation in the anterior inferior frontal gyrus. The researchers interpreted the data as an indication that dyslexic readers demonstrate a functional disruption in extensive posterior cortex areas, encompassing both traditional language regions and portions of the association cortex centered about the angular gyrus. The latter region is considered pivotal in carrying out cross-modal integrations necessary for reading (i.e., mapping the visual percept of the print onto phonologic structures of the language). Thus, disruption within the neural systems that serve to link visual representations of letters to the phonological structures they represent are a possible locus of developmental and acquired disorders affecting reading.

Rich evidence has been accumulating from a number of regional cerebral blood flow studies that have confirmed reduced activation of posterior brain regions in dyslexia ,primarily fusiform gyrus and angular gyrus; BA 37,39 (Brunswick, McCrory, Price, Frith, & Frith, 1999; Paulesu et al., 1996; Rumsey et al., 1992, 1997b; Shaywitz, 1998), along with over-activation of anterior regions, mainly the inferior frontal gyrus; BA 6/44, 44-45 (Sandak, Mencel, Frost, & Pugh, 2004; Shaywitz & Shaywitz, 2005). The hypoactivation of the left angular gyrus, found among dyslexic individuals, has been associated with difficulties mapping visual input (print) onto suitable phonological representations (Shaywitz & Shaywitz, 2005).

The activation of the anterior regions, mainly Broca's area, has been associated with articulatory coding (Demonet et al., 1992). The over-activation of this region among dyslexic subjects has been interpreted as an effortful compensation used for phonological assembly during explicit reading, due to a possible lack of access to automated articulatory routines. This compensation is thought to impose an extra computational load on articulation during sublexical processing in dyslexics (Hagoort et al., 1999; Sandak et al., 2004; Shaywitz & Shaywitz, 2005).

Another pattern potentially corresponding to a compensatory mechanism among dyslexics was found in functional connectivity studies that examined the covariance between brain regions involved in the reading process. Pugh et al. (2000b) found that during phonological assembly dyslexic individuals show the opposite activation pattern to the one found among normal readers; no evidence of functional connectivity within posterior regions of the left hemisphere, and strong connections between homologues right hemisphere regions. These findings have been interpreted as evidence that right posterior regions may serve a compensatory role in mediating phonological performance. Sandak and her associates (2004) have also used functional connectivity analysis to examine dyslexic and normal readers' response during pseudo- and real-word reading. Results illustrated that while normal readers showed a strong connectivity between the occipitotemporal area and Broca's area, connectivity among dyslexic readers was observed between the occipitotemporal area and areas in right prefrontal cortex. These findings imply that dyslexic individuals have difficulty integrating orthographic and phonological processing, and are thus forced to rely on word recognition strategies involving long-term memory recall.

The apparent convergence of evidence indicated in functional imaging and post mortem studies regarding cerebral abnormalities in dyslexics' posterior left language regions, together with findings suggesting a decrease in hemispheric asymmetry may reflect right hemisphere compensation for left hemisphere malfunction (Milne, Syngenotis, Jackson, & Corballis, 2002). This shift of activation from left to posterior right hemisphere regions, might indicate a word recognition strategy that relies on visuo-semantic processes. The increased connectivity to anterior regions might further suggest an effortful attention-guided reading strategy (Sandak et al., 2004).

Support for the compensatory role of the posterior regions of the right hemisphere together with the left inferior frontal gyrus, as well as for the dysfunctional core around the left angular gyrus, was found in a three-case fMRI study conducted by Milne et al. (2002). In this study, patterns of brain activity were examined during phonological assembly processes induced by lexical decision tasks that made progressively stronger demands on grapheme-to phoneme conversion. The findings from this research show increased activation of the anterior frontal gyrus (BA 44/6) in the left hemisphere, increased activation of the parietal cortex (BA 7) and occipital cortex (BA 18) in the right hemisphere, and in the cerebellum in the phonological dyslexic subject, as phonological demands were systematically increased.

In a further analysis of the Shaywitz (1998) data, Pugh et al. (2000a) turned their attention to the functional connectivity of the angular gyrus. Their reasons were twofold: First, the (left) angular gyrus is considered pivotal in mapping visually presented inputs onto phonologic representations. Second, dyslexic males have been reported to show a functional disconnection between the left angular gyrus and related posterior regions during reading (Horwitz, Rumsey, & Donohue, 1998). However, it could not be determined whether this disruption was specific to phonological decoding engaged by reading tasks. The re-analyzed data by Pugh et al. (2000a) revealed significant correlations between angular gyrus and occipital and temporal lobe sites on pseudoword rhyme and semantic category judgments in controls, but not in the dyslexic group. In the right hemisphere, corresponding correlations were significant for both reading groups. Thus, this pattern of results suggests a breakdown in left-hemisphere connectivity in reading, when substantial phonological decoding (or "phonological assembly," Pugh et al., 2000a, p.51) was required, whereas right-hemisphere homologues seem to work in a compensatory manner for dyslexic readers.

Comparable evidence for an atypical left-hemisphere brain activation pattern thought to reflect fundamental disruption of phonological processing in poor reading has been taken from the PET study by Brunswick et al. (1999). The researchers compared six non-impaired adult readers with six readers with a childhood history of developmental dyslexia (all right-handed males) on word and pseudoword naming. Dyslexic individuals showed less activation in ventral occipito-temporal sites and greater engagement of left inferior frontal gyrus than non-impaired controls. In the same laboratory, using identical sets of stimuli, verbal repetition was tested in eight dyslexic men and six controls (McCrory, Frith, Brunswick, & Price, 2000). In this case, the dyslexic group demonstrated a decreased hemodynamic response compared with the control group in the right superior temporal and right post-central gyri. As studies in healthy individuals indicate that attending to the phonetic structure of speech is associated with a decrease in right-hemisphere processing, McCrory and his colleagues concluded that reduced right-hemisphere activation in the dyslexic group indicates an attentional bias towards phonetic elements of the auditory input. That is, less processing of non-phonetic aspects of speech may receive greater salience than the phonological structure of attended speech for dyslexic readers. With respect to findings of atypical brain activation profiles observed either in the left hemisphere (Brunswick et al., 1999) or the right (McCrory et al., 2000), the authors proposed that the neural manifestation of phonological disruption in dyslexia is task-specific, i.e., functional rather than structural in nature.

Bringing together results from print tasks tapping phonological processing, we can see that dyslexic adults have shown normal or enhanced activity in left-hemisphere frontal-lobe language regions, but reduced or absent activity in left temporo-parietal language areas (Brunswick et al., 1999; Paulesu et al., 1996; Rumsey et al., 1997a; Shaywitz, 1998). Furthermore, the left angular gyrus has been found to be functionally disconnected from related temporal and occipital regions (Horwitz et al., 1998; Pugh et al., 2000a).

In order to clarify whether atypical cerebral responses in individuals with dyslexia reflect a fundamental deficit of phonological processing or rather a compensation for poor reading in adulthood, Temple et al. (2001) conducted an fMRI study in children. Whole-brain imaging data were acquired from 24 dyslexic and 15 normally reading children (8-12 years old) during phonological and orthographic tasks of rhyming and matching visually presented consonant letter pairs (e.g., "*Do T and D rhyme?*" and "*Are P and P the same?*", respectively). During letter rhyming, activity in left frontal-lobe regions was evident in both groups, though the dyslexic children displayed larger activation than their normally reading peers. Activity in left temporo-parietal cortex associated with phonological processing was only observed in normally reading controls, however. During letter matching, the control group demonstrated activity throughout the extrastriate cortex, whereas the dyslexic group showed reduced extrastriate occipital responses to orthographic processing. Thus, altered temporo-parietal activation probed by rhyme letters in dyslexic children parallels prior findings in dyslexic adults, pointing to core phonological deficits. Moreover, childhood dyslexia may be characterized by impaired extrastriate activity thought to be important for orthographic processing.

To complete the overview of functional neuroimaging research on phonological processing in dyslexia, the second fMRI study (Georgiewa et al., 1999) conducted in young developmental dyslexics should be briefly mentioned here. Thirty-four (German) dyslexic and normal literate adolescents with an average age of 14 years (all right-handed) were scanned while silently performing several tasks, including viewing of letter strings, reading of nonwords (e.g., *bnams*) and frequent words (e.g., *blume,* engl.: *flower*), and phonological transformation ("*Move the first letter to the end of the word and add the common German suffix '-ein'*; e.g., *blume* ➔ *lume-bein*). Dyslexic adolescents showed reduced activation in inferior frontal regions (in particular Broca's area) and in left-hemisphere inferior temporal-lobe sites during tasks that invoked substantial grapheme-phoneme conversions and phonological awareness (i.e., nonword reading and phonological transformation). Neither group displayed temporo-parietal activity, however. These results differed from the brain activation pattern observed in dyslexic children (Temple et al., 2001) as well as from the previously cited findings in adult subjects. As suggested by Temple and her associates (2001), task differences (covert behavioral response in the adolescent study versus overt response in the other studies) and the variation in image analysis procedures (only a limited number of brain regions were imaged in the adolescents) might have played a significant role in accounting for the deviant findings of Georgiewa et al. (1999).

Hagoort et al. (1999) examined the neural correlates of reading and the phonological conversion of legal letter strings with or without meaning among adult German speaking subjects. Increased activation of the lingual gyri during silent reading was found, in comparison with activation during viewing a fixation cross. Comparison between the reading of words and pseudowords suggested the involvement of the middle temporal gyri in retrieving both the phonological and semantic codes of words. It is suggested that this area might be involved in the sublexical conversion of orthographic input strings into phonological output codes. The middle fusiform gyrus was activated in response to pseudoword reading, a finding that fits previous findings regarding its role in processing letter strings. Premotor areas were activated both in silent reading and in reading aloud, with differential activation observed between word-reading pseudoword-reading. The left medial premotor cortex showed increased blood flow for pseudowords as compared to words, whereas the reading and pronunciation of words resulted in increased blood flow to the SMA as compared to pseudowords. It was hypothesized that these differences could be attributed to frequency differences between the syllables in the words and pseudowords employed in the current study, as the words were comprised of mainly high frequency syllables and the pseudowords contained more low frequency syllables. The researchers assumed that the articulation of high frequency syllables requires the retrieval of their associated articulatory gestures from the SMA, while low frequency syllables recruit the left medial premotor cortex.

This review of functional neuroimaging studies involving phonological tasks illustrated that there is a reduced activation of the left posterior brain regions in dyslexia, accompanied by a shift of activation to analogous regions in the right hemisphere and an over-activation of anterior regions (Paulesu et al., 1996; Rumsey et al., 1992, 1997a; Sandak et al., 2004; Shaywitz, 1998, Shaywitz et al., 2003). As stated throughout this chapter, a common interpretation of these finding was to say that they reflect a compensation strategy. However, as pointed out by Katzir, Misra and Poldrack (2005), interpreting the results should also take into account the differences between various types of phonological tasks; namely between phonological and print-mediated phonological tasks. In their study, Katzir et al. employed phonological tasks that did not involve orthography to skilled readers. Their study suggested that phonological processing that is not mediated by print relies primarily on frontal language processing areas. Contrary to the studies reviewed in this chapter, Katzir et al. did not find any evidence of activation in the angular gyrus or nearby temporo-parietal areas, and when visual complexity of the stimuli was accounted for, activations in the striate and extrastriate cortices were eliminated as well. The possible confound of orthographic processing with phonological processing in the previous literature might be an important trail to follow in future studies involving dyslexic populations.

One such attempt was an MEG study by Parviainen, Helenius, and Salmelin (2005). These researchers investigated the auditory cortical activation induced by dyslexic and normal readers in response to speech and non-speech sounds, not mediated by print. Speech stimuli were comprised of Finnish vowels and CV syllables. Non-speech stimuli were complex non speech sounds and simple sine wave tones, spectrally and temporally matched with the speech sounds. Ten normal readers and 10 dyslexic readers passively listened to sound stimuli, presented monaurally to the right ear, while watching a silent movie. For both subject groups, the N100m evoked was stronger to speech than non-speech sounds in the left, but not in the right, auditory cortex. Dyslexic readers however showed a delayed left-hemisphere response and a weaker right than left-hemisphere response to both stimuli types. Control subjects' response was earlier in left than right hemisphere, and a similar level of activation was detected in both hemispheres. These results cannot be easily compared to previous findings elaborated in this review, due to the different stimuli and terms of presentation used here. Parviainen et al. (2005) suggested an explanation based on the notion of a general auditory deficit. According to the authors, the altered hemispheric balance seen among dyslexics reflects an abnormality within the left planum temporale, or deficient communication between this region and the primary auditory cortex.

3.2.2 Functional Neuroimaging Findings in Word Processing

Helenius et al. (2002) used a MEG technique to elucidate the cortical activation associated with the segmentation of spoken words in dyslexic and non-reading-impaired adults. Subjects listened to binaurally presented sentences, which had either semantic-appropriate or semantic-inappropriate final words. Half of the inappropriate final words shared two or three initial phonemes with highly expected semantically appropriate words. Two temporal and functional peak response patterns were detected in the superior temporal lobe. One, which had no sensitivity to the semantic appropriateness of the final word, occurred at 100 msec (N100m) approximately in the supra-temporal plane. Dyslexics exhibited an abnormally strong presemantic N100m response. The other peak response activation occurred at 400 msec (N400m) in the superior temporal cortex, in the vicinity of the auditory cortex. This peak appeared to be greater in response to inappropriate sentence endings and was delayed in all subjects for word endings with phoneme beginnings similar to expected words, until acoustic-phonetic dissimilarity emerged. An enhanced delay of approximately 50 msec in this semantic auditory activation of the left hemisphere was seen in the dyslexic subjects. Helenius indicates that the subtle delay in semantic processing supports the notion of initial reliance on phonemic acoustic features in lexical access. The additional delay among dyslexics was attributed to the presemantic-phonological deficits reflected in the abnormal N100m response.

McCandliss and Nobles (2003) referred in their review to two cortical areas demonstrating dysfunctions in dyslexia; the superior temporal gyrus (STG), associated with phonological processing, and the visual word form area (VWFA), associated with visuo- orthographic aspects of word processing. The VWFA is located near the middle portion of the fusiform gyrus, in the left occipito-temporal extra-striate visual system. This region has been associated with the development of a form of visual expertise allowing to rapidly identify words as an integrated unit. The VWFA typically shows an increase in activity in response to word-like stimuli, compared to letter-strings, false-letters or auditory words. The VWFA seems to also be sensitive to conventions of the writing system, responding more vigorously to familiar words and letter strings that do not violate patterns of the writing system (for reviews see: McCandliss & Nobles, 2003; Rayner & Pollatsek, 1995). Dyslexic readers, however, seem to under-activate this region when required to rapidly read words, or differentiate real words from false-letter words (Brunswick et al., 1999). This difference between normal and dyslexic readers was also demonstrated in a cross-cultural study, comparing alphabetic languages with different degrees of letter-to-sound mapping complexities (Paulesu et al., 2001).

Siok, Perfetti, Jin, and Tan (2004) further examined the universal biological origin notion, often raised regarding dyslexia, using Chinese script; a logographic rather than an alphabetic system. Unlike alphabetic orthographies, in which the mapping of graphemes onto phonemes has been shown to be crucial to reading development, the Chinese logographic system maps graphic forms onto morphemes, involving also an inherent connection between orthography and semantics. Siok et al. performed two experiments using the fMRI technology with reading impaired Chinese children, and their matched control group. The first experiment involved a homophone judgment task, and the second, a character decision task (a form of a lexical decision). Findings indicated that unlike reading impairments in alphabetic languages, in which left temporo-parietal regions have been found to be impaired, Chinese reading difficulty is associated with reduced activation in the left middle frontal gyrus, a region related to working memory of visuo-spatial and verbal information. These results suggest that cross-cultural studies should take into account the fundamental characteristics of different orthographic systems. The manifestation of reading difficulties may be attributed to the specific interplay between biological deficits and the way the specific characteristics of the orthographic system (influencing the cognitive strategies) tune the cortex.

3.2.3 Neuroimaging Findings in Letter Processing

In an fMRI study conducted by Temple and her colleagues (Temple, Poldrack, Salidis, et al., 2001), differential patterns of activity during processing of single letters (match letters vs. match lines) were found between dyslexics and normally reading children. Normally reading children showed activity in the exrastriate region, while the reading-impaired group did not show any activity in this area. This finding has been interpreted as support for the hypothesis raised by Wolf and Bowers (1999), which proposes large group differences between children with dyslexia and children who read normally, in the brain regions involved in orthographic processing of single letters.

Salmelin and Helenius (2004) reviewed studies which used the MEG technology to provide temporal estimations of the processes involved in word recognition. Two word-perception stages were identified during the first 200 msec following word presentation; a low-level visual analysis, insensitive to content and occurring over the first 100 msec, and a letter-string specific activation, about 50 msec later, occurring around the left occipitotemporal (OT) cortex. Salmelin and Helenius postulated that the reading sequence diverges from the normal course in the left inferior occipitotemporal cortex at about 150-170 msec after word presentation. The first visual analysis stage was found to be intact among dyslexic individuals, however, an abnormal weak activation was observed among participants with dyslexia during the second stage of letter-string analysis. Attempting to interpret the nature of the occipitotemporal deficit, Salmelin and Helenius turned to studies exploring the activation of this region during non-letter stimuli. Previous studies found that faces also evoke a stimulus-specific response in the inferior OT cortex, within the same time framework as do letter-strings. In response to processing of faces, however, participants with dyslexia showed similar activation to the patterns observed among normal readers in the OT region. Hence, the underactivation of the left inferior OT region during the reading tasks was interpreted to reflect a specific impairment in reading letter-strings. The authors inferred the deficits in the OT region to mean that the setting apart of letter-string stimuli from other objects has not been fully established among dyslexic readers, leading to a slower reading pace.

Whitney and Cornelissen (2005) discussed in their review the ways by which auditory and visual deficits may lead to abnormal processing of letter strings in dyslexia. The dorsal magnocellular pathways have been associated with letter encoding ability and visual attention difficulties. Whitney and Cornelissen suggested that the allocation of visual attention to fixated letters aids in the formation of reliable graphoneme representations. These representations in turn pressure the system to induce faster left-to-right letter processing and eventually string-specific processing is learned. The notion raised by Salmelin & Helenius (2004), according to which dyslexic readers process letter-strings and objects in a similar way, is explained here in terms of magnocellular and visual attention deficits.

3.2.4 Brain Activation During Auditory Temporal Processing Tasks

Employing PET, Rumsey et al. (1994) contrasted brain activation in 15 right-handed dyslexic men and 18 normal readers during performance of a tonal matching task. The task required participants to press a button if paired tonal sequences (3-4 tones) were identical to one another. During tonal matching, dyslexic and normally reading adults displayed similar left-hemisphere temporal activation, but the dyslexic group exhibited reduced blood flow in right fronto-temporal regions. Along with this physiological difference, the dyslexic group was significantly impaired in performing the task. Since the task involved fast-paced stimulus presentation (16 tonal pairs/mm), the authors considered the impaired right-hemisphere activation to be consonant with hypothesized deficits in rapid temporal processing in dyslexia. As many of the subjects had participated in the Rumsey et al. (1992) PET study of phonological processing (see above), Rumsey and her colleagues proposed that dyslexic individuals may have more widespread deficits encompassing left- as well as right-hemisphere temporal cortex.

In a recent fMRI study, Temple, Poldrack, Protopapas, et al. (2000) examined whether adults with dyslexia exhibit deviances in the neural response to rapidly changing acoustic information. The stimuli employed were non-speech analogues of consonant-vowel-consonant syllables with either brief (= rapid) or temporally extended (= slow) acoustic transitions. In each stimulus condition, subjects were asked to press a key for high-pitched but not for low-pitched sounds. While normal readers displayed increased activity in the left prefrontal cortex in response to rapid relative to slow non-speech analogues, dyslexic individuals showed no differential left-frontal activity for the two stimulus types. Furthermore, differential left-frontal responsiveness was inversely correlated with rapid auditory processing performance (i.e., the lower the threshold ISI needed for sequencing three 20-ms tones, the greater the difference between activity for rapid compared with slow stimuli). According to Temple and her colleagues, these results point to the role of left prefrontal regions in normal mediation of rapid auditory processing and attest to the disruption of these regions in dyslexic readers. In supporting their conclusion, the researchers cite a PET study by Belin et al. (1998) on healthy right-handed men. Using comparable non-verbal stimuli, they found left prefrontal activation in response to rapidly changing stimuli relative to a resting baseline, but no activation in response to slow stimuli relative to rest. Additional support for these findings comes from a recent MEG study preformed by Renvall and Hari (2002), which displayed weaker reactivity to acoustical changes, in particular to noise/square-wave transitions, in the auditory cortices of both hemispheres in dyslexic subjects. According to these researchers, their results demonstrate a deficit in processing acoustic changes presented in rapid succession among dyslexics, which might be related to a lack of automatic auditory triggering originating from a general deficiency of the magnocellular system.

The two studies described above (Rumsey et al., 1994; Temple et al., 2000) yielded contrasting results. However, differences between the studies in imaging technologies, stimulus materials, tasks, and brain regions of interest, as well as the lack of further research, prevent concluding remarks on neuronal responses to auditory temporal processing in dyslexia.

3.2.5 Brain Activation During Reading and Reading-related Tasks

Backes et al. (2002) used fMRI to examine differences between dyslexic and normally reading children in patterns and locations of brain activation during reading-related processes. The children performed tasks that varied in visuospatial, orthographic, phonological, and semantic processing demands. Enhanced activation of the left extrastriate cortex was found during all tasks in the dyslexic group. During both orthographic processing and the visuospatial task, dyslexic children showed activation predominantly in the right prefrontal cortex. Normal readers also showed activation in the left prefrontal cortex. Dyslexic children showed less activation of both the temporal and the prefrontal cortex during phonological processing. These results suggest that dyslexic readers fail to use brain areas that are normally specialized for language processing, and use areas that underlie visuospatial processing instead.

In the Temple et al. (2001) cited earlier, results regarding phonological processing revealed a selective impairment in the phonological (rhyme) judgments and reduced left-hemisphere temporo-parietal brain activity among dyslexic children during this task. ROI analysis indicated that dyslexic children failed to activate this area at all above base line. Dyslexic children had a greater extent of activation in the left IFG and a different location of activation in comparison with normally reading children, who showed more posterior activity than dyslexics. This latter finding differs from current results from studies that have used different methodological and different imaging analysis techniques.

Results regarding the orthographic processing task (match letters vs. match lines) revealed activity throughout the extrastriate cortex, especially in the occipito-parietal regions, in the normal subjects and reduced activity in these areas among the dyslexic subjects during performance of the task. The study indicates that dyslexia is characterized by disruption in phonological and orthographic neural systems. The existence of these disruptions in childhood supports the belief that these altered neural responses are causal rather than compensatory responses.

Paulesu et al. (2001) examined the different areas of activation during reading and reading-related tasks among dyslexic and normal adult readers in deep (English & French) and shallow (Italian) orthographies, in an attempt to explore similarities and differences at both the behavioral and neurophysiological levels. Behavioral measures consisted of reading tests (word/non-word reading speed), digit naming, short term memory, phoneme manipulations (spoonerism) and the Wechsler Adult Intelligence Scale (WAIS). Results revealed better performances by Italian dyslexics on reading tasks, as compared to English and French dyslexics. This was attributed to the shallow orthography of Italian, which facilitates reading. All dyslexics were equally impaired relative to controls on reading and phonological tasks. Neurofunctional data were collected using PET, in order to link the psychological findings to brain physiology. Two rCBF/PET activation experiments were conducted during implicit and explicit reading of single words, among 72 participants (6 control groups and 6 dyslexics groups). The patterns of rCBF revealed greater activation of the left superior temporal regions (areas which have been associated with processing phonemes) among the Italian control subjects and greater activation in the left posterior inferior temporal gyrus (areas which have been associated with word retrieval during reading and naming tasks) among English controls. All the dyslexic subjects from all three countries, showed reduced and restricted activation compared to controls in the left hemisphere perisylvian areas, with peak differences in the middle temporal gyrus and in the inferior and superior temporal gyri and middle occipital gyrus. No areas with significantly greater activation were found in dyslexic subjects, as compared to controls. The researchers interpreted these patterns of activity as evidence of the existence of a neurocognitive basis for dyslexia and as support for the conception that reading performance differences among dyslexics from different countries are due to different orthographies.

Silani et al. (2005) conducted an MRI study utilizing a voxel-based morphometry method with the same subjects that participated in Paulesu et al.'s (2001) PET study. The aim of this study was to examine whether abnormal activation patterns, induced during reading tasks in the PET study, could be also reflected in a structural abnormality of grey and white matter density in specific brain regions. Results indicated a between-group difference in the middle temporal region, expressed as a reduced grey matter density among the dyslexic group. A within group correlation was found among the dyslexic group alone; the higher the grey matter density, the more impaired were the dyslexic subjects on the reading tasks. Silani et al. (2005) suggested that these abnormalities reduced the connectivity between near-by regions. Reduction of white matter was also found among dyslexic readers within the arcuate fasiculus, supporting Paulesu et al.'s (1996) notion of deviant neural connectivity between language areas.

Ingvar et al. (2002) used a regional cerebral blood flow technique to elucidate differences between dyslexic and control subjects in cerebral activation patterns during reading. Their findings indicated specific differences between the two groups as a function of the language task. Minor qualitative differences in the dominant hemisphere were found when the visual route for language information was used. During pseudoword reading, a reading task of greater complexity, greater activations were found among the dyslexic subjects in the left frontal region and in a minor region in the extrastriate lateral occipital cortex (BA19). Reduced activations in dyslexic subjects were seen in the right angular gyrus, the right dorsolateral prefrontal cortex, and the right pallidum. These results indicate that dyslexics use cerebral areas that controls do not, and that reading skill is correlated with the level of activity in the right frontal cortex.

Shaywitz et al. (2003) examined in an fMRI study the differences in brain activation between three different groups of adults: normal readers, compensated dyslexics (accurate but slow readers) and non-compensated dyslexics (slow and inaccurate readers). All groups performed a pseudoword rhyming task and a semantic task (deciding whether two words belong to the same category or not). The findings show that compensated readers, who are accurate but not fluent, demonstrate a relative decrease in activation in posterior neural reading systems located in left parietotemporal and occipitotemporal regions while performing the rhyming task. This data is consistent with functional brain imaging studies showing failure of left hemisphere posterior brain systems to function properly in both adults and children with dyslexia while they perform reading tasks (see Shaywitz & Shaywitz, 2005, for a review). In contrast, left posterior reading systems were activated during reading real words in both the non-compensated and non-impaired readers. No differences were found in the insula. The researchers concluded that there are two systems involved in the development of skilled reading. One system involves word analysis, operates on individual units of words such as phonemes, and processes information slowly. The second system operates on the whole word and processes information rapidly. The data from this study indicate that both the non-impaired readers and non-compensated dyslexics rely on the visual areas in the occipitotemporal system for word recognition but the non- impaired readers develop this system through the phonological route while the non-compensated dyslexics rely on memory. The information comes from the connections, from left occipital areas to left frontal areas (language areas) in the non-impaired readers, and from left occipital areas to right frontal areas (associated to memory) in the non-compensated dyslexics. Behavioral data was consistent with this hypothesis: the non-compensated dyslexics could pronounce high frequency words but not low frequency ones. The compensated dyslexics were found to have higher cognitive skills, which presumably help them overcome their reading problems.

Shaywitz et al. (2001) suggest a neural model for reading. They point out that previous hypotheses and findings suggest that a few posterior brain regions are critical for reading, including the angular gyrus and the supramarginal gyrus in the inferior parietal lobule and the posterior aspect of the superior temporal gyrus. Extensive literature on acquired reading disabilities has pinpointed the angular gyrus as a crucial region for mapping visual percepts to print onto phonological structures. Recent findings have concluded that another posterior brain region, the ventral occipito-temporal area, serves as a visual word form area that appears to respond preferentially to rapidly presented stimuli. These dorsal and ventral areas differ in their chronometry and in their response latencies, with the occipito- temporal area responding early (between 150 and 80 ms) and the temporo-parietal responding later in time (approximately 250 ms) (Salmelin, Service, Kiesilae, & Uutela, 1996; Tarkiainen, Helenius, Hansen, Cornelissen, & Salmelin, 1999) during reading of words and pseudowords. Another neural circuit employed in reading involves the inferior frontal gyrus (Broca's area), which is associated with articulation and serves an important function in silent reading and naming. Shaywitz et al. (2001) assume that dyslexics suffer from a disruption of the left posterior reading systems and, in attempt for compensation, shift to other ancillary systems, for example anterior sites such as the IFG and right posterior sights. The anterior sites may help dyslexics develop an awareness of the sound structures of words through articulation, thereby allowing them to read but in a slower and less efficient manner. The right posterior regions may be used to facilitate visual pattern recognition, compensating for the poor left posterior word analysis system. These shifts may support accurate, though not fluent and automatic, word reading.

The fluency aspect of reading has been receiving a growing amount of attention in recent years within the field of reading research. Some of the fluency studies have provided indications suggesting that reading rate may be considered an independent variable, associated with a possible second core deficit, not explained by phonological awareness (Breznitz, 2002; Wolf & Bowers, 2000). Corresponding to this view, a line of research conducted by Breznitz (Breznitz, 1987; Breznitz & Share, 1992; Breznitz, DeMarco, Shammi, & Hakerem, 1994) has illustrated an "acceleration phenomenon", according to which the acceleration of the reading speed has the power to improve reading accuracy and comprehension. In a recent fMRI study conducted by Karni et al. (2005) the acceleration paradigm was examined using two presentation rates: a rate 20% slower than each subject's self-paced rate ("slow"), and a fast rate. Eight dyslexic and 8 normal readers performed three tasks under these 3 presentation conditions: a non-word task (NW; homophonic judgment), a single word task (SW; concrete/abstract judgment), and a sentences task (SNT; plausibility judgment). The largest difference between the groups was found in the NW slow presentation condition. As observed in previous studies (Shaywitz et al., 2001; Shaywitz & Shaywitz, 2005), dyslexic readers activated the left IFG and operculum, whereas the control subjects activate the visual processing areas (extra-striate cortex). In the fast presentation condition, however, no differences were found between the groups in accuracy and comprehension measures, as well as in brain activation patterns. The opposite pattern was found when comparing responses evoked in response to the two presentation rates in the SW and SNT tasks. However, when data of all three tasks was pooled together, the difference between the two presentation rates resembled the one seen on the NW task. Karni et al. (2005) suggested that the accelerated conditions may have the power to "push" the dyslexic brain to process grapheme information in a manner much closer to the one employed by normal readers. The remarkable "normalizing effect" observed following acceleration in dyslexics' brain activation may point to the potential benefits intervention programs may bring.

4. INTERVENTION PROGRAMS

As illustrated throughout this chapter, atypical brain activity was found among dyslexic individuals during reading tasks. Among other things, decreased activity in the left temporoparietal cortex was observed during phonological processing (Temple et al., 2003), as well as in the left inferior frontal area, left inferior temporal/occipital area and the cerebellum (Demonet, Taylor, & Chaix, 2004). Different types of intervention programs, employing behavioral measures, have managed to remediate, to some extent, the reading skills of dyslexic children. What remains unknown is the extent to which the neural response disruptions observed in dyslexia can also be changed through remediation. The nervous system is plastic in nature and can be altered on the basis of development and experience. Learning a skill through training is one of the triggers of plasticity. Training can change relevant cerebral representations and increase cerebral activity according to a given task (Breznitz, 2006).

Training tends to be associated with increases in cerebral activity, or expansion of activity areas. Increases generally occur after extensive exposure to stimuli and a period of consolidation before brain imaging is performed again (Callan et al., 2003). Decreases in cerebral activity, however, can also occur as a result of training. Decreases are thought to reflect a sharpening of responses. The decrease is present when a minority of neurons fire more robustly, while the majority of neurons show decreased firing. Decreases generally occur when training and exposure to the stimuli are less extensive and when imaging is conducted shortly after training (Poldrack, 2000; Callan et al., 2003). Shifts refer to an activity observed after training in regions where it was not present before training. Shifts are thought to reflect the use of new neural pathways or representations. The nature of brain plasticity; increases, decreases or shifts, is determined by various factors such as task type, the extent of learning, and the brain region involved (Poldrack, 2000).

Two proposed patterns of training-induced activity may be used to interpret these effects (Simos et al., 2002): The compensatory hypothesis refers to interventions that result in the establishment of a new pathway for reading that is not present in normal readers. The normalization hypothesis, on the other hand, refers to interventions that show a "correction" of the functionally deviant brain circuit observed among dyslexic readers, whilst establishing a pathway that is practically identical to the one typically found in the brain of regular readers.

A few studies have examined the effects of reading intervention programs in terms of both behavioral and brain-activity measures. These studies were interested in the nature of training-induced changes in the brain areas previously reported as deficient in children with dyslexia. Examining the functional reorganization occurring over the course of an intervention has the potential of providing us with new insights into the mechanisms that allow a given intervention to achieve its goals.

Most intervention studies utilizing measures of brain activity have integrated some sort of phonological instruction and practice within their intervention programs. However, the programs differed in quite a few variables, such as the emphasis put on phonics instruction and reading within a contextual framework, the type of comparison group chosen, subjects' characteristics and the measures used to evaluate progress.

Simos and associates (2002) employed two training programs; The Phono-Graphix program (Read America, Orlando, FL) and the Lindamood Phonemic-Sequencing program, on a group of 8 children, aged 7 to 17 years with severe reading difficulties. Six of these children were also diagnosed as having ADD. The training programs included 80 hours of one-to-one phonological processing and decoding instruction for 1 to 2 hours daily for 8 weeks. Before and after intervention a visual pseudo-word rhyme-matching task was performed, during which MSI scans were obtained. Task stimuli included four blocks of 25 pairs of pseudo-words. Children were asked to indicate whether the stimuli in each pair rhymed or not. Eight age-matched children who had never experienced reading problems were also tested on two separate occasions, with an 8-week interval, during which they received regular reading instruction at school.

Data collected from the dyslexic group of children before receiving intervention showed the typical dyslexia-specific profile; smaller responses over the left posterior superior temporal gyrus regions (STGp) and inferior parietal areas, and strong activation of homologous regions in the right hemisphere. The reading program administered yielded significant improvements in phonological decoding abilities.

Normalization of the brain activation profile was also found; the most pronounced change was found in the posterior portion of the left

STP. In most children these changes rendered the brain activation associated with word reading virtually identical to that found in the age-matched control group children. However, the temporal features of the activation profiles indicated that the initial engagement of the left STGp may not occur as fast as in regular readers. This may suggest that despite an impressive brain plasticity activation pattern, correlated with improved reading skills, the posterior temporal circuit established by training may not be as efficient as that found in regular readers.

Richards and associates (2000) used a different technique to investigate the effect of phonology-based treatment on brain response to language stimuli. During a phonological task dyslexic boys tended to show a greater area of brain lactate elevation in the left frontal quadrant of the brain compared with regular readers. This area contains portions of the frontal operculum, inferior frontal gyrus, and anterior temporal lobe, related to motor aspects of speech, as well as sections of the frontal lobe, associated with executive functions. Richards et al. (2000) used a proton echo-planar spectroscopic imaging technique to measure lactate changes in these brain regions, produced by a temporary delivery-consumption mismatch of oxygen in response to neuronal activation. A 3-week intervention program was implemented on a group of 8 dyslexic boys, aged between 10 and 13. Treatment consisted of 15 group sessions of two hours each. The first hour was dedicated to a phonologically driven instruction at all levels of language (from sub-words sound games to oral text reading), and the second hour was devoted to hands-on science activities, in which guest scientists lectured about their field of expertise. Follow-up sessions were held over several months to maintain the improvements. Brain lactate metabolism was measured at two time points, 1 year apart, during four different cognitive tasks; rhyming and lexical decision conditions, a tone judgment task, used to activate auditory non-linguistic functions of the brain, and control tasks of passive listening. Behavioral measures of reading skills were administered immediately after treatment. Brain and behavioral measures was also administered to a group of 7 age-matched non-dyslexic readers, receiving no treatment.

Results indicated that while before treatment the dyslexic boys showed the typical profile of greater lactate elevation in the left anterior quadrant of the brain, after treatment, brain lactate elevation in these regions during the same phonological task did not differentiate the two groups. Behaviorally, the dyslexic participants reached age level achievements in phonological decoding and text oral reading. Approximately 1 year after the initial images were obtained, six out of eight participants maintained their age-level phonological awareness. Also, no differences were found between the groups in lactate elevation in the left frontal quadrant during the same phonological task.

Regarding the lexical access task, lactate metabolic activation increased for the dyslexic participants compared with the control participants. Richards et al. (2000) have interpreted this result arguing that despite the normalizing brain-effects found for phonological processing; a brain signature may remain making some linguistic processes difficult for people with dyslexia.

Not all intervention studies have focused on improving accuracy of decoding ability. Shaywitz et al. (2004) utilized a functional magnetic resonance imaging technique to study the effects of a phonologically based reading intervention on brain organization and reading fluency. This study differed from previous studies not only in the fluency measure but also in the large sample of children used, and in the inclusion of three experimental conditions. Seventy-seven children aged 6.1–9.4 years (49 with reading disability and 28 control subjects), were divided between three experimental conditions. The experimental intervention (**EI**) was adapted from a model previously used in a remedial study (Blachman et al., 2003). Intervention consisted of individual, explicit and, systematic instruction of phonological knowledge and the alphabetic principle. This intervention provided practice opportunities combining word-level skills with text reading to support fluency and comprehension. This condition provided children with an average of 105 hours of tutoring throughout 8 months. The community intervention condition (**CI**) provided dyslexic children with a variety of interventions commonly offered within the school setting (remedial reading, special education, speech and language therapy etc.). Systematic and explicit phonologically based interventions were not included. The community intervention was provided 1-4 days a week lasting between 15 to 50 minutes. The community control condition (**CC**) consisted of regular readers receiving no intervention.

fMRI images were obtained before and immediately after treatment, while performing a cross-modal letter-identification task. Twenty-five children of the EI condition were also imaged a year later. A standardized reading fluency test was also administered before and after intervention. Results showed that gains in reading fluency made by the EI group were significantly greater than those made by the CI group. The two other comparisons (CC/EI; CC/CI) did not yield significant results. Increased activation was found immediately after treatment both for EI and CC participants in left hemisphere regions, including the inferior frontal gyrus and the posterior parts of middle temporal gyrus. One year following treatment the EI subjects were activating bilateral inferior frontal gyri, left superior temporal sulcus, and occipito-temporal regions, cited as critical for the development of an automatic word recognition system. Results also illustrated how a year-long phonologically based intervention can eliminate the need to rely on the right-sided compensatory systems previously used; the right middle temporal gyrus and the right caudate nucleus.

The normalization effect following intervention received further support from a study by Aylward and colleagues (2003). This study provided 10 children with dyslexia, aged about 11.6 years, with 28 hours of instruction. Intervention included the instruction of linguistic awareness, alphabetic principle skills, fluency and reading comprehension elements. A control group, consisting of 11 age-matched regular readers, received no intervention. Both groups were scanned (fMRI) before and after intervention while performing phoneme- and morpheme-mapping tasks.

At the behavioral level, the experimental group exhibited significant improvements on the Woodcock word reading test, on a morphological mapping test and on an oral reading test of words with and without suffixes. Imaging results showed that brain activation patterns of dyslexic children changed to resemble the pattern of regular readers. However, the authors suggest that an increase in activation among dyslexic children together with a practice effect among controls (decreased activation) may have led to the lack of group differences following intervention. Brain activation was also found to be specific to each of the language mapping tasks. Treatments-related activation changes for the phoneme-mapping task involved the inferior and middle frontal gyrus and the superior parietal lobe. Treatment-related changes for the morpheme-mapping task were found in the right fusiform gyrus and superior parietal lobe.

Temple and his associates (2003) utilized a different type of intervention program, namely, a program built on the assumption that phonological processing difficulties reflect a basic deficit in processing and integration of rapid auditory sequences. Fast ForWord Language (FFW-L; Scientific Learning Corporation, Oakland, CA) is a computerized intervention program that uses nonlinguistic and linguistic speech and acoustically modifies it by slowing down and amplifying rapid frequency transitions. FFW-L is composed of seven exercises designed to improve auditory and oral language processing, including auditory attention, discrimination, memory, phonological processing and listening comprehension.

Twenty children with dyslexia (8–12 years old) participated in the FFW-L remediation program during an 8-week period. Training lasted about 100 min a day, 5 days per week, for an average of 27.9 training days. Before and after attending the program these children underwent fMRI and behavioral testing. Twelve regular reading children, serving as a control group, also underwent two fMRI testing sessions but did not attend the FFW-L. Behavioral tests included a phonological processing task, a non-phonological task, and a non-letter base-line task.

On the behavioral level, children with dyslexia improved significantly on tests of real word reading, pseudo-word decoding, and passage comprehension. These improvements raised the dyslexic participants into the normal range. fMRI data illustrated a normalization effect; the left hemisphere temporo-parietal cortex and inferior frontal gyrus, previously under-activated, were now showing increased activity. The intervention-induced activity in the temporo-parietal region, however, did not reach the normal range seen in regular readers. The authors suggested that this normalizing effect reflects a partial but not a complete amelioration of the disrupted temporo-parietal response.

Data also indicated a compensatory effect, namely, right inferior, middle and superior frontal gyri, and middle temporal gyrus not activated by the regular reader, showed increased activation in the dyslexic brain. Such an effect was also found in bilateral anterior cingulate gyrus, a region associated with increased attention, and in the left hippocampal gyrus, a region associated with memory. The left inferior temporal gyrus, a region sensitive to visual processing of words, also showed increased activation following remediation. Additional areas showing a compensatory effect included the left lingual gyrus, right precuneus/posterior cingulate, right parieto-occipital sulcus, and bilateral thalamus.

Kujala et al., 2001 extended the assumption underlying the FFW-L training program by maintaining that the phonological difficulties faced by dyslexic readers reflect a general deficit in auditory and visual perception. Hence, this study was aimed at examining whether audiovisual training without linguistic material could have a remediating effect on reading skills and central auditory processing in dyslexic children. Forty-eight 7-year-old reading impaired children were pseudorandomly divided into two groups; a training group participating in the audiovisual training, and a control group. The training procedure consisted of a computer game presenting abstract, nonverbal tasks that require audiovisual matching. Stimuli were sound patterns varying in pitch, duration, and intensity, graphically represented on a computer screen. Subjects were required to recognize, match or follow the audio-visual patterns presented. Intervention included 14 training sessions, lasting about 10 min each, twice a week for a period of 7 weeks.

Brain activity was measured using the event-related potentials technique (ERP) while performing a tone-pair discrimination task. Recordings of the mismatch negativity (MMN) were then obtained, cited as reflecting auditory discrimination without biasing factors as attention, decision-making, or motor response. In addition, reading-skill measures were administered including, counting the syllables of words, deleting the first phoneme of words, and reading short words (correctness and speed).

Despite having equivalent reading scores prior intervention, the training group correctly read more words than the control group, and was nearly significantly faster in reading after training. In addition, the earlier parts of the MMN response were enhanced in the training group as compared to those of the control group. These results are important because they suggest that perceptual nonlinguistic training can cause plastic changes in the neural substrate of sound discrimination that may transfer to linguistic material and improve reading skills.

5. CONCLUSION

While there is not yet a consensus regarding the specific nature of neurophysiological deficits in dyslexia, it is clear from the aforementioned findings that the neural functioning of dyslexic individuals differs in distinctive ways from that of normal readers. Results from post-mortem, structural and functional imaging, and intervention studies comparing the brains of dyslexic subjects to those of normal readers, converge to show abnormalities in a variety of areas including anterior and posterior language areas, thalamic structures, visual cortex, the cerebellum and the *corpus callosum*. These findings lend support to the idea that systems involved in all levels of the reading process, from processing sensory input to higher-level analysis of phonological information, may be affected in dyslexia.

Though extensive research has been collected, many questions remain unanswered. Neural changes clearly accompany dyslexia, but the specific relationships defining these changes are still not clear. Do they represent developmental deficits that lead directly to the difficulties witnessed in dyslexic individuals or are they the result of these difficulties (e.g., compensation mechanisms)? Are they representative of inefficient or damaged functioning in normal reading systems, or can they be viewed as indications of alternative processing routes in dyslexia? Can they be used to differentiate between the varying behavioral deficits viewed among dyslexics? Future research in this field will address these and other issues as the attempt to uncover the structural and functional neural correlates of dyslexia continues.

REFERENCES

Adams, M. J. (1990) Beginning to read: Thinking and learning about print. Cambridge, MA: MIT Press.

Aylward, E. H., Richards, T. L., Berninger, V. W., Nagy, W. E., Field, K. M, Grimme, A. C., et al. (2003). Functional magnetic resonance imaging changes in brain activation as a result of instructional treatment in children with dyslexia, *Neurology*, *61*, 212-219.

Backes, W., Vuurman, E., Wennekes, R., Spronk, P., Wuisman, M., van Engelshoven, J., et al. (2002). Atypical brain activation of reading processes in children with developmental dyslexia. *Journal of Child Neurology*, *17*, 867-871.

Beaton, A. A. (1997). The relation of planum temporale asymmetry and morphology of the corpus callosum to handedness, gender, and dyslexia: A review of the evidence. *Brain and Language*, *60*, 255-322.

Belin, P., Zilbovicius, M., Crozier, S., Thivard, L., Fontaine, A., Masure, M. C., et al. (1998). Lateralization of speech and auditory temporal processing. *Journal of Cognitive Neuroscience, 10*, 536-540.

Best, M., & Demb, J. B. (1999). Normal planum temporale asymmetry in dyslexics with a magnocellular pathway deficit. *Neuroreport*, *10*, 607-612.

Blachman, B. A., Schatschneider, C., Fletcher, J. M. & Clonan, S. M. (2003). Early reading intervention: A classroom prevention study and a remediation study. In: Foorman, B. R., Editor, 2003. *Preventing and Remediating Reading Difficulties: Bringing Science to Scale*, York Press, Timonium, MD, pp. 253-271.

Breznitz, Z. (1987). Increasing first-graders' reading accuracy and comprehension by accelerating their reading rates. *Journal of Educational Psychology*, *79*, 236-242.

Breznitz, Z. (2001). The determinants of reading fluency: A comparison of dyslexic and average readers. In M. Wolf (Ed.), *Dyslexia, fluency and the brain*, (pp. 245-276). Cambridge, MA: York Press.

Breznitz, Z. (2002). Asynchrony of visual-orthographic and auditory-phonological word recognition processes: An underlying factor in dyslexia. *Reading and Writing, 15*, 15-42.

Breznitz, Z. (2006). *Fluency in Reading: Synchronization of Processes.* Mahwah, NJ: Lawrence Erlbaum Associates.

Breznitz, Z., DeMarco, T., Shammi, P., & Hakerem, G. (1994). Self-paced versus fast-paced reading rates and their effect upon comprehension and event-related potentials. *The Journal of Genetic Psychology*, *155*, 397-407.

Breznitz, Z., & Share, D. L. (1992). The effect of accelerated reading rate on memory for text. *Journal of Educational Psychology*, *84*, 193-200.

British Psychological Society (1999). Dyslexia, Literacy and Psychological Assessment. Leicester, UK: British Psychological Society.

Brunswick, N., McCrory, E., Price, C. J., Frith, C. D., & Frith, U. (1999). Explicit and implicit processing of words and pseudowords by adult developmental dyslexics. *Brain*, *122*, 1901-1917.

Callan, D. E., Tajima, K., Callan, A. M., Kubo, R., Masaki, S., & Akahane-Yamada, R. (2003). learning-induced neural plasticity associated with improved identification performance after training of a difficult second-language phonetic contrast. *NeuroImage*, *19*, 113-124.

Chi, J. G., Dooling, E. C., & Gilles, F. H. (1977). Left-right asymmetries of the temporal speech areas of the human fetus. *Archives of Neurology*, *34*, 346-8.

Cohen, M., Campbell, R., & Yaghmai, F. (1989). Neuropathological abnormalities in developmental dysphasia. *Annals of Neurology*, *25*, 567-570.

Dalby, M. A., Elbro, C., & Stodkilde-Jorgensen, H. (1989). Temporal lobe asymmetry and dyslexia: An in vivo study using MRI. *Brain and Language*, *62*, 51-69.

De LaCoste, M. C., Kirkpatrick, J. B., & Ross, E. D. (1985). Topography of the human corpus callosum. *Journal of Neuropathology and Experimental Neurology*, *44*, 578-91.

Demonet, J. F., Celsis, P., Nespoulous, J. L., Viallard, G., Marc-Vergnes, J. P., & Rascol, A. (1992). Cerebral blood flow correlates of word monitoring in sentences: Influence of semantic incoherence: A SPECT study in normals. *Neuropsychologia*, *30*, 1-11.

Duara, R., Kushch, A., Gross-Glenn, K., Barker, W. W., Jallad, B., Pascal, S., Loewenstein, D. A., Sheldon, J., Rabin, M., & Levin B. (1991). Neuroanatomic differences between dyslexic and normal readers on magnetic resonance imaging scans. *Archives of Neurology*, *48*, 410-416.

Eckert, M. A. & Leonard, C. M. (2000). Structural imaging in dyslexia: The planum temporale. *Mental Retardation and Developmental Disabilities Research Reviews*, *6*, 198-206.

Eckert, M. A., Lambardino, L. J., & Leonard, C. M. (2001). Planar asymmetry tips the phonological playground and environment raises the bar. *Child Development*, *72*, 988-1002.

Eckert, M. A., Leonard, C. M., Richards, T. L., Aylward, E. H., Thomson, J., & Berninger, V. W. (2002). Anatomical correlates of dyslexia: frontal and cerebellar findings. *Brain*, *126(Pt 2)*, 482-94.

Filipek, P. A. (1995). Neurobiologic correlates of developmental dyslexia: How do dyslexics' brains differ from those of normal readers? *Journal of Child Neurology*, *10(Suppl 1)*, S62-S69.

Filipek, P. A. (1999). Neuroimaging in the developmental disorders: The state of the science. *Journal of Child Psychology and Psychiatry and Allied Disciplines*, *40*, 113-128.

Finch, A. J., Nicolson, R. I., & Fawcett, A. J. (2002). Evidence for a neuroanatomical difference within the olivo-cerbellar pathway of adults with dyslexia. *Cortex*, *38*, 529-539.

Flowers, D. L. (1993). Brain basis for dyslexia: A summary of work in progress. Journal *of Learning Disabilities*, *26*, 575-582.

Galaburda, A. M. (1988). The Pathogenesis of Childhood Dyslexia, In: F. Plum (Ed.), *Language, communication and the brain,* New York: Raven Press.

Galaburda, A. M. (1989). Ordinary and extraordinary brain development: Anatomical variation in developmental dyslexia. *Annals of Dyslexia*, *39*, 67-80.

Galaburda, A. M. (1993). Neuroanatomic basis of developmental dyslexia. *Neurologic-Clinics*, *11*, 161-173.

Galaburda, A. M. (1994). Developmental dyslexia and animal studies: At the interface between cognition and neurology. *Cognition*, *50*, 133-149.

Galaburda, A. M., Corsiglia, J., Rosen, G. D., & Sherman, G. F. (1987). Planum temporale asymmetry, reappraisal since Geschwind and Levitsky. *Neuropsychologia*, *25*, 853-68.

Galaburda, A., & Livingstone, M. (1993). Evidence for a magnocellular defect in developmental dyslexia. In P. Tallal, A. M. Galaburda, R. R. Llinas, & C. von Eurler (Eds.), *Temporal information processing in the nervous system. Annals of the New York Academy of Sciences*, *682*, 70-82.

Galaburda, A. M., Menard, M. T., & Rosen, G. D. (1994). Evidence for aberrant auditory anatomy in developmental dyslexia. *Proceedings of the National Academy of Sciences, 91*, 8010-8013.

Galaburda, A. M., Rosen, G. D., & Sherman, G. F. (1990). Individual variability in cortical organization: Its relationship to brain laterality and implications to function. *Neuropsychologia*, *28*, 529-546.

Galaburda, A. M., Sherman, G. F., Rosen, G. D., Aboitiz, F., & Geschwind, N. (1985). Developmental dyslexia: four consecutive patients with cortical anomalies. *Annals of Neurology*, *18*, 222-33.

Georgiewa, P., Rzanny, R., Hopf, J. M., Knab, R., Glauche, V., Kaiser, W. A., et al. (1999). fMRI during word processing in dyslexic and normal reading children. *Neuroreport*, *10*, 3459-3465.

Geschwind, N., & Levitsky, W. (1968). Human brain: Left-right asymmetries in temporal speech region. *Science*, *161*, 186-187.

Hagoort, P., Indefrey, P., Brown, C., Herzog, H., Steinmetz, H., & Seitz, R. J. (1999). The neural circuitry involved in the reading of German words and pseudowords: A PET study. *Journal of Cognitive Neuroscience*, *11*, 383-98.

Heiervang, E., Hugdahl, K., Steinmetz, H., Inge Smievoll, A., Stevenson, J., Lund, A., et al. (2000). Planum temporale, planum parietale and dichotic listening in dyslexia. *Neuropsychologia*, *38*, 1704-13.

Helenius, P., Salmelin, R., Service, E., Connolly, J. F., Leinonen, S., & Lyytinen, H. (2002). Cortical activation during spoken-word segmentation in nonreading – impaired and dyslexic adults. *Journal of Neuroscience*, *22*, 2936-2944.

Hiemenz, J. R., & Hynd, G. W. (2000). Sulcal/gyral pattern morphology of the perisylvian language region in developmental dyslexia. *Brain & Language*, *74*, 113-133.

Horwitz, B., Rumsey, J. M., & Donohue, B. C. (1998). Functional connectivity of the angular gyrus in normal reading and developmental dyslexia. *Proceedings of the National Academy of Science* U.S.A., *95*, 8939-8944.

Humphreys, P., Kaufmann, W. E. & Galaburda, A. M. (1990). Developmental dyslexia in women: Neuropathological findings in three patients. *Annals of Neurology*, *28*, 727-738.

Hynd, G. W., & Semrud-Clikeman, M. (1989). Dyslexia and brain morphology. *Psychological Bulletin*, 106, 447- 482.

Hynd, G. W., Semrud-Clikeman, M., Lorys, A. R., Novey, E. S., & Eliopulos, D. (1990). Brain morphology in developmental dyslexia and attention deficit disorder/hyperactivity. *Archives of Neurology*, *47*, 919-926.

Hynd, G. W., Hall, J., Novey, E. S., Elipulos, D., Black, K. C., Gonzales, J. J., et al. (1995). Dyslexia and corpus callosum morphology. *Archives of Neurology*, *52*, 32-38.

Ingvar, M., af Trampe, P., Greitz, T., Eriksson, L., Stone-Elander, S., & von Euler, C. (2002). Residual differences in language processing in compensated dyslexics revealed in simple word reading tasks. *Brain and Language*, *83*, 249-267.

Jenner, A. R., Rosen, G. D., & Galaburda, A. M. (1999). Neuronal asymmetries in primary visual cortex of dyslexic and nondyslexic brains. *Annals of Neurology*, *46*, 189-196.

Karni, A., Morcoz, I. A., Bitan, T., Shaul, S., Kushnir, T., & Breznitz, Z. (2005). An fMRI study of the differential effects of word presentation rates (reading acceleration) on dyslexic readers' brain activity patterns. *Journal of Neurolinguistics*, *18*, 197-219.

Katzir, T., Misra M., & Poldrack R.A. (2005). Imaging phonology without print: Assessing the neural correlates of phonemic awareness using fMRI. *Neuroimage*, *27*, 106-115.

Kujala, T., Karma, K., Ceponiene, R., Belitz, S., Turkkila, P., Tervaniemi, M., & Naatanen R. (2001). Plastic neural changes and reading improvement caused by audiovisual training in reading-impaired children. *PNAS*, *98*, 10509- 10514.

Kushch, A., Gross-Glenn, A. K., Jallad, B., Lubs, H., Rabin, M., Feldman, E., & Duara, R. (1993). Temporal lobe surface area measurements on MRI in normal and dyslexic readers. *Neuropsychologia*, *31*, 811-821.

Lambe, E. K. (1999). Dyslexia, gender, and brain imaging. *Neuropsychologia*, *37*, 521-536.

Landau, W., Goldstein, R., & Kleffner, F. (1960). Congenital aphasia: A clinicopathologic study. *Neurology*, *10*, 915-921.

Larsen, J. P., Hoien, T., Lundberg, I., & Odegaard, H. (1990). MRI evaluation of the size and symmetry of the planum temporale in adolescents with developmental dyslexia. *Brain & Language, 39*, 289-301.

Larsen, J. P., Hoeien, T., & Oedegaard, H. (1992). Magnetic resonance imaging of the corpus callosum in developmental dyslexia. *Cognitive Neuropsychology*, *9*, 123-134.

Leonard, C. M., Voeller, K. S., Lombardino, L. J., Morris, M. K., Hynd, G. W., Alexandria, A. W., et al. (1993). Anomalous cerebral structure in dyslexia revealed with magnetic resonance imaging. *Archives of Neurology*, *50*, 461-469.

Leonard, C. M., Eckert, M. A., Lombardino, L. J., Oakland, T., Kranzler, J., Mohr, C. M., et al. (2001). Anatomical risk factors for phonological dyslexia. *Cerebral Cortex*, *11*, 148-157.

Livingstone, M. S., Rosen, G. D., Drislane, F. W., & Galaburda, A. M. (1991). Physiological and anotomical evidence for a magnocellular deficit in developmental dyslexia. *Proceedings of the National Academy of Sciences*, *88*, 7943-7947.

Lovett, M. W. (1987). A developmental approach to reading disability: Accuracy and speed criteria of normal and deficient reading skill. *Child Development*, *58*, 234-260.

McCandliss B. D., & Noble, K. G. (2003) The development of reading impairment: A cognitive neuroscience model. *Mental Retardation and Developmental Disabilities Research Reviews*, *9*, 196- 205.

McCrory, E., Frith, U., Brunswick, N., & Price, C. (2000). Abnormal functional activation during a simple word repetition task: A PET study of adult dyslexics. *Journal of Cognitive Neuroscience*, *12*, 753-762.

Milne, R. D., Syngeniotis, A., Jackson, G., & Corballis, M. C. (2002). Mixed lateralization of phonological assembly in developmental dyslexia. *Neurocase*, *8*, 205-209.

Pandya, D. N., & Seltzer, B. (1986). The topography of the commissural fibers. In F. LePore, M. Petito, & H. H. Jasper (Eds.), *Two-hemispheres-one brain: functions of the corpus collosum* (pp. 47-73). New York: Alan R, Liss. Inc.

Parviainen, T., Helenius, P., & Salmelin, R. (2005). Cortical differentiation of speech and nonspeech sounds at 100 ms: Implications for dyslexia. *Cerebral Cortex, 15*, 1054-1063.

Paulesu, E., Demonet, J. F., Fazio, F., McCrory, E. Chanoine, V., Brunswick, N., et al. (2001). *Dyslexia Cultural Diversity and Biological Unity. Science, 291*, 2165-2167.

Paulesu, E., Frith, U., Snowling, M., & Gallagher, A. (1996). Is developmental dyslexia a disconnection syndrome? Evidence from PET scanning. *Brain, 119*, 143-157.

Poldrack, R. A. (2000). Comments and controversies. Imaging brain plasticity: Conceptual and methodological issues - A theoretical review. *NeuroImage, 12*, 1-13.

Preis, S., Jaencke, L., Schittler, P., Huang, Y., & Steinmetz, H. (1998). Normal intrasylvian anatomical asymmetry in children with developmental language disorder. *Neuropsychologia, 36*, 849-855.

Preis, S., Steinmetz, H., Knorr, U., & Jaencke, L. (2000). Corpus callosum size in children with developmental language disorder. *Cognitive Brain Research, 10*, 37-44.

Pugh, K. R., Mencl, W. E., Shaywitz, B. A., Shaywitz, S. E., Fulbright, R. K., Constable, R. T., et al. (2000a). The angular gyrus in developmental dyslexia: Task-specific differences in functional connectivity within posterior cortex. *Psychological Science, 11*, 51-56.

Pugh, K. R., Mencl, W. E., Jenner, A. R., Katz, L., Frost, S. J., Lee, J., et al. (2000b). Functional neuroimaging studies of reading and reading disability (developmental dyslexia). *Mental Retardation and Developmental Disabilities Research Reviews, 6*, 207-213.

Rayner K., & Pollatsek A. (1995). *The Psychology of Reading*. Englewood Cliffs, NJ: Erlbaum.

Rae, C., Harasty, J. A., Dzendrowskyj, T. E., Talcott, J. B., Simpson, J. M., Blamire, A. M., et al. (2002). Cerebellar morphology in developmental dyslexia. *Neuropsychologia, 40*, 1285-1292.

Renvall, H., & Hari, R. (2002). Auditory Cortical Responses to Speech-Like Stimuli in Dyslexic Adults. *Journal of Cognitive Neuroscience, 14*, 757-768.

Richards, T L., Corina, D., Serafini, S., Steury, K., Echelard, D. R., Dager, S. R., et al. (2000). Effects of a phonologically driven treatment for dyslexia on lactate levels measured by proton MR spectroscopic image. *American Journal of Neurobiology, 21*, 916-922

Robichon, F., & Habib, M. (1998). Abnormal callosal morphology in male adult dyslexics: Relationships to handedness and phonological abilities. *Brain and Language, 62*, 127-146.

Robichon, F., Levrier, O., Farnarier, P., & Habib, M. (2000). Developmental dyslexia: Atypical cortical asymmetries and functional significance. *European Journal of Neurology, 7*, 35-46.

Rosen, G. D., Sherman, G. F., & Galaburda, A. M. (1989). Interhemispheric connections differ between symmetrical and asymmetrical brain regions. *Neuroscience, 33*, 525-33.

Rumsey, J. M., Andreason, P., Zametkin, A. J., Aquino, T., King, C., Hamburger, S. D., et al. (1992). Failure to activate the left temporal cortex in dyslexia: An oxygen 15 positron emission tomographic study. *Archives of Neurology, 49*, 527-534.

Rumsey, J. M., Andreason, P. Zametkin, A. J., King, A. C., Hamburger, S. D., Aquino, T., et al. (1994). Right frontotemporal activation by tonal memory in dyslexia, an O-1-5 PET study. *Biological Psychiatry, 36*, 171-180.

Rumsey, J. M., Casanova, M., Mannheim, G. B., & Patronas, N. (1996). Corpus callosum morphology, as measured with MRI, in dyslexic men. *Biological Psychiatry, 39*, 769-775.

Rumsey, J. M., Donohue, B. C., Brady, D. R., Nace, K., Giedd, J. N., & Andreason, P. (1997a). A magnetic resonance imaging study of planum temporale asymmetry in men with developmental dyslexia. *Archives of Neurology, 54*, 1481-1489.

Rumsey, J. M., Dorwart, R., Vermess, M., Denckla, M. B., Kruesi, M. J., & Rapoport J. L. (1986). Magnetic resonance imaging of brain anatomy in severe developmental dyslexia. *Archives of Neurology, 43*, 1045-1046.

Rumsey, J. M., Nace, K., Donohue, B., Wise, D., Maisog, M., & Andreason, P. (1997b). A positron emission tomographic study of impaired word recognition and phonological processing in dyslexic men. *Archives of Neurology, 54*, 562-573.

Salmelin, R., Service, E., Kiesilae, P., & Uutela, K. (1996). Impaired visual word processing in dyslexia revealed with magnetoencephalography. *Annals of Neurology, 40*, 157-162.

Salmelin, R., & Helenius, P. (2004). Functional neuroanatomy of impaired reading in dyslexia. *Scientific Studies of Reading, 8*, 257-272.

Sandak, R. Mencel, W. E., Frost, S. J., & Pugh, K. R. (2004). The neurobiological basis of skilled and impaired reading: Recent findings and new directions. *Scientific Studies of Reading, 8*, 273-292.

Schultz, R. T., Cho, N. K., Staib, L. H., Kier, L. E., Fletcher, J. M., Shaywitz, S. E., et al. (1994). Brain morphology in normal and dyslexic children: the influence of sex and age. *Annals of Neurology, 35*, 732-42.

Shapleske, J., Rossell, S. L., Woodruff, P. W. R., & David, A. S. (1999). The planum temporale: A systematic, quantitative review of its structural, functional and clinical significance. *Brain Research Reviews, 29*, 26-49.

Shankweiler, D. P., Katz, L., Lacadie, C., & Gore, J.C. (2000). The angular gyrus in developmental dyslexia: Task-specific differences in functional connectivity within posterior cortex. *Psychological Science, 11*, 51-56.

Shaywitz, S. E. (1998). Current concepts: Dyslexia. *New England Journal of Medicine, 338*, 307-312.

Shaywitz S. E., & Shaywitz, B. A. (2005). Dyslexia (specific reading disability). *Biological Psychiatry, 57*, 1301-1309.

Shaywitz, B. A., Shaywitz, S. E., Pugh, K. R., Fulbright, R. K., Mencl, W. E., Constable, R. T., et al. (2001). The Neurobiology of dyslexia. *Clinical Neuroscience Research, 1*, 291-299.

Shaywitz, S. E., Shaywitz, B. A., Fulbright, R. K., Skudlarski, P., Mencl, W. E., Constable, R. T., et al. (2003). Neural systems for compensation and persistence: Young adult outcome of childhood reading disability. *Biological Psychiatry, 54*, 25-33.

Shaywitz B. A., Shaywitz, S. E., Blachman, B. A., Pugh, K. R., Fulbright, R. K., Skudlarski, P., et al. (2004). Development of left occipitotemporal systems for skilled reading in children after a phonologically based intervention. *Biological Psychiatry*; *55*, 926-933.

Sherman, G. F., & Galaburda, A. M. (1999). Neuronal migration abnormalities in auto-immune mice: Implications for developmental dyslexia. *Developmental Neuropsychology, 16*, 355-357.

Silani, G., Frith U., Demonet, J. F., Fazio, F., Perani, D., Price, C., et al. (2005). Brain abnormalities underlying altered activation in dyslexia: A voxel based morphometry study. *Brain, 123*, 2453-2461.

Simos, P. G., Fletcher, J. M., Bergman E., Breier, J. I., Foorman, B. R. Castillo, E. M., et al. (2002). Dyslexia-specific brain activation profile becomes normal following successful remedial training. *Neurology, 58*, 1203-1213.

Siok, W. T., Perfetti, C. A., Jin, Z., & Tan, L. H. (2004). Biological abnormality of impaired reading is constrained by culture. *Nature, 431*, 71-76.

Stanovich, K. E. (1991). Word recognition: *Changing perspectives. Handbook of Reading Research Volume 2.* Mahwah, NJ: Lawrence Erlbaum Ass. Inc.

Tarkiainen, A., Helenius, P., Hansen, P. C., Cornelissen, P. L., & Salmelin, R. (1999). Dynamics of letter string perception in the human occipitotemporal cortex. *Brain 122*, 2119-2132.

Temple, E., Deutsch, G. K., Poldrack, R. A., Miller, S. L., Tallal, P., Merzenich, M. M, et al. (2003). Neural deficits in children with dyslexia ameliorated by behavioral remediation: Evidence from functional MRI. *PNAS, 100*, 2860-2865.

Temple, E., Poldrack, R. A., Salidis, J., Deutsch, G. K., Tallal, P., Merzenich, M. M., et al. (2001). Disrupted neural responses to phonological and orthographic processing in dyslexic children: an fMRI study. *Neuroreport, 12*, 299-307.

Temple, E., Poldrack, R. A., Protopapas, A., Nagarajan, S., Salz, T., Tallal, P., et al. (2000). Disruption of the neural response to rapid acoustic stimuli in dyslexia: Evidence from functional MRI. *PANS, 97*, 13907-13912.

Terepocki, M., Kruk, R. S., & Willows, D. M. (2002). The incidence and nature of letter orientation errors in reading disability. *Journal of Learning Disabilities, 35*, 214- 233.

Wada, J. A., Clarke, R., & Hamm, A. (1975). Cerebral hemispheric asymmetry in humans: Cortical speech zones in 100 adult and 100 infant brains. *Archives of Neurology, 32*, 239-246.

Whitney, C., & Cornelissen, P. (2005). Letter-position encoding and dyslexia. *Journal of Research in Reading, 28*, 274-301.

Wolf, M., & Bowers, P. G. (1999). The double-deficit hypothesis for the developmental dyslexias. *Journal of Educational Psychology, 91*, 415-438.

Wolf, M., & Bowers, P. (2000). The question of naming-speed deficits in developmental reading disabilities: An introduction to the double-deficit hypothesis. *Journal of Learning Disabilities, 33*, 322-324.

Wolf, M., & Katzir-Cohen, T. (2001). Reading fluency and its intervention. *Scientific Studies of Reading, 5*, 211-238.

2

EVENT-RELATED POTENTIALS (ERPS) IN THE STUDY OF DYSLEXIA

A Review

Shelley Shaul

Neurocognitive Research Laboratory, Faculty of Education, University of Haifa, Haifa 31905 Israel

Abstract: Electrophysiological methods are based on Electroencephalogram (EEG) data, and EEG methods are used to assess on-line processing of cognitive activity focusing on the measurement of Event-Related Potentials (ERP). This method permits direct observation of information processing at different levels of analysis; it can provide crucial information regarding real-time imaging of the neural system's responses to sensory stimulation (Bentin, 1989). This chapter will review the different ERP components which are relevant to reading and language processing, in order to aid us in understanding the different stages of processing that occur in the brain during reading. In addition, the differences in ERP components between regular and dyslexic readers will be discussed with the aim of understanding the manner in which reading ability affects brain activity. This information, which has been collected during the past few years, constitutes a stepping stone toward the development of diagnostic tools for the early identification of individuals at risk for dyslexia as well as the development of intervention programs for its remediation.

Key words: Event Related Potentials, reading, developmental dyslexia

1. INTRODUCTION

Investigation of cerebral activity in cognitive processing has recently received impetus in scientific research. Based on the development of new technologies, there are methods that are able to trace brain activity as well as to identify the localization of processes in reading. The most common technology is functional Magnetic

Resonance Imaging (fMRI). However, when investigating a cognitive temporal activity such as reading the fMRI technique has some disadvantages which derive from the time resolution of this method. fMRI allows sampling of brain activity data only within large frames of time measurement. The reading process is based on the information processing system (Brandeis & Lehmann, 1994; Johnson, 1995) which is characterized by limitations of capacity and rapid decay (Baddeley, Vallar, & Wilson, 1987). Moreover, this process is also based on stages of activation from perception to processing and finally to output. In order to trace the activation of the brain on-line during reading, the time units of the brain sample must be smaller. Thus, the technology recently adopted in reading research, which is capable of overcoming some of these time resolution limitations is electro-encephalogram (EEG) utilizing the Evoked Reponses Potential (ERP) methodology. EEG collects electrical signals during brain activity every 3.9 milliseconds and the systems existing today are capable of incorporating 128 or more brain sites. This method permits direct observation of information processing at different levels of analysis, and can provide crucial information by means of real-time imaging of the neural system's responses to sensory stimulation (Bentin, 1989).

ERPs are extracted from EEG data by means of averaging the brain responses to a number of equivalent trials in a given experiment. ERPs consist of various discrete components, or brain waves, that can be related to different stages of information processing in terms of amplitude and/or latency variations. The components are usually designated by their polarity (P, N) and by the latency of their maximal amplitudes in milliseconds. Areas of brain specialization can be identified by observing variations of amplitude and latency in ERP components across different scalp locations (see Halgren, 1990). ERP components reflect the time course of sensory and cognitive processes with millisecond resolution and the data is complementary to behavioral data in cognitive research.

Several ERP components have been identified in different studies, which appear to be characteristic of certain types of brain activity during the reading process. The components are: P100-N100, P200, N200, P300, N400, P600 and MMN. Each component is considered to be associated with a specific stage of activation in the reading process within an explicit time window. Any deviation in the process of reading might exhibit changes in ERP amplitudes and latencies.

2. RESEARCH EVIDENCE ON THE ERP COMPONENTS

2.1 The P100-N100 component

The P100 is a positive and N100 a negative evoked potential with a typical latency of about 100 ms (Hyde, 1997). The P100-N100 is assumed to represent an exogenic response, or sensory activity, to elicited stimuli (Johnstone, Barry, Anderson, & Coyle, 1996; Tonnquist-Uhlen, 1996). The N100 is more commonly observed among regular readers, and the scalp topographic distributions for N100 are usually frontal-central, with maximal amplitude on the Fz electrode (Hyde, 1997; Johnstone, et al., 1996; Picton, Hillyard, Krausz, & Galambos, 1974). Research on the visual N100 using pattern reversal stimuli (e.g. Hennighausen, Remschmidt, & Warnke, 1994) indicates that N100 appears earliest at the occipital sites (25-190 ms), and then moves towards the central and frontal sites (approximately 110-215 ms). Attention to spatial location has been found to enhance the amplitudes of N100 in response to both verbal and nonverbal stimuli (Wijers, Mulder, Van-Hooff, & Lange, 1993) and verbal (word) stimuli (McCarthy & Nobre, 1993). Research on the auditory N100 employing a three-tone oddball paradigm has shown that with increasing age, N100 peaks increase at the midline and become less diffusely distributed across the scalp, and then tend to develop a left bias. Furthermore, small amplitude increases to rare attended tones are significant among adults, but not children (Oades, Dittmann-Balcar, & Zerbin, 1997). The N100 latency has been reported to decrease with age by some researchers (e.g., Martin & Lovegrove, 1988) but not others (e.g., Polich, Howard, & Starr, 1985).

Research carried out using linguistic (word) tasks indicates that the N100 to visually presented words typically occurs over the front of the head at around 80-180 ms and the back of the head (occipital and temporal leads) at around 150-200 ms. The N100 to aurally presented words occurs in approximately the same time frame, but is more broadly distributed (Hagoort & Kutas, 1995). Nobre and McCarthy (1995) found that N100 in response to terminal words in visually presented normal and anomalous sentences peaked at 182 ms over the lateral posterior sites and was largest over the left hemisphere.

The N100 component is thought to index the initiation of an attention like process (Oades, Dittmann-Balcar, & Zerbin, 1997; Novak, Ritter, Vaughan, & Wiznitzer, 1992). Some researchers maintain that N100 amplitudes are related to arousal/attentional factors (Leppanen & Lyytinen, 1997). Others have suggested that N100 reflects selective attention. Evidence in this direction is derived from studies demonstrating that the N100 amplitude is increased by prior preparation for a demanding task (Harter & Aine, 1984; Näätänen & Picton, 1987). Other research on the auditory N100-P200 complex indicates that it can be evoked by almost any perceptible change in any feature of the acoustic environment (for instance, amplitude or frequency modulation). For this reason, it has been suggested that this complex can provide an objective measure of distractibility or discriminate different stimuli changes. Furthermore, empirical evidence suggests that both the N100 and P200 are important neurophysiological correlates of central auditory pathophysiology that may have clinical utility in the study of abnormal function and its development (see Hyde, 1997, for review).

The N100 has been found to appear in the left lateral occipital scalp area (visual word form area) at about 165 ms following a word presented in a familiar alphabet as compared to a similar component, which appears in the right homologous area for an unknown alphabet (Proverbio & Zani, 2004). A similar component was found by Wong, Gauthier, Woroch, DeBuse, and Curran (2005) at about 170 ms following presentation of different kinds of letters, with a larger amplitude for familiar letters.

Maurer, Brem, Kerstin, and Brandeis (2005) compared adult readers and children prior to the acquisition of reading. In this study, all subjects, adult and children, detected repetitions of visually presented words, pseudowords, symbol strings, and pictures during ERP mapping. Adult subjects could reliably differentiate words as indicated by the appearance of the occipito-temporal N100 component before 150msec as compared to children, who exhibited a later, more mid-occipital N100 component with marginal word-symbol differences.

Moreover, children with greater letter knowledge revealed stronger sensitivity to letter strings, which was confined to right occipito-temporal sites, unlike children with low letter knowledge for whom the N100 component did not distinguish word-symbol differences and adults for whom the specialization was stronger. The researchers suggested that their findings indicate the existence of a critical degree of early literacy, which induces some immature, but fast, specialization for letter strings before word reading becomes possible.

Among dyslexic readers this line of investigation has focused partly on the examination of the magnocellular deficit hypothesis (Stein, 2001). Therefore, all reports are on the visual P100 and mixed results have been obtained. Mecacci, Sechi, and Levi (1983) and Solan, Sutija, Ficarra, and Wurst (1990) reported smaller P100 amplitudes in Reading Disabled (RD) as compared to control children using pattern reversal stimuli. Brannan, Solan, Ficarra, and Ong (1998) also obtained evidence of lower VEP (P100) amplitudes among dyslexic readers in response to sinusoidal checkerboard patterns of a spatial frequency arc at 1, 4, and 8 Hz, as well as for an 8 Hz flicker fusion stimulus. These results were obtained in both high and low luminance conditions. Latency differences in P100 have also been reported. Brecelj, Strucl, and Raic (1996), for instance, found a significant prolongation of the P100 wave in dyslexic children when responding to high-contrast, small-checked patterns. On the other hand, Lehmkuhle, Garzia, Turner, and Hash (1993) found that both P100 and N100 latencies of visual evoked potentials among dyslexic children were longer in response to low, but not high, spatial frequency targets. A flickering background for these stimuli was found to increase the latency and the amplitudes of these components among regular readers, but to affect only amplitude among RD children. Livingstone, Rosen, Drislane, and Galaburda (1991) obtained similar results. Visually evoked potentials between 70-170 ms post-stimulus were delayed among dyslexics over the occipital areas when processing rapidly changing patterns with low spatial frequencies and low contrast.

The scarce data available suggests that the N100 component may differ among dyslexic and regular readers, although the direction of this difference is not yet clear. In a study by Harter, Anllo-Vento, and Wood (1989), it was found that reading disabled boys had a larger N100 than regular boys on a visual target detection paradigm.

Conversely, Hennighausen, Remschmidt, and Warnke, (1994) found that a sample of highly selected dyslexic children evidenced lower N100 amplitudes in the left-central region (C3) when fixating on a reversing checkerboard pattern. On the whole, the N100 component was significantly more absent among dyslexics as compared to controls, but more frequent in dyslexics with low spelling scores. In another study, Neville, Coffey, Holcomb, and Tallal (1993) observed a lower N100 amplitude and longer latency among dyslexics as compared to regular readers during simple auditory and visual recognition tasks. Leikin, and Breznitz (2001) examined the difference in brain activity between dyslexic and regular adult readers while processing sentence components with different grammatical functions. A higher N100 amplitude and longer N100 latency were found among the dyslexic readers as compared to the regular readers while reading sentences at their own and at an accelerated pace (the words were presented at an average and fast rate of presentation). In addition, the N100 is related to the search process and to identification of core points in sentences requiring information and focusing of attention. Thus, the shorter latencies found in the fast paced condition of this experiment may be interpreted as maximization of attention in reading due to decreased susceptibility to distractions.

The N100 is the most prominent peak of auditory ERPs elicited by simple repetitive stimuli such as tones or syllables. Differences in latency or amplitude of the auditory N100 have been reported in children with reading difficulties (Brunswick & Rippon, 1994; Neville, Coffey, Holcomb, & Tallal, 1993; Pinkerton, Watson, & McClelland, 1989) as well as in children with language impairments (Dawson, Finley, Phillips, & Levy, 1989; Lincoln, Courchesne, Harms, & Allen, 1995; Neville et al., 1993; Tonnquist-Uhlen, Borg, Persson, & Spens, 1996). Amplitude reduction of the N100 was found in a group of 14 boys with difficulties in reading, writing, and spelling (designated 'poor readers') as compared to 18 'good readers' (all 8-9 years old) in a study by Pinkerton et al. (1989). Cortical auditory ERPs were recorded in response to 2000-Hz tone bursts while participants watched silent films. Reduced N100 amplitudes (around 160 ms) in poor readers were observed in three of four scalp locations. For the whole sample, the N100 amplitude was correlated positively with performance IQ, spelling scores, reading accuracy and comprehension, as well as arithmetic. In interpreting the data, Pinkerton and colleagues suggested that the decreased N100 magnitude could be associated with impaired processes mediating selective attention.

Brunswick and Rippon (1994) contrasted 15 dyslexic boys (7-11 years old) and 15 regular reading controls (8-10 years old) on ERPs to stop consonant-vowel syllables presented in a dichotic listening paradigm. The participants were asked to report simultaneously presented syllables as accurately as possible. No significant group differences were observed either in the right or in the left ear responses. However, regular reading children exhibited larger N100 amplitudes in left temporal-electrode sites as compared to dyslexic children who showed less lateralized temporal N100 magnitude. N100 lateralization was also found to be positively related to performance on a phonological awareness task, rhyme oddity detection among words differing in their final sounds (e.g., pin, win, sit, fin; Bradley & Bryant, 1983). According to Brunswick and Rippon (1994), the deviances in N100 laterality are associated with abnormal cerebral lateralization of language fluctuations in dyslexia. The failure of the dichotic listening task to discriminate between dyslexic and normal readers in spite of the N100 laterality differences was suggested to indicate that laterality does not affect processing of the stimuli per se but appears to be associated with later aspects of phoneme analysis. However, in view of the fact that the N100 has been considered a basic index of adequate sensory registration, Leppanen and Lyytinen (1997) proposed that an altered N100 response might reflect inaccurate tuning of sensory information resulting in less reliable auditory representations that are, in turn, manifested in poor performance on language tests.

Moisescu-Yiflach and Pratt (2005) compared a group of 14 adult dyslexic students to 14 regular readers on two different auditory discrimination tasks (linguistic and non linguistic stimuli), they found delayed N100 latencies to all 4 types of stimuli among the dyslexic readers, differences in the current density distribution was also found, with left dominance for the regular readers and alternations between the two hemispheres among the dyslexic readers.

Yingling, Galin, Fein, Peltzman, & Davenport (1986), on the other hand, did not find any differences between 38 severely dyslexic boys (mean age 13.3 years) and their 38 non-impaired peers in ERPs following stimulation with auditory clicks. Bernal et al. (2000) observed no deviances in the N100 to pure tones in a group of 20 poor readers (10-12 years old), but reported larger amplitudes in two later components, the N200 and the P200 as compared to 20 regular reading children.

In a recent study, Molfese (2000) presented evidence that auditory ERPs recorded within 36 hours of birth discriminated between newborns who 8 years later would be classified as dyslexic, poor, or regular readers. The auditory ERPs analyzed by Molfese included that the N1-P2-N2 waves elicited by speech and non-speech syllables with mean peak latencies of 174ms, 309ms, and 458ms, respectively. The left-hemisphere N100 latency at birth was found to be shortest for the regular reading children and longest for the poor readers. Neither the dyslexic nor the poor readers displayed a well-defined N100 component. Right-hemisphere N200 peak amplitudes were largest for the dyslexic children and smallest for the poor readers. In particular the group differences in the N100 latency might point, as suggested by Molfese, to an underlying perceptual mechanism upon which some aspects of later developing verbal and cognitive processes are based.

As for SLI, Dawson, et al. (1989) reported atypical hemispheric asymmetry of N100 in response to a simple speech stimulus. In this study, 10 children with SLI ranging from 6 to 15 years were compared to 10 children with autism and 10 language-normal controls (aged 8-13 years). Children were presented with a series of auditory stimuli involving 80% clicks, 10% syllables (viz., /da/), and 10% piano chord stimuli and asked to indicate whenever the /da/ stimulus occurred. Based on the analysis of right-hemisphere-minus-left-hemisphere scores, both the SLI and autistic group showed the reversed pattern of N100 asymmetry characterized by the controls (i.e., smaller left-than-right amplitude and shorter left-than-right latency). Furthermore, in children with autism, language abilities were associated with right-hemisphere activity measures, while performance on three out of six verbal tests correlated positively with the N100 latency, correctness on all six tests was negatively related to the N100 amplitude. In children with SLI, on the other hand, impaired performance on four of the language measures was associated with longer left-hemisphere N100 latency. No statistical relationship between N100 and language measures was obtained for the control children. According to Dawson and colleagues, the pattern of hemispheric activity found in children with SLI coincides with a deficit in processing sequential information, for which the left hemisphere is thought to be pivotal.

Lincoln et al. (1995) studied children with SLI, autism, or regular language skills (10 in each group; aged 8-14 years) running two experiments. The first experiment involved passive listening to series of pure tones which differed in frequency and intensity (1000 Hz/60dB vs. 70 dB and 3000 Hz/63 dB vs.73 dB, all with equal probability). No group differences in latency or amplitude of the auditory N100 were obtained. However, unlike the children with autism or SLI, the control participants did show an increase in N100 amplitude to increases in stimulus intensity. In the second experiment, two pure tones were presented with the following variation on the so-called oddball paradigm in two different conditions. The active or response condition required the child to press one button to each frequent tone (probability = 70%) and another button to each infrequent tone (probability = 30%). In the passive or no-response condition, children simply listened to the stimuli. Both in the active and passive condition, N100 amplitude was found to be generally larger in SLI children compared to control subjects (and nearly significant larger compared to autistic children). The N100 latencies were similar in autistic and control children, but differed from the SLI group. Lincoln and colleagues concluded that the N100 deviations are consistent with theories of SLI related to ineffective regulation of sensory input. They speculated that the brief (50 ms) duration of the tones employed in their study may have been too short for full processing without SLI children having to allocate further attentional resources as mirrored by the enhanced N100. Alternatively, the increased N100 peak is possibly associated with impaired encoding of auditory information in short-term memory. Thus, for some of the SLI children the 2-second ISI might be too long to maintain the internal reference indicating whether the tone designated the frequent or infrequent stimulus.

Neville et al. (1993) reported N100 deviations in a subset of SLI children who exhibited deficits in auditory temporal processing. Twenty-two SLI children with concomitant reading disability (RD) and 12 controls with regular language development and academic achievement (all 8-10 years old) were compared on auditory and visual ERPs. The auditory paradigm involved an active oddball task in which a 1000-Hz tone was presented as the target stimulus

(10% probability) among 2000-Hz standard stimuli at one of three ISIs (200 ms, 1000 ms, and 2000 ms) and at one of three different stimulus positions (left ear, both ears, and right ear). Since no group differences were obtained for the auditory ERPs to either stimulus, the SLI/RI children were classified into two subgroups according to their performance on an auditory rapid sequencing test (see under 'Auditory temporal processing deficit', this chapter). SLI/RI children performing below the median level were classified as 'low repetition' (i.e., displaying auditory temporal processing problems) while those scoring above were classified as 'high repetition'. Subsequently, the N140 component to standard tones was found to be significantly diminished over the right hemisphere at the shortest ISI in the low-repetition group compared to both the language-normal controls and the high-repetition SLI/RD group. In addition, the latency of the standard N140 was significantly delayed in the low-repetition SLI/RI group especially over temporal and parietal sites of the left hemisphere. Neville and co-workers considered the N140 component equivalent to the adult N100. A contralateral (to the stimulated ear) and anterior distribution of the N140 response suggested to them reflection of activity generated in the superior temporal gyrus encompassing primary and secondary auditory areas. Hence, these findings were assumed to indicate that in SLI/RD children with auditory temporal processing problems, the reduced and slowed activity within these cortical sites contributed to their language symptoms. The authors' interpretation is not to be taken as a single-factor account of the deficits of language- and reading-impaired children, however. Thus, various deviations in visual ERPs to both language and non-language stimuli were also reported for either the whole SLI/RD group or only a subset of it.

Finally, Tonnquist-Uhlen et al. (1996; see also Tonnquist-Uhlen, 1996) observed a significantly delayed N100 latency and a tendency towards a higher incidence of unusual topographic maps in 20 children with severe SLI (9-15 years old) when contrasted to an age- matched control group (n = 20). Using a passive listening paradigm, pure-tone stimuli of 500 Hz were delivered to the left and right ear separately. The peak latency of the vertex-recorded N100 was longer in the SLI children (on average 110ms) than in the regular controls (on average 100 ms) following right-ear stimulation. Both left-ear and right-ear elicited N100 responses tended to decline with increasing age in the control children but not in the SLI group. While the delayed N100 latencies were presumed to be due to slower processing in central auditory pathways, the lack of an age-related latency decrease was considered to indicate that the disturbance persists rather than reflects a pure maturational delay. Furthermore, the SLI children showed a trend towards a greater number of deviating or non-focal topographical maps after left-ear stimulation. According to Tonnquist-Uhlen et al. (1996), atypical N100 topography may be accounted for by a lack of synchronization that is due to immature or poor connections between different cortical areas and deeper structures.

Taken together, the auditory ERP studies cited above indicate differences in N100 features between groups of children designated SLI, dyslexia, or poor readers and regular controls. While latency deviations in language-based learning impairments may be associated with a common timing deficit, N100 amplitude differences have been related to attentional factors or inadequate sensory processing. Great individual subject variability coupled with recording techniques using only a limited number of electrodes have often led to negative results or only non-significant trends.

2.2 The P200 Component

In the normal course of processing, the P200 is a positive-going waveform whose peak latency ranges from 150-275 ms. Some research examining the auditory P200 has shown that the scalp distribution of this component tends to be frontal-central with maximum amplitude at the vertex (see Hyde, 1997 for a review; Oades et al., 1997; Picton et al., 1974). Other research examining auditory P200s using pure tones indicates that the P200 amplitude in response to target stimuli has a strongly parietal distribution, while the P200 in response to standard stimuli is characterized by maximum amplitudes at parieto-central sites (Dunn, Gomes, & Sebastian, 1996). Other researchers (e.g., Oades et al., 1997) found that auditory P200 maxima tend to be more posterior among children, but are more centrally localized among adults when employing a three-tone auditory oddball task. That is, P200 loci shift anteriorly to the vertex with increasing age. These researchers also found that P200 amplitudes increased with age, and that P200 latencies decreased markedly at lateral sites with increasing age. Other researchers, however, reported different developmental trends. Martin and Lovegrove (1988) found that N100-P200 amplitudes increased up to age 14 years, but Johnson (1989) reported no such change. Oades and colleagues (1997) suggested that these inconsistent results may imply that P200 measures are unreliable for inferring developmental change.

The visual P200 has been less well-investigated. However, research on visual VEPs in nonlinguistic tasks among children carried out by Hennighausen et al. (1994) using pattern reversals indicates that P200 appeared earliest at the occipital sites (75-225 ms), and then moved towards the central and frontal sites (approximately 170-265 ms). Research using linguistic stimuli (words) indicates that the P200 component occurs to both visually and aurally presented words at around 180-250 ms. In the visual modality, the P200 can be observed across the head, but is larger over the frontal-central leads. The P200 is larger in response to visually as compared to aurally presented words (Hagoort & Kutas, 1995).

Research suggests that P200 is not merely an exogeneous component, but may also be related to endogneous or cognitive processing variables (Dunn, Dunn, Languis, & Andrews, 1998; McDonough, Warren, & Don, 1992). P200 is thought to index mechanisms of feature detection (e.g., Luck & Hillyard, 1994), selective attention (e.g., Hackley, Woldorff, & Hillyard, 1990), and other early sensory stages of item encoding (Dunn et al., 1998). Other researchers have obtained data indicating that a P200-like component is associated with short-term memory storage (e.g., Chapman, McCrary, & Chapman, 1978) and retrieval (e.g., Chapman et al., 1978; Friedman, Vaughn, & Erlenmeyer-Kimling, 1981; Taylor, Smith, & Iron, 1990), as well as working memory functions (e.g., Raney, 1993; Smith, 1993; Stelmak, Saxe, Noldy-Cullum, Campbell, & Armitage, 1988). It has been suggested that anterior and posterior P200s index different aspects of stimulus feature detection and encoding. Recent research suggests that P200s may be differentiated on the basis of their location. Dunn and colleagues (1998) proposed that frontal P200s may be related to early item encoding, whereas posterior (and possibly central) P200s may be related to partial or complete word retrieval from long-term memory into working memory.

Very little data has been reported on the P200, among dyslexics readers although the available data suggests that a similar pattern may characterize both young and adult dyslexic readers, at least at the linguistic level in the visual modality. Harter, Diering, and Wood (1988) found smaller P20040 amplitudes in the left hemisphere as compared to the right among dyslexic and compared to regular children during a letter recognition task (an intralocation selective attention paradigm). Naylor, Wood, and Harter (1995) obtained similar results with adult readers. These researchers obtained evidence of a smaller P200 at left central sites among dyslexic adults using the same task. Subjects exhibited a general reduction in positivity beginning at around 150 ms until about 500 ms. However, adult dyslexics appear to be characterized by more diffuse, bilateral reduction in electrophysiological responses.

2.3 The N200 Component

The N200 is a negative component typically occurring at approximately 200 ms after stimulus onset, and is usually characterized by a frontal-central scalp distribution (Oades et al., 1997). Research on visual N200s among children using pattern reversal stimuli (in which the subject was merely required to fixate, but not to respond) has shown that this component appears at the occipital sites around 190-440 ms, the central sites at 215-260 ms, and the frontal sites at approximately 205-390 ms (Hennighausen et al., 1994). Work on the auditory N200 indicates that this component peaks fronto-centrally at the Fz electrode when using two-tone oddball paradigms (Enoki, Sanada, Yoshinaga, Oka, & Ohtahara, 1993; Johnstone, Barry, Anderson, & Coyle, 1996). Other work on the auditory N200 using a three-tone oddball task revelaed that N200 amplitudes and N200 latencies tend to decrease with age, and exhibit a right bias from about 14 years of age. Around this age, larger midline responses to common versus rare tones also develop. Frontal maxima appear for non-target processing at all ages, but only become marked for target processing around age 17. N200 latencies have been found to be longer at frontal rather than posterior sites (Oades et al., 1997). The N200 is often held to represent the event-related, endogenous response (Tonnquist-Uhlen, 1996), although it has also been considered as exogeneous and stimulus-related (Jirsa & Clontz, 1990; Korpilahti & Lang, 1994).

In visual word tasks, Nobre & McCarthy (1995) observed two ERP features at 288 ms which were associated with orthographically legal stimuli (including pseudowords) with a left-mastoid focus and a midline-occipital focus. These authors suggested that the midline-occipital focus may reflect the preferential activation of a visual area in response to a word form. They also suggested that this component may be related to lexical search or access of function words. (These authors attributed a similar role to the N330 in response to content words).

While the N200 is generally considered to be a processing negativity associated with focused attention, stimulus classification and discrimination (Näätänen & Picton, 1986; Ritter, Simson, Vaughan, & Macht, 1982; Vaughan & Kurtzberg, 1992), it may also be elicited in unattended situations (Picton, 1995). Research has shown that the N200 amplitude typically increases with task difficulty and in response to deviant stimuli. N200 latencies appear to be shorter during focused rather than diffused attention and shorter after deviant as compared to standard stimuli (Oades et al., 1995; Oades et al., 1997). Other work has shown that the N200 is the first index of target detection (Potts et al., 1998). Research carried out using word paradigms indicated that the N200 in word tasks may be elicited by physically unexpected stimuli (for discussion, see Deacon, Breton, Ritter & Vaughan, 1991; Herning, Speer & Jones, 1987; Polich, 1985).

It has been proposed that the N200 is associated with "mismatch detection" (typically sensory, see Niznikiewicz & Squires, 1996 for a review). Research showing that the N200 is related to the degree of mismatch between a stimulus template of a neuronal model supports this view (Näätänen & Picton, 1986; Ritter et al., 1982). Additional research carried out on visual spatial attention and letter target detection suggests that the N200 may reflect an early, partly automatic process of template matching (Wijers, Lange, Mulder, & Mulder, 1997).

The N200 has been found to appear in the left visual word form area at about 285 ms post stimulus during the processing of words rather than pseudowords in skilled readers, supporting the view that the visual word form area discriminates words on the basis of their familiarity, and is alphabetic-specific based on the shaping of familiar letters (Proverbio & Zani, 2006).

An N200 component was found to appear when a sentence with a word category violation was presented (word order changed such as:

Max's of). It seems that the reader had a very fast syntactic diagnosis process, and the error elicited the component at about 200ms mainly in the anterior areas (Lau et al., 2006). In addition, Brunelliere, Hoen, & Dominey (2005) suggested that the N280 is an anterior negative event-related potential profile associated with the lexical categorization of grammatical function words versus content words. They found that the N280 effect is related to an index of grammatical complexity.

In general, the limited studies reporting on the N200 component indicate that N200 latencies may occur later among dyslexic as compared to regular readers. No group differences in N200 amplitude were reported. This appears to be true in both the visual and auditory modalities. In the auditory domain, Fawcett et al. (1993) found evidence of later N200s among dyslexic readers in response to target tones in an oddball paradigm. Comparatively more studies examined this component using visual stimuli. In a study by Taylor and Keenan (1990), later N200 latencies among dyslexics with visual processing impairment were found in response to both linguistic (letters, words and nonwords) and nonlinguistic (symbols) stimuli. In another study using a visual recognition paradigm, Neville et al. (1993) reported attenuated N20030 latencies among language-disabled dyslexic readers. Taylor and Keenan (1999) examined dyslexic children with auditory processing deficits and regular children on three visual target detection tasks; orthographic (targets were letters with closed loops), phonological (targets were letters that rhymed with v) and semantic (3-letter animal names). The results indicated that N200 latencies were longer on the semantic task among dyslexic as compared to regular children.

2.4 The P300 component

The P300 component is an endogeneous, prominent, positive-going wave. P300's maximal amplitude on the scalp typically has a centro-parietal distribution, and a latency range of 280-600 ms in tasks that require active discrimination, such as the oddball (Dunn et al., 1998; Wilson, Swain, & Ullsperger, 1998). In passive procedures (i.e., tasks that do not require an intentional discrimination response) P300-like waveforms tend to have a frontal-central scalp distribution, and can occur much earlier or later than 300 ms, and typically decrease in amplitude over relatively few trials (Polich, 1989; Polich & Heine, 1996). Recent research indicates that there is a trend towards a more equipotential distribution of P300 with increasing age, as evidenced by a significant increase in the ratio of P300 at Fz to Pz (e.g., Johnstone, et al., 1996.) This is apparent in both auditory tasks (e.g., Friedman & Simpson, 1994; Iragui, Kutas, Mitchener, & Hillyard, 1993; Johnstone et al., 1996) and visual P300s (Wijker et al., 1989). Although P300s in the auditory and visual modalities show similar (but not identical) scalp topographies, in general, the P300 appears to be smaller and shorter in latency in response to auditory as opposed to visual stimuli (Polich & Heine, 1996). Other research using language tasks has shown that the P300 is larger over the left hemisphere (McCarthy & Nobre, 1993; Nobre & McCarthy, 1995).

The P300 latency and amplitude are modified as a function of psychological parameters that reflect information processing of the stimulus (Erez & Pratt, 1992). For this reason, it been suggested that the P300 is a valid index of central information processing during task-related decision making (Palmer, Nasman, & Wilson, 1994). Included among the different processes held to be associated with the P300 are the dynamic updating of information held in working memory (Donchin & Israel, 1980; Fitzgerald & Picton, 1983), cognitive resource allocation and task involvement (Kramer, Strayer, & Buckley, 1991), and mental effort, or workload (Humphrey & Kramer, 1994; Wilson, et al., 1998). The P300 latency is believed to reflect higher-order cognitive processes such as stimulus evaluation and categorization (Polich, 1987; Polich & Heine, 1996). Consequently, it has been suggested that the P300 latency can serve as a temporal measure of neural activity underlying the speed of attention allocation and immediate memory operations (Cohen & Polich, 1997; Polich & Heine, 1996). The P300 amplitude is thought to be related to the task relevance (Hillyard & Picton, 1987), and probability, or expectancy (Comerchero & Polich, 1999; Duncan-Johnson & Donchin, 1981; Gehring, et al., 1992; Johnson, 1988) of the eliciting stimulus. Another notable feature of the P300 is its sensitivity to task/decision difficulty (Palmer et al., 1994). For instance, P300 amplitudes are larger and latencies are longer during oddball as opposed to single-stimulus recognition procedures (Polich & Heine, 1996). The P300 amplitude appears to be inversely related to decision confidence) Hillyard, Squires, Bauer, & Lindsay, 1971; Ruchkin, Sutton, & Stega, 1980), decision difficulty and stimulus discriminabilit (Johnson, 1986). However, the interactions between these variables have yet to be precisely determined (Wilson et al., 1998).

Research carried out using word stimuli indicates that word type may affect the P300. Nobre & McCarthy (1995) found that compared to other word types, exemplars elicited a larger P300 (maximal over the parietal sites). The P300 amplitude and distribution did not differ across the other word types.

A number of investigators distinguished between P300a and P300b components. These components are held to differ in both brain sources and physiological correlates (Cycowicz, Friedman, & Rothstein, 1996). The traditional auditory or visual P300b typically has a central/parietal distribution with a latency range of about 280-350 ms. P300a components are usually found in fronto-central areas, have a relatively short peak latency, and habituate rapidly (Comerchero & Polich, 1999; Dunn et al., 1998; Knight, 1996; Squires, Squires, & Hillyard, 1975). For both the visual and auditory modalities, novel (target) stimuli appear to elicit a frontal-central maximum P300 (or P300a), while frequent (nontarget) stimuli elicit a central/parietal P300 (or P300b) (Comerchero & Polich, 1999; Verbaten, Huyben, & Kemner, 1997). In regular subjects, the P300a is evoked primarily by novel stimuli suggesting that it may be associated with a passive shift of attention, or the orienting response (Comerchero & Polich, 1999; Cycowicz et al., 1996; Halgren & Marinkovik, 1995; Halgren, & Marinkivic, 1998). This component has been interpreted as reflecting frontal lobe function (Friedman, & Simpson, 1993; Friedman & Simpson, 1994; Knight, 1996). Several researchers have obtained evidence indicating that the decrease in novelty P300 amplitude is associated with a change to more parietally focused activity when novel items are repeated (Friedman & Simpson, 1994; Kazmerski & Friedman, 1995). It has been hypothesized that this change may reflect categorization of the initially uncategorized events (Courchesne, 1978) and/or the reduction of the orienting response to stimuli that were initially unexpected (Friedman & Simpson, 1994; Kazmerski & Friedman, 1995).

The P300b has been hypothesized to reflect the controlled or conscious processing of an event (such as stimulus evaluation), particularly the completion of that processing (Cycowicz et al., 1996; Hoffman, 1990). For instance, the P300b is evident only if the stimulus has captured the subject's attention and has been apprehended. P300b onset occurs at about the same latency as the specification of the subject's response, suggesting that the P300b may begin when the stimulus has been sufficiently processed to be accurately perceived (Halgren et al., 1998). Other researchers have suggested that the P300b may be the manifestation of a categorization response (Cycowicz et al.,1996).

Additional research supports the view that the P300a may be more closely related to attentional processes and the P300b with categorization (Comerchero & Polich, 1999). Comerchero & Polich (1999) demonstrated that the ease of perceptual discrimination affects the P300a and P300b. These investigators employed 3-stimulus auditory and visual paradigms in which the subjects responded to a target with a button press. The target was a frequently occurring stimulus, and the nontarget was an infrequently occurring stimulus. The auditory stimuli were tones, and the visual stimuli were solid blue shapes. The results indicated that regardless of discrimination difficulty, the target stimulus in both modalities elicited a P300b that was largest over the parietal sites. When perceptual discrimination between the target and nontarget was difficult (i.e., the target was very similar to the standard), the P300b amplitude decreased and latency lengthened in response to target stimuli. The nontarget stimuli in difficult discrimination conditions in both modalities elicited a P300 that was largest over the frontal sites, and whose latency was much shorter than the latency for targets. Hence, the P300 elicited by infrequently occurring nontargets in both modalities was very similar to the P300a found in "novel" stimulus paradigms. These authors suggest that these results may indicate that frontal lobe functions (e.g., attentional focus) are associated with the P300a.

Other work employing a three-tone auditory oddball task (e.g., Oades et al., 1997) revealed that the centro-parietal peak becomes larger in size with increasing age. The late P300 appears to decrease in size with age, especially in target-processing waveforms. In this study, young children (age 10) exhibited larger temporal and smaller, long-latency frontal responses than older children (age 14) and adults (17-21 years). When processing targets, the youngest children showed a frontally extending P300, whereas right-biased posterior maxima were characteristic of adults. The P300b latencies decreased with age more rapidly at the frontal as compared to the posterior sites. Oades and colleagues interpreted these results as reflecting the increasing efficiency of maturing attentional processes controlled by a central executive in the frontal lobe. Supporting this view is research such as that carried out by Hohnsbein, Falkenstein, and Hoorman (1995) using auditory and visual choice reaction time tasks. These researchers found evidence of two P300 subcomponents that appeared to be time-related to stimulus evaluation and response selection, respectively.

Many investigators reported that the P300 component among dyslexic subjects exhibited smaller amplitudes and longer latencies in response to both linguistic and nonlinguistic auditory and visual stimuli (Barnea, Lamm, Epstein & Pratt, 1994; Duncan et al., 1994; Erez & Pratt, 1992; Fawcett et al., 1993; Holcomb, Ackerman & Dyskman, 1985, 1986; Harter, Anllo-Vento, Wood & Schroeder, 1988; Harter, Deiring, & Wood, 1988; Johannes, Mangun, & Munte, 1994; Taylor & Keenan, 1990; 1999). Nevertheless, not all studies showed evidence of differences in both parameters concurrently in a particular task.

In the auditory domain, for instance, several investigators found evidence of smaller but not longer P300s among dyslexic children when using simple auditory stimuli (Holcomb, Ackerman & Dykman, 1986; Lovirch & Stamm, 1983). Other investigators found the reverse pattern. Fawcett et al. (1993), for instance, observed longer P300 latencies but no differences in P300 amplitudes to target tones among dyslexic adolescents performing a selective choice reaction (oddball) task.

A similar pattern of results is characteristic of studies carried out employing visual stimuli. Neville et al. (1993), for instance, found that language impaired reading disabled children had significantly smaller P300 amplitudes relative to regular children in response to visual stimuli in target detection tasks. Duncan et al. (1994) obtained evidence of reductions in visual P300s among dyslexic as compared to regular men with increasing task demands. However, additional analyses revealed that group differences were accounted for by dyslexic readers with many symptoms of ADHD in childhood.

Other researchers reported evidence of differences in P300 latencies. Johannes et al. (1994), for example, examined visual P300s among dyslexic and regular children using a simple visual discrimination task. These investigators found that while the P300 amplitude did not differ in the two groups, the P300 latencies were longer among dyslexic readers. Furthermore, the distribution of this component over the two hemispheres was almost symmetrical among dyslexic readers, but appeared primarily in the left hemisphere among regular readers.

Taylor & Keenan (1990) found evidence that dyslexics with a visual processing deficit exhibited longer latency P300s to nonlinguistic symbols, letters and words on an oddball task. In a later study, Taylor and Keenan (1999) found that dyslexic children exhibited longer P300 latencies on phonological and semantic tasks, but not on orthographic tasks. The P300 appeared to be more posterior located among dyslexic readers across the three tasks.

Differences in processing linguistic versus nonlinguistic stimuli were also reported using different types of tasks. Generally, non-linguistic visual stimuli (symbols) were found to elicit P300s of greater amplitude and longer latencies than linguistic visual stimuli (words) in dyslexic readers (Barnea et al., 1994; Holcomb et al., 1985). Barnea, Lamm, Epstein & Pratt (1994) compared ERPs in dyslexic and regular children on a short-term memory task for lexical (digits) and nonlexical (characters) visual stimuli and found smaller P300 amplitudes to lexical stimuli among dyslexics. In addition, response to probes was more prominent over the right scalp in dyslexics, and over the left scalp in regular readers.

Silva-Pereyra et al. (2001) compared the P300 on verbal and nonverbal working memory tasks among 3rd grade dyslexics and regular readers. On the verbal task (Sternberg's task) the P300 latency was longer among the dyslexic children, with no significant difference in amplitude, on the non verbal task a smaller P300 was found among poor readers over occipital regions and a larger amplitude over central regions. The poor readers' latencies were longer than the controls.

The authors concluded that a later P300 on both linguistic and nonlinguistic tasks is due to difficulty in temporal visual processing. A higher amplitude on the linguistic task may reflect a higher degree of difficulty for the dyslexics on this task.

Results were reported when comparing verbal and nonverbal auditory stimuli. Erez and Pratt (1992) compared dyslexic and regular children on target detection tasks and observed both smaller P300 amplitudes and longer P300 latencies in response to verbal (nonsense monosyllables) as compared to nonverbal (pure tones) stimuli. The P300 apex orientation tilted to the right among dyslexics, but to the left among normal readers. Barnea and colleagues (1994) suggested that this general pattern of results may indicate that dyslexic readers relate more to physical features of stimuli, while regular readers may rely more on linguistic features.

In addition, Leikin & Breznitz (2001) examined the difference in brain activity between dyslexic and regular adult readers while processing sentence components with different grammatical functions. Higher P300 amplitude and longer P300 latencies were found among the dyslexic readers as compared to the regular readers while reading sentences at their own and at an accelerated pace (the words were presented at an average and fast rate of presentation). In addition, the P300 is associated with operations involving classification of target words and updating in short-term memory (Brandeis & Lehmann, 1994). Thus, the P300 findings in the self-paced condition showed that syntactic interpretation of words seemed to be a more significant and complex task among dyslexic readers than regular controls, and as such may demand greater short-term memory resources.

Miller-Shaul & Breznitz (2004) found a delay in the P300 latency among dyslexic adults and children on a lexical decision task while processing words and pseudowords. Moreover, as their age increased, the discrepancy between dyslexic and regular readers was maintained or increased. These results support the notion that the dyslexia phenomenon is characterized by inaccurate and slow word recognition skills.

2.5 The N400 component

The N400 is a negative-going wave occurring around 300-600 ms post-stimulus (Hagoort & Kutas, 1995). The N400 is usually broadly distributed across the scalp, and is often slightly larger over the right than the left. The N400 is usually regarded as a manifestation of lexical integration and is associated with different aspects of semantic processing (Neville et al., 1993). While this component does not appear to change in response to the physical characteristics of stimuli (see Nobre & McCarthy, 1995 for review), it does appear to be affected by attention. Larger N400s have been elicited in response to attended, but not unattended, words. For attended words, the N400 appears to be smaller for semantically primed or repeated words (McCarthy & Nobre, 1993).

The N400 appears to be elicited by any stimulus with a semantic representation, such as pictures (Holcomb & McPherson, 1994; Pratarelli, 1994; Rugg & Doyle, 1992). Pseudowords (nonwords that obey orthographic and pronunciation rules) and pseudo-objects also elicit an N400-like component (Bentin, 1987; 1989; Holcomb & McPherson, 1994; Rugg & Doyle, 1992; van Petten & Kutas, 1991). N400s in response to pseudowords have been shown to be similar to or larger in magnitude than N400s elicited by words, whether they are written or spoken (Bentin, 1987,1989; Holcomb & Neville, 1990; Holcomb, Coffey, & Neville, 1992; Rugg, 1987). Conversely, phonologically or orthographically illegal nonwords fail to produce N400s (Holcomb & Neville, 1990; Rugg & Nagy, 1987). Pseudowords and words are typically characterized by a negativity, and true nonwords by a large positivity (Hagoort & Kutas, 1995). Nobre & McCarthy (1995), who also found that pseudowords failed to produce an N20080 component) suggested that orthographic or phonological analysis may be necessary to engage the language-related processes reflected in these components.

The N400 amplitude seems to be inversely related to semantic content (i.e., the less context, the greater the N400 amplitude (Dunn et al., 1998; Kutas & Van Petten, 1988; Kutas & Hillyard, 1989). For instance, if a target word is preceded by a semantically unrelated word, a smaller N400 is elicited than when it is preceded by a semantically related word (e.g. Bentin, McCarthy, & Wood, 1985; Kutas & Hillyard, 1989). It has also been demonstrated that the N400 varies with the amount of search needed to retrieve the meaning of a stimulus from long-term memory (e.g., Picton, 1988).

The N400 is largest when elicited by content words in sentences (Kutas, Van-Petten, & Besson, 1988), whereas words serving grammatical functions elicit N400s of smaller amplitude (Kutas et al., 1988; Neville, Mills, & Lawson, 1992; van Petten & Kutas, 1991). The magnitude of the N400 appears to reflect the degree of association between the content words in sentences (Kutas & Hillyard, 1989). The findings that word lists are affected by semantic priming (e.g., Bentin, 1987; 1989; Holcomb & Anderson, 1993; Rugg & Doyle, 1992) support the idea the semantic relationship among words determines the N400 amplitude (Nobre & McCarthy, 1993).

It has been suggested that anterior and posterior N400s may index different semantic processes (Dunn et al., 1998). Research has shown that frontal N400s are obtained during phonological and orthographic matching tasks (Rugg, 1985), picture naming tasks (Stuss, Picton, & Cerri, 1986), simple lexical decision tasks (Bentin et al., 1985), and category decision tasks (Neville, Kutas, Chesney, & Schmidt, 1986). Central-parietal N400s often occur when sentences or text are processed (Kutas & Hillyard, 1980). On the basis of such data, Stelmack and Miles (1990) argued that anterior N400s index word recognition in short-term memory, whereas posterior N400s indicate elaborative semantic processes in long-term memory. These two types of N400 may also be distinguished in terms of their latencies: The frontal N400 usually appears earlier, whereas the central-parietal N400 typically occurs later (Dunn et al., 1998; Nobre & McCarthy, 1995).

Research has shown that the N400 differs in sentence tasks as opposed to word list tasks. In sentence tasks, the N400 appears to be largest in the central-parietal regions of the scalp, and somewhat larger and more prolonged over the right as compared to the left hemisphere (Kutas et al., 1988). In word tasks, the N400 appears to have a more anterior distribution, with the highest ampitudes over the frontal or central sites (Bentin, 1987; McCarthy & Nobre, 1993). Other studies have reported a greater left as compared to right scalp distribution for word tasks (Boddy, 1986; McCarthy & Nobre, 1993).

According to lexical theories, the N400 is held to reflect the activation of the lexical and/or semantic representations of a word (e.g., Fischler & Raney, 1989; Van Petten & Kutas, 1987). This theory is primarily supported by data obtained from sentence processing paradigms showing that the N400 is not affected by physical or grammatical manipulations (Neville, Nicol, Barss, & Forster, 1991; Osterhout & Holcomb, 1990; 1994), yet the N400 amplitude is reliably reduced by semantic priming (Besson, Kutas, & Van-Petten, 1992; Kounios & Holcomb, 1992).

The post lexical hypothesis argues that the N400 reflects an associative process that integrates word representations with ongoing context (Holcomb, 1993; Neville et al., 1991; Rugg & Doyle, 1992). Data from word-list paradigms provide the main support for this view. Such studies have demonstrated that the N400 amplitude in response to words depends on selective attention (McCarthy & Nobre, 1993), the level of processing required by the task (Bentin, 1987; 1989, Kutas & Hillyard, 1989), and subject strategy (Bentin, 1987). According to

Nobre & McCarthy (1995), the fact that no mnemonic role has been identified for the N400 poses a problem for this position. Nobre & McCarthy (1995) found that the time window typically associated with the N400 contains multiple ERP features with distinct spatial distributions over the scalp. These authors found different distributions in response to target words in sentences vs word list paradigms. Furthermore, even in the absence of sentence constraints (e.g., in a single word paradigm) content and function words were found to elicit different N400 distributions.

Several researchers reported differences between dyslexic and regular readers on the N400 component. Lovrich, Cheng, Velting, & Kazmerski, (1997) compared regular and reading impaired college students on auditory rhyme decision and semantic decision tasks. The results indicated a relatively larger negativity at around 480 ms for RD as compared to regular readers during word rhyming tasks. This was particularly pronounced at the C3 electrode. No differences were found between the groups in N400 when they were required to make semantic decisions. However, within group analyses revealed that the N480 amplitude was larger for semantic as compared to rhyme tasks among regular readers, but not for the impaired readers. Similar findings were reported by Lovrich, Cheng, & Velting, (1996) when comparing dyslexic and regular children.

Ackerman, Dykman, & Oglesby (1994) found that compared to slow readers and children with ADD, dyslexic children exhibited an attenuated N450 peak when performing a visual rhyme decision task in which the first of two sequentially presented stimuli was a real word, and the second was either an orthographically similar word or a non-word. Reading disabled children did not show the N400 reduction for rhyming stimuli characteristic of regular children.

McPherson, Ackerman, Oglesby, and Dykman (1996) examined dyslexic adolescents in a paradigm which required them to decide whether two sequentially presented pictures were objects with names that rhymed. Phonetic dyslexics (i.e., the better decoders) showed a N400 priming effect, but dysphonetics (poorer decoders) did not. The priming effect was calculated on the basis of the mean N450 of the rhyming targets subtracted from the non-rhyming targets. In a later study, McPherson, Ackerman, Holcomb, and Dykman (1998) examined disabled and regular readers on visual and auditory rhyme decision tasks using single syllable, real words. It was found that phonetic dyslexics exhibited reduced auditory priming for the N450, while dysphonetic dyslexics displayed reduced visual priming.

Miles, and Stelmack (1994) also used a priming paradigm and found that reading disabled children displayed an absence in the usual left hemisphere asymmetry in the frontal N450 amplitude to unprimed spoken words. However, the same was true of arithmetic disabled and combined reading/arithmetic disabled subgroups.

Studies using sentence paradigms also reported differences in the N400. Brandeis, Vitacco & Steinhausen (1994) found evidence of delayed N400 among dyslexic as compared to regular children during the silent reading of correct and incorrect sentence endings. Neville et al. (1993) reported that dyslexic readers exhibited both higher amplitude and later N400s in response to unexpected words at the end of sentences. In a study performed by Robichon, Besson, and Habib (2002), researchers found a larger N400 among dyslexic as compared to regular adults while reading sentences which appeared word by word on a computer screen at a rate of 100 ms per word, in congruous and incongruous sentences. They did not find any differences in the P300 and assumed that the adults dyslexics have difficulties integrating the meaning of words into a sentence, and not only a pure sensory deficit.

Plante, Van-petten, & Senkfor, (2000) studied the differences between adult learning disabled (reading and language disabilities) as compared to regular adult readers. They used a cross model experiment with one visual and one auditory stimulus, which were connected or not connected semantically. There were pairs of words and pairs of non verbal stimuli (picture and sound). No differences were found in the early components, the N400 amplitude was smaller among the LD group, and it appeared only after the non verbal stimuli in this group. In addition, there was a different scalp distribution for the component, a higher amplitude in the right hemisphere for the LD group on verbal and non verbal stimuli, while for the controls the right hemisphere was dominant for words and the left for non verbal stimuli. Even though there were no differences in the behavioral data, it was assumed that the two groups used different physiological mechanisms to accomplish the task of semantic associations.

2.6 P600 Component

This component has two functionally different interpretations, one associated with memory processes and another related to memory (Key, Dove, & Maguire, 2005). The component is most apparent when the stimulus is unfamiliar such as infrequent words. It is also believed that this component is associated with searching for words in memory (Allan, Wilding, & Rugg, 1998), with processing words that are syntactically inappropriate (Van Herten, Kolk & Chwilla, 2005) and processing pseudowords or any irregular word (Osterhout & Hagoort, 1999). The P600 is connected to the "new-old effect", a larger P600 occurs in response to old stimuli previously presented to the participant compared to new stimuli that have never been experienced before (Rugg & Doyle, 1992; Smith, 1993). Almost all of the studies on the P600 involve visual stimuli. Studies such as Wilding & Rugg (1996, 1997) presented auditory words and then tested them visually and found the same old-new effect. These findings suggest that the component is not modality specific.

The P600 also appears after different syntactic violations and syntactic ambiguity. It has been found in different languages such as: English, Dutch, German and Italian. It is considered to reflect additional syntactic processing in response to parsing failure. It has been found in morphosyntactic, semantic and orthographic violations as well (Key et al., 2005).

Balconi & Pozzoli (2005) found the P600 component in visual and auditory tasks in which sentences had an incorrect grammatical final word. Casado, Martín-Loeches, Muñoz, & Fernández-Frías, (2005) also found the P600 component after sentence reading, and suggested that this component is an indicator of the syntactic processing costs incurred by the variation of word order, reflecting the phrase structure reallocation processes.

Few studies have dealt with the P600 component among dyslexics. One study that examined processing of new/old words by comparing words presented a number of times to the subject as opposed to new words presented for the first time found a P600 gap appearing among regular readers in response to reading a word (new or old) in the left hemisphere only. The amplitude of this component was higher when reading old words before new words. This gap was not found in the left hemisphere of dyslexics. The researchers claimed that this finding is the result of memory failure among dyslexics when retrieving words from the lexicon (Russeler, Probst, Johannes, & Munte, 2003).

In addition, Rispens, Been, & Zwarts (2006) investigated the presence and latency of the P600 component in response to subject-verb agreement violations in spoken language in people with and without developmental dyslexia. The two groups performed at-ceiling level on judging the sentences on their grammaticality, but the ERP data revealed subtle differences between them. The P600 tended to peak later in the left posterior region in the dyslexic group compared with the control group. In addition, the group of dyslexic subjects did not show a P600 in response to sentences with a plural subject. These results suggested that brain activation involved in syntactic repair is more affected by linguistic complexity in developmental dyslexia compared with non-dyslexic individuals.

Shaul (2005) found a delayed P600 among dyslexic adults on different lexical decision tasks as compared to regular readers. The P600 appeared later while processing words and pseudowords which were presented to the center of the visual field and both to the right and left visual field. These findings are supported by previous results showing that the cerebral processing of dyslexics is slower during visual tasks (Breznitz, 2002; 2003; 2005; Barnea & Breznitz, 1998; Breznitz & Misra, 2003; Miller-Shaul & Breznitz, 2004). In addition, it was assumed there are differences in the time it takes the regular readers compared to the dyslexic readers to find the meaning of a word in the long term memory.

2.7 The MMN Component

The MMN is a fronto-centrally negative component of the auditory ERP, usually peaking between 100 and 250 ms post-stimulus onset. It is thought to reflect a pre-attentive neuronal change-detection mechanism, occurring when an infrequent physically 'deviant' sound encounters a well-established sensory memory trace of a frequently presented 'standard' sound (e.g., Näätänen, 2001).The MMN is a subtraction of the brain's response to the standard stimuli from that of the deviant stimuli. The repetitive aspects of the auditory stimulation are encoded in their sensory neural representation or memory trace. If a stimulus does not fully match this representation a MMN is elicited (Kujala & Näätänen, 2001). The MMN can be elicited by any perceptible change in an auditory stimulus sequence. In addition to any simple stimulus features such as pitch, duration and intensity or a more complex feature such as phonetic change, or order reversal of two tones. (Näätänen, Tervaniemi, Sussman, Paavilainen, & Winkler, 2001). The larger the difference between the two stimuli the larger and earlier the MMN becomes (Tiitinen, Sinkkonen, May, Näätänen, 1994). Furthermore, there is usually a good correspondence between the MMN elicitation and behavioral discrimination accuracy (Amenedo & Escera, 2000). Masking studies have shown that if a masking stimulus is presented shortly (20-50 ms) after the offset of each auditory stimulus, then no MMN is elicited and if the interval is larger than 150 ms then the MMN is elicited (Winkler, Paavilainen, & Näätänen, 1992). The MMN has its major generator source in the auditory cortex, but frontal-lobe sources have also been reported (Alho, 1995). The MMN can even be obtained without the subjects attention to auditory stimuli, It is usually measured when the subject is engaged in some other activity such as reading a book or watching a movie, therefore, it is possible to study infants or patients who have problems in communication or performing tasks (Näätänen, 1991).

The MMN has proven to be a suitable tool for studying auditory discrimination in both adults and children (for a review see e.g., Cheour, Leppaenen, & Kraus, 2000; Kraus & Cheour, 2000; Näätänen, 2001). In addition, there is a large amount of evidence that the MMN can serve as an index of learning associated neural plasticity for verbal and non verbal stimuli (Heim et al., 2000). The MMN emerged among subjects who learned to discriminate between two sounds and not among subjects who could not discriminate (Näätänen, Paavilainen, Tiitinen, Jiang, & Alho, 1993), and the same occurred with speech discrimination (Tremblay, Kraus, & McGee, 1998).

The MMN is relatively mature at the age of 6 (Cse'pe, 1995; Kraus, Koch, McGee, Nicol, & Cunningham, 1999). Response of this kind was reported in neonates (e.g., Cheour, Tabbene, Khiari, & Douki, 1999) and even in pre-term infants (Cheour-Luhtanen, Alho, Sainio, Rinne, & Reinikainen, 1996). The MMN has been demonstrated as a sensitive measure for distinguishing individuals with language-based learning impairments from regular peers (e.g., Baldeweg, Richardson, Watkins, Foale, & Gurzelier, 1999; Holopainen, Korpilahti, Juottonen, Lang, & Sillanpaeae, 1998; Korpilahti & Lang, 1994; Schulte-Koerne,

Deimel, Bartling, & Remschmidt, 1998, 2001; Schulte-Koerne, Bartling, Deimel, & Remschmidt, 1999; Kujala et al., 2000; for a review see Kujala & Näätänen, 2001).

Recently the MMN was applied to studying phonological and auditory dysfunctions in dyslexia and the results are very promising. (Kujala & Näätänen, 2001). Schulte-Korene et al. (1998) examined the differences in processing tones and syllables among adolescent dyslexic and regular readers, and found no differences with the non-verbal stimuli or the syllables (/ba/ - deviant and /da/ - standard). The researchers found that the MMN amplitude was smaller among the dyslexics and interpreted this result as reflecting a phonological deficit and not a general failure in processing auditory information.

Other studies such as Baldeweg et al. (1999) found differences in tone discrimination as well (1000 Hz – standard and 1015,1030, 1060 Hz – deviation). Among adult dyslexics, the MMN amplitude was lower, and their behavioral discrimination was less accurate. In addition, the MMN and discrimination performance correlated with the degree of impairment of phonological skills.

Csepe, Szucs, Lukacs, & Osman Sagi, (2001) showed that dyslexics have difficulties in processing small rather then large stimulus differences, which is reflected in the discrimination of stop-consonants separated from each other by acoustically minor sound differences. Schulte-Koerne et al. (1999) found that changes in the temporal order of pattern elements also elicited a smaller MMN among dyslexic as compared to regular readers. These results might imply that that sound elements are masked or interrupted by surrounding sounds or sound sequences in dyslexics. Kujala, Belitz, Tervaniemi, & Näätänen, (2003) found that dyslexic subjects had diminished MMN to tone order reversal, which strengthens this assumption.

Differences in MMN were also found in at risk children. Children who have a family member with dyslexia due to the genetic factor of dyslexia (Pennington, 1995), as compared to children with no risk of dyslexia. Leppanen et al. (2002) found several differences between the groups, duration changes elicited a different MMN in amplitude and scalp distribution between the two groups, the amplitude was lower over the left hemisphere among the at risk children. A small difference in duration elicited a MMN in control but not in at risk children. These results indicate that with the MMN, dysfunctions of phonological/auditory processing in dyslexia can be determined in infants as young as 6 months old.

Kujala et al. (2001) showed that children who underwent a phonological training program and improved their phonological processing, had their MMN amplitude changed and correlated with their improvement on the reading skill measures. Heim et al. (2000) showed similar results with language impaired children, for whom the MMN looked more like that of the control group following a phonological training program.

3. STUDIES EMERGING FROM THE NEUROCOGNITIVE RESEARCH LABORATORY

In recent years, several comprehensive research projects have been carried out at the Center for Brain Research and Learning Disabilities at the University of Haifa. These studies sought to investigate the underlying cause of the dyslexia phenomenon in terms of lower level visual and auditory processing as well higher order orthographic and phonological processing using electrophysiological parameters among different age groups. The majority of experiments found two main ERP components among all subjects regardless of age: the P200 and P300 (Breznitz & Meyler, 2003; Breznitz & Misra, 2003; and Breznitz, 2006 for review).

Results of these research projects indicated longer latencies for both components in young as well as adult readers in the visual and auditory modalities in response to non-linguistic (flashes/tones) and linguistic stimuli (letters/words/sentences).

In these studies, the P200 component appeared at approximately 200 msec post stimulus onset among adult regular readers as compared to children for whom the component appeared later at approximately 240 msec post stimulus onset. Among the dyslexic readers, the P200 component appeared at approximately 225 msec for adults and 280 msec for children in both the visual and auditory lower level non-linguistic tasks. A similar pattern was found for the P300 component. Among regular adults, this component appeared at approximately 330 msec following stimulus presentation as compared to approximately 350 msec among regular reading children. In contrast, it appeared later among dyslexic readers, at approximately 360 msec for adults and 380 for children during performance of lower level non-linguistic tasks. The results of the P200 and P300 components emphasize the processing slowness that characterizes dyslexics.

In terms of the high order processing tasks, when processing words and pseudowords, regular readers exhibited a P200 appearing approximately 235 msec for children and 200 msec for adults following stimulus onset. Among dyslexic children, the P200 appeared at approximately 270 msec while among adults it appeared at approximately 240 msec. Similarly, the P300 component appeared at approximately 360 msec for regular adults as opposed to 430 for regular children while among dyslexic adults it appeared at approximately 450 msec and for dyslexic children at approximately 500 msec. Thus, it can be argued that the most significant difference exists with regards to the P300 during higher order linguistic processing where the dyslexics, adults and children, exhibit the greatest difficulty.

4. SUMMARY

In the past few years, an abundance of evidence has accumulated concerning the reading process through the use of electrophysiological measures. This information has provided insight into the different stages of the reading process on-line from the stage of letter perception to the higher order processing of semantic meaning of words and sentences. Consequently, we have been able to compare the regular reading process to the impaired reading of dyslexic subjects and gain a better understanding of the underlying difficulties associated with the dyslexics' slow and inaccurate reading. This contribution constitutes a stepping stone toward the development of diagnostic tools for the early identification of people at risk for dyslexia as well as the development of intervention programs for its remediation.

Future research in this field will address these and other issues as the attempt to uncover the structural and functional neural correlates of dyslexia continues.

REFERENCES

Ackerman, P. T., Dykman, R. A., & Oglesby, D. M. (1994). Visual event-related potentials of dyslexic children to rhyming and nonrhyming stimuli. *Journal of Clinical and Experimental Neuropsychology, 16*, 138-154.

Alho, K. (1995). Cerebral generators of mismatch negativity (MMN) and its magnetic counterpart (MMNm) elicited by sound changes. *Ear and Hearing, 16*, 38-51.

Allan, K., Wilding, E. L., & Rugg, M. D. (1998). Electrophysiological evidence for dissociable processes contributing to recollection. *Acta Psychologica, 98*, 231-252.

Amenedo, E., & Escera, C. (2000). The accuracy of sound duration representation in the human brain determines the accuracy of behavioral perception. *European Journal of Neuroscience, 12,* 2570-4.

Baddeley, A., Vallar, G., & Wilson, B. (1987). Sentence comprehension and phonological memory: Some neuropsychological evidence. In M. Coltheart (Ed). *Attention and performance 12: The psychology of reading* (pp. 509-529). Hillsdale, NJ: Lawrence Erlbaum Associates, Inc.

Balconi, M., & Pozzoli, U. (2005). Comprehending semantic and grammatical violations in Italian N400 and P600 comparison with visual and auditory stimuli. *Journal of Psycholinguistic Research, 34*, 71-98.

Baldeweg, T., Richardson, A., Watkins, S., Foale, C., & Gurzelier, J. (1999). Impaired auditory frequency discrimination in dyslexia detected with mismatch evoked potentials. *Annals of Neurology, 45*(4), 495-503.

Balgor, A. (1980). *The Frequency of words in Hebrew*. Hapoalem Library, Tel Aviv, Israel.

Barnea, A., Lamm, O., Epstein, R., & Pratt, H. (1994). Brain potentials from dyslexic children recorded during short-term memory tasks. *International Journal of Neuroscience, 74*, 227-237.

Barnea, A. & Breznitz, Z. (1998). Phonological and orthographic processing of Hebrew words: Electrophysiological aspects. *Journal of Genetic Psychology, 159*, 492-504.

Bentin, S. (1987). Event-related potentials, semantic processes, and expectancy factors in word recognition, *Brain and Language, 31*, 308-327.

Bentin, S. (1989). Electrophysiological studies of visual word perception, lexical organization, and semantic processing: A tutorial review. *Language and Speech, 32,* 205-220.

Bentin, S., McCarthy, G., & Wood, C. C. (1985). Event-related potentials, lexical decision, and semantic priming. *Electroencephalography and Clinical Neurophysiology, 60*, 343-355.

Bernal, J., Harmony, T., Rodriguez, M., Reyes, A., Yanez, G., Fernandez, T., et al. (2000). Auditory event-related potentials in poor readers. *International Journal of Psychophysiology, 36*, 11-23.

Besson, M., Kutas, M., & Van-Petten, C. (1992). An event-related potential (ERP) analysis of semantic congruity and repetition effects in sentences. *Journal of Cognitive Neuroscience, 4*(2), 132-149.

Boddy, J. (1986). Event related potentials in chronometric analysis of primed word recognition with different stimulus onset asynchronies. *Psychophysiology, 23*, 232-245.

Bradley, L., & Bryant, P. E. (1983). Categorizing sounds and learning to read - A causal connection. *Nature, 301,* 419-421.

Brandeis, D., & Lehmann, D. (1994). ERP mapping: a tool for assessing language disorders. In H. J. Heinze, T. F. Mante, & G. R. Mangun (Eds.), *Cognitive electrophysiology* (pp. 242-250). Boston: Birkhauser.

Brandeis, D. L., Vitacco, D., & Steinhausen, H. C. (1994). Mapping brain electric microstates in dyslexic children during reading. *Acta Paedopsychiatrica, 56*, 239-247.

Brannan, J. R., Solan, H. A., Ficarra, A. P., & Ong. E. (1998). Effect of luminance on visual evoked potential amplitudes in normal and disabled readers. *Optom Visual Science, 75*, 279-83.

Brecelj, J., Strucl, M., & Raic, V. (1996). Do visual neurophysiological tests reflect magno-cellular deficit in dyslexic children? *Pfluegers Archive, 431*[6 Suppl 2], R299-300.

Breznitz, Z. (2002). Asynchrony of visual-orthographic and auditory-phonological word recognition processes: An underlying factor in dyslexia. *Reading and Writing, 15*(1-2), 15-42.

Breznitz, Z. (2003). Speed of phonological and orthographic processing as factors in dyslexia: Electrophysiological evidence. *Genetic, Social and General Psychology Monographs, 129*, 183-206.

Breznitz, Z. (2005). Brain activity during performance of naming tasks: Comparison between dyslexic and regular readers. *Scientific Studies of Reading, 9*, 17-42.

Breznitz, Z. (2006). *Reading Fluency: Synchronization of Processes*. Lawrence Erlbaum and Associates. Mahwah, NJ, USA.

Breznitz, Z., & Meyler, A. (2003). Speed of lower-level auditory and visual processing as a basic factor in dyslexia: Electrophysiological evidence. *Brain & Language, 85*, 166-184.

Breznitz, Z., & Misra, M. (2003). Speed of processing of the visual-orthographic and auditory-phonological systems in adult dyslexics: The contribution of "asynchrony" to word recognition deficits. *Brain & Language, 85*, 486-502.

Brunelliere, A., Hoen, M., & Dominey, P. F. (2005). ERP correlates of lexical analysis: N280 reflects processing complexity rather than category or frequency effects. *Neuroreport, 16*, 1435-1438.

Brunswick, N., & Rippon, G. (1994). Auditory event-related potentials, dichotic listening performance and handedness as indices of lateralisation in dyslexic and normal readers. *International Journal of Psychophysiology, 18*, 265-275.

Casado, P., Martín-Loeches, M., Muñoz, F., & Fernández-Frías, C. (2005). Are semantic and syntactic cues inducing the same proceses in the identification of word order? *Cognitive Brain Research, 24*, 526-543.

Chapman, R. M., McCrary, J. W., & Chapman, J. A. (1978). Short-term memory: The "storage" component of human brain responses predicts recall. *Science, 202*, 1211-1214.

Cheour, M., Tabbene, K., Khiari, G., & Douki, S. (1999). Influence of personality disorder on the course of manic-depressive illness. *Encephale, 25*, 73-76.

Cheour, M., Leppaenen, P. H. T., & Kraus, M. (2000). Mismatch negativity (MMN) as a tool for investigating auditory discrimination and sensory memory in infants and children. *Clinical Neurophysiology, 111*, 4-16.

Cheour-Luhtanen, M., Alho, K., Sainio, K., Rinne, T., & Reinikainen, K. (1996). The ontogenetically earliest discriminative response of the human brain. *Psychophysiology, 33*, 478-481.

Cohen, J., & Polich, J. (1997). On the number of trials needed for P300. *International Journal of Psychophysiology, 25*, 249-255.

Comerchero, M. D., & Polich, J. (1999). P3a and P3b from typical auditory and visual stimuli. *Clinical Neurophysiology, 110*, 24-30.

Courchesne, E. (1978). Changes in P3 waves with event repetition: Long-term effecgs on scalp distribution and amplitude. *Electroencepthography and Clinical Neurophysiology, 45*, 754-766.

Csepe, V. (1995). On the origin and development of the mismatch negativity. *Ear and Hearing, 16*, 91-104.

Csepe,V., Szucs, D., Lukacs, A., & Osman Sagi, J. (2001). The role of reading acquisition methods in phoneme representation as shown by MMN changes. *International Journal of Psychophysiology, 41*(3): 209.

Cycowicz, Y. M., Friedman, D., & Rothstein, M. (1996). An ERP study of repetition priming by auditory novel stimuli. *Psychophysiology, 33*, 680-690.

Dawson, G., Finley, C., Phillips, S., & Lewy, A. (1989). A comparison of hemispheric asymmetries in speech-related brain potentials of autistic and dysphasic children. *Brain and Language, 37*, 26-41.

Deacon, D., Breton, F., Ritter, W., & Vaughan, H. G. (1991). The relationship between N2 and N400: Scalp distribution, stimulus probability, and task relevance. *Psychophysiology, 28*, 185-200.

Donchin, E., & Israel, J. B. (1980). Event-related brain potential and psychological theory. In: H. H. Kornhuber and L. Deecke (Eds.), *Motivation, motor and sensory processes of the brain: Electrical potentials, behavior and clinical use* (pp. 697-715). Amsterdam: Elsevier.

Duncan, C. C., Rumsey, J. M., Wilkniss, S. M., Denckla, M. B., Hamburger, S. D., & Odou-Potkin, M. (1994). Developmental dyslexia and attention dysfunction in adults: Brain potential indices of information processing. *Psychophysiology, 31*, 386-401.

Duncan-Johnson, C. C., & Donchin, E. (1982). The P300 component of the event related brain potential as an index of information processing. *Biological Psychology, 14*[1-sup-2], 1-52.

Dunn, M., Gomes, H., & Sebastian, M. (1996). Prototypicality of responses of autistic, language disordered, and normal children in a word fluency task. *Child Neuropsychology, 2*, 99-108.

Dunn, B. R., Dunn, D. A., Languis, M., & Andrews, D., (1998). The relation of ERP components to complex memory processing. *Brain and Cognition, 36*, 355-376.

Enoki, H., Sanada, S., Yoshinaga, H., Oka, E., & Ohtahara, S. (1993). The effects of age on the N200 component of the auditory event-related potentials. *Cognitive Brain Research,* 161-167.

Erez, A., & Pratt, H. (1992). Auditory event-related potentials among dyslexic and normal-reading children: 3CLT and midline comparisons. *International Journal of Neuroscience, 63*, 247-264.

Fawcett, A. J., Chattopadhyay, A. K., Kandler, R. H., Jarrat, J. A., Nicolson, R. I., & Proctor, M. (1993). Event-related potentials and dyslexia. In P. Tallal, A. M. Galaburda, R. R. Llinas, & C. von Eurler (Eds.), *Temporal information processing in the nervous system. Annals of the New York Academy of Sciences, 682,* 342-345.

Fischler, I., & Raney, G. E. (1989). Language by eye: Behavioral, autonomic and cortical approaches to reading. In J. R. Jennings & M. G. H. Coles (Eds.), *Handbook of cognitive psychology: Central and autonomic nervous system.* (pp. 511-577). New York: Wiley.

Fitzgerald, P. G., & Picton. T. W. (1983). Event-related potentials recorded during the discrimination of improbable stimuli. *Biological Psychology, 17*, 241-276.

Friedman, D., Vaughan, H., & Erlenmeyer-Kimling, L. (1981). Multiple late positive potentials in two visual discrimination tasks. *Psychophysiology, 18*, 635-649.

Friedman, D., Simpson, G. V., & Hamburger, M. (1993). Age-related changes in scalp topography to rare and target stimuli. *Psychophysiology, 30*, 383-396.

Friedman, D., & Simpson, G. V. (1994). ERP amplitude and scalp distribution to target and novel events: Effects of temporal order in young, middle-aged and older adults. *Cognitive Brain Research, 2*, 49-63.

Gehring, W. T., Gratton, G., Coles, M. G. H., & Donchin, E. (1992). Probability effects on stimulus evaluation and response processes. *Journal of Experimental Psychology: Human Perception and Performance, 18*, 198-216.

Hackley, S. A., Woldorff, M., & Hillyard, S. A. (1990). Cross-modal selective attention effects on retinal, myogenic, brainstem, and cerebral evoked potentials. *Psychophysiology, 27*, 195-28.

Hagoort, P., & Kutas, M. (1995). Electrophysiological insights into language deficits. In F. Boller and J. Grafman (Eds.), *Handbook of neuropsychology*, (pp. 105-134). Amsterdam: Elsivier.

Halgren, E. (1990). Insights from evoked potentials into the neuropsychological mechanisms of reading. In A. B. Scheibel & A. F. Wechsler (Eds.), *Neurobiology of higher cognitive function.* New York: Guilford Press.

Halgren, E., & Marinkovic, K. (1995). Neurophysiological networks integrating human emotions. In Gazzaniga (Ed.), *The Cognitive Neurosciences*, (pp. 1447). Boston: The Mit Press.

Halgren, E., Marinkovik, K., & Chauvel, P. (1998). Generators of late cognitive potentials in auditory and visual oddball tasks. *Electroencephalography and Neurophysiology, 106,* 156-164.

Harter, M. R., & Aine, C. J. (1984). Brain mechanisms of visual selective attention. In R. Parasuraman & D. R. Davies (Eds.), *Varieties of attention* (pp. 293-321). New York: Academic Press.

Harter, M. R., Anllo-Vento, L., & Wood, F. B. (1989). Event-related potentials, spatial orienting, and reading disabilities. *Psychophysiology, 26,* 404-421.

Harter, M. R., Anllo-Vento, L., Wood, F. B., & Schroeder, M. M. (1988). Separate brain potential characteristics in children with reading disability and attention deficit disorder: Color and letter-relevance effects. *Brain and Cognition, 7,* 115-140.

Harter, M. R., Deiring, S., & Wood, F. B. (1988). Separate brain potential characteristics in children with reading disability and attention deficit disorder: Relevance-independent effects. *Brain and Cognition, 7,* 54-86.

Heim, S., Eulitz, C., Kaufmann, J., Fuchter, I., Pantev, C., Lamprecht-Dinnesen, A., et al. (2000). Atypical organisation of the auditory cortex in dyslexia as revealed by MEG. *Neuropsychologia*, 38, 1749-59.

Hennighausen, K., Remschmidt, H., & Warnke, A. (1994). Visually evoked potentials in boys with developmental dyslexia. *European Child and Adolescent Psychiatry, 3*(2), 72-81.

Herning, R. I., Speer, M. & Jones, R. T. (1987). Event-related potentials to spoken equations: is the N400 really a late N200? *Electroencephalography and Clinical Neurophysiology, Suppl. 40*, 394-8.

Hillyard, S. A., Squires, K. C., Bauer, J. A., & Lindsay, P. H. (1971). Evoked potential correlates of auditory signal detection. *Science, 172*(3990), 1357-1360.

Hillyard, S., and T. W. Picton. (1987). Electrophysiology of cognition. In F. Plum (Ed.), *Handbook of physiology section 1: The nervous system.* Vol. 5, *Higher functions of the brain* (pp. 519-584). Bethesda: American Physiological Society.

Hoffman, J. E. (1990). Event-related potentials and automatic and controlled processes. In J. W. Rohrbaugh & R. Parasuraman (Eds.), *Event-related brain potentials: Basic issues and applications* (pp. 145-157). New York: Oxford University Press.

Hohnsbein, J., Falkenstein, M. & Hoorman, J. (1995). Effects of attention and time-pressure on P300 subcomponents and implications for mental workload research. *Biological Psychology, 40*(1-2), 73-81.

Holcomb, P. J. (1993). Semantic priming and stimulus degradation: Implications for the role of the N400 in language processing. *Psychophysiology, 30*(1), 47-61.

Holcomb, P. J., Ackerman, P. T., & Dykman, R. A. (1985). Cognitive event-related brain potentials in children with attention and reading deficits. *Psychophysiology, 22,* 656-667.

Holcomb, P. J., Ackerman, P. T., & Dykman, R. A. (1986). Auditory event-related potentials in attention and reading disabled boys. *International Journal of Psychophysiology, 3,* 263-273.

Holcomb, P. J. & Anderson, J. (1993). Cross-modal semantic priming: A time course analysis using event related potentials. *Language and Cognitive Processes, 8* (4), 379-411.

Holcomb, P. J., Coffey, S. A., & Neville, H. J. (1992). Visual and auditory sentence processing: A developmental analysis using event-related brain potentials. *Developmental Neuropsychology, 8,* 203-241.

Holcomb, P. J. & McPherson, W. B. (1994). Event-related brain potentials reflect semantic priming in an object decision task. *Brain and Cognition, 24*(2), 259-276.

Holcomb, P. J., & Neville, H. (1990). Auditory and visual semantic priming in lexical decision: A comparison using event-related potentials. *Language and Cognitive Processes, 5,* 281-312.

Holopainen, I. E., Korpilahti, P., Juottonen, K., Lang, H., & Sillanpaeae, M. (1998). Abnormal frequency mismatch negativity in mentally retarded children and in children with developmental dysphasia. *Journal of Child Neurology, 13*, 178-183.

Humphrey, D. G., & Kramer, A. F. (1994). Toward a physiological assessment of dynamic changes in mental workload. *Human Factors, 36*, 3-26.

Hyde, M. (1997). The N1 response and its applications. *Audiology and Neuro-Otology, 2,* 281-307.

Iragui, V. J., Kutas, M., Mitchener, M. R., & Hillyard, S. A. (1993). Effects of aging on event-related potentials and raction time in an auditory oddball task. *Psychophysiology, 30*, 10-22.

Jirsa, R. E., & Clontz, K. (1990). Long latency auditory event related potentials in children with auditory processing disorders. *Ear and Hearing, 11*, 222-232.

Johannes, S., Mangun, G. R., & Muente, T. F (1994). Developmental dyslexia and cerebral lateralization: Electrophysiological findings. *Nervenarzt, 65*, 859-864.

Johnson, R. (1986). A triarchic model of P300 amplitude. *Psychophysiology, 24,* 367-384.

Johnson, R. (1988). The amplitude of the P300 component of the event-related potential: Review and synthesis. In: P. Ackles, J. R. Jennings, and M. G. H. Coles (Eds). *Advances in psychophysiology: A research annual, Vol 3.* (pp. 69-138). JAI Press: Greenwich, CT.

Johnson, R. (1989). Developmental evidence for modality-dependent P300 generators: A normative study. *Psychophysiology, 26*, 651-667.

Johnson, R. (1995). Effects of color on children's naming of pictures. *Perceptual and Motor Skills, 80,* 1091-1101.

Johnstone, S. J., Barry, R. J., Anderson, J. W., & Coyle, S. F. (1996). Age-related changes in child and adolescent event-related potential component morphology, amplitude and latency to standard and target stimuli in an auditory oddball task. *International Journal of Psychophysiology, 24*, 223-238.

Kazmerski, V. A., & Friedman, D. (1995). Repetition of novel stimuli in an ERP oddball paradigm: Aging effects. *Journal of Psychophysiology, 9*, 298-311.

Key, A. P. F., Dove, G. O., & Maguire, M. (2005). Linking brainwaves to the brain: An ERP primer. *Developmental Neuropsychology, 27*(2): 183-215.

Knight, R. T. (1996). Contribution of human hippocampal region to novelty detection. *Nature, 383,* 256-259.

Korpilahti, P., & Lang, H. A. (1994). Auditory ERP components and mismatch negativity in dysphasic children. *Electroencephalography and Clinical Neurophysiology, 91*(4), 256-264.

Kounios, J., & Holcomb, P. J. (1992). Structure and process in semantic memory: Evidence from event-related brain potentials and reaction times. *Journal of Experimental Psychology: General, 121*, 459-479.

Kramer, A. F., Strayer, D. L., & Buckley, J. (1991). Task versus component consistency in the development of automatic processing: A psychophysiological assessment. *Psychophysiology, 28*, 425-437.

Kraus, N., & Cheour, M. (2000). Speech sound representation in the brain. *Audiology and Neuro-Otolog., 5*, 140-150.

Kraus, N., Koch, D. B., McGee, T. J., Nicol, T. G., & Cunningham, J. (1999). Speech-sound discrimination in school-age children: Psychophysical and neurophysiological measures. *Journal of Speech, Language, and Hearing Research, 42*(5): 1042-1060.

Kujala, T., Belitz, S., Tervaniemi, M. & Näätänen, R. (2003). Auditory sensory memory disorder in dyslexic adults as indexed by the mismatch negativity. *European Journal of Neuroscience, 17*, 1323-1327.

Kujala, T., Karma, K., Ceponiene, R., Belitz, S., Turkkila, P., Tervaniemi, M., et al. (2001). Plastic neural changes and reading improvement caused by audio-visual training in reading-impaired children. *Proceedings of the National Academy of Sciences*, 98, 10509-10514.

Kujala, T., Myllyviita, K., Tervaniemi, M., Alho, K., Kallio, J., & Näätänen, R. (2000). Basic auditory dysfunction in dyslexia as demonstrated by brain activity measurements. *Psychophysiology, 37*, 262-266

Kujala, T., & Näätänen, R. (2001). The mismatch negativity in evaluating central auditory dysfunction in dyslexia. *Neuroscience and Biobehavioral Reviews, 25*, 535-543.

Kutas, M., & Hillyard, S. A. (1980). Reading senseless sentences: Brain potential reflect semantic incongruity. *Science, 207,* 203-205.

Kutas, M., & Hillyard, S. A. (1989). Brain potentials during reading reflect word expectancy and semantic association. *Nature, 307*, 161-163.

Kutas, M., & Van Petten, C. (1988). Event-related potential studies of language. In P. K. Ackles, J. R. Jennings, & M. G. H. Coles (Eds.), *Advances in psychophysiology.* Greenwich, CT: Jai Press.

Kutas, M., Van-Petten, C., & Besson, M. (1988). Event-related potential asymmetries during the reading of sentences. *Electroencephalography and Clinical Neurophysiology, 69*, 218-233.

Lau, E., Stroud, C., Plesch, S., & Phillips, C. (2006). The role of structural prediction in rapid syntactic analysis. *Brain and Language, 98*, 74-88.

Lehmkuhle, S, Garzia, R.P., Turner, L., & Hash, T. (1993). A defective visual pathway in children with reading disability. *New England Journal of Medicine, 328*, 989-996.

Leikin, M., & Breznitz, Z. (2001). Effects of accelerated reading rate on syntactic processing of Hebrew sentences among normal readers: Electrophysiological evidence *Genetic, Social and General Psychology Monographs, 127,* 193-211.

Leppaenen, P. H. T., & Lyytinen, H. (1997). Auditory event-related potentials in the study of developmental language related disorders. *Audiology and Neuro-Otology, 2*, 308-340.

Leppaenen, P. H. T., Richardson, U., Pihko, E., Eklund, K. M., Guttorm, T. K., Aro, M., et al. (1997). Brain responses to changes in speech sound durations differ between infants with and without familial risk for dyslexia. *Developmental Neuropsychology, 22*(1): 407-422.

Lincoln, A. J., Courchesne, E., Harms, L., & Allen, M. (1995). Sensory modulation of auditory stimuli in children with autism and receptive developmental language disorder: Event related brain potential evidence. *Journal of Autism and Developmental Disorders. 25*, 521-539.

Livingstone, M. S., Rosen, G. D., Drislane, F. W., & Galaburda, A. M. (1991). Physiological and anotomical evidence for a magnocellular deficit in developmental dyslexia. *Proceedings of the National Academy of Sciences, 88,* 7943-7947.

Lovrich, D., & Stamm, J. S. (1983). Event-related potential and behavioral correlates of attention in reading retardation. *Journal of Clinical Neuropsychology, 5*(1), 13-37.

Lovrich, D., Cheng, J. C., & Velting, D. M., (1996). Late cognitive brain potentials, phonological and semantic classification of spoken words, and reading ability in children. *Journal of Clinical and Experimental Neuropsychology, 18,* 161-177.

Lovrich, D., Cheng, J. C., Velting, D. M., & Kazmerski, V. (1997). Auditory ERPs during rhyme and semantic processing: Effects of reading ability in college students. *Journal of Clinical and Experimental Neuropsychology, 19*, 313-330.

Luck, S. J., & Hillyard, S. A., (1994). Electrophysiological correlates of feature analysis during visual search. *Psychophysiology, 31*, 291-308.

Martin F., & Lovegrove, W. J. (1988). Uniform-field flicker masking in control and specifically disabled readers. *Perception, 17*, 203-214.

Maurer, U., Brem, S., Kerstin, B., & Brandeis, D. (2005). Emerging neurophysiological specialization for letter strings. *Journal of Cognitive Neuroscience, 17*, 1532-1552.

McCarthy, G., & Nobre, A. C. (1993). Modulation of semantic processing by spatial selective attention. *Electroencephalography and Clinical Neurophysiology, 88*, 210-219.

McDonough, E. B., Warren, C. A., & Don, N. S., (1992). Event related potentials in a guessing task: The gleam in the eye effect. *International Journal of Neuroscience, 66*, 209-219.

McPherson, W. B. Ackerman, P. T., Oglesby, M., & Dyckman, R. A. (1996). Event-related brain potentials elicited by rhyming and non-rhyming pictures differentiate subgroups of reading disabled adolescents. *Integrative Physiological and Behavioral Science, 31*, 3-17.

McPherson, W. B., Ackerman, P. T., Holcomb, P. J,. & Dykman, R. A. (1998). Event-related brain potentials elicited during phonological processing differentiate subgroups of reading disabled adolescents. *Brain and Language, 62*, 163-185.

Mecacci, L., Sechi, E., & Levi, G. (1983). Abnormalities of visual evoked potentials by checkerboards in children with specific reading disability. *Brain and Cognition, 2*, 135-143.

Miles, J., & Stelmack, R. M. (1994). Learning disability subtypes and the effects of auditory and visual priming on visual event-related potentials to words. *Journal of Clinical and Experimental Neuropsychology, 16*, 43-64.

Miller-Shaul, S., & Breznitz, Z. (2004). Electrocortical Measures during a Lexical Decision Task: A Comparison between Elementary School-Aged Children Normal and Dyslexic Readers and Adult, Normal and Dyslexics Readers. *Journal of Genetic Psychology, 165*, 399-424.

Moisescu-Yiflach, T., & Pratt, H. (2005). Auditory event related potentials and source current density estimation in phonologic/auditory dyslexics. *Clinical Neurophysiology, 116*, 2632-47.

Molfese, D. L. (2000). Predicting dyslexia at 8 years of age using neonatal brain responses. *Brain and Language, 72*, 238-245.

Näätänen, R. (1991). Mismatch negativity outside strong attentional focus: A commentary on Woldorff et al. (1991). *Psychophysiology, 28*, 478-484.

Näätänen, R. (2001). The perception of speech sounds by the human brain as reflected by the mismatch negativity (MMN) and its magnetic equivalent (MMNm). *Psychophysiology, 38*, 1-21

Näätänen, R., Paavilainen, P., Tiitinen, H., Jiang, D., & Alho, K. (1993). Attention and mismatch negativity. *Psychophysiology, 30*, 436-450.

Näätänen, R., & Picton, T. W. (1986). N2 and automatic versus controlled processes. Cerebral Psychophysiology: Studies in Event-Related Potentials (EEG Suppl. 38), 169-171.

Näätänen, R., & Picton, T. W. (1987). The N1 wave of the human electric and magnetic response to sound: A review and an analysis of the component structure. *Psychophysiology, 24*, 375-425.

Näätänen, R., Tervaniemi, M., Sussman, E., Paavilainen, P. & Winkler, I. (2001) "Primitive intelligence" in the auditory cortex. *Trends in Neurosciences, 24*, 283-288.

Naylor, C. E., Wood, F. B., & Harter, M. R. (1995). Event-related potentials in adults diagnosed as reading disabled in childhood. Special issue: M. Russell Harter memorial issue: Progress in visual information processing. *International Journal of Neuroscience, 80*, 339-352.

Neville, H. J., Coffey, S. A., Holcomb, P. J., & Tallal, P. (1993). The neurobiology of sensory and language processing in language-impaired children. *Journal of Cognitive Neuroscience, 5*, 235-253.

Neville, H. J., Kutas, M., Chesney, G., & Schmidt, A. (1986). Event-related brain potentials during initial encoding and subsequent recognition memory of congruous and incongruous words. *Journal of Memory and Language, 25*, 75-92.

Neville, H. J., Mills, D. L., & Lawson, D. S. (1992). Fractionating language: Different neural subsystems with different sensitive periods. *Cerebral Cortex, 2*, 244-258.

Neville, H. J., Nicol, J. L., Barss, A., & Forster, K. I. (1991). Syntactically based sentence processing classes: Evidence from event-related brain potentials. *Journal of Cognitive Neuroscience, 3*(2), 151-165.

Niznikiewicz, M., & Squires, N. K., (1996). Phonological processing and the role of strategy in silent reading: Behavioral and electrophysiological evidence. *Brain and Language, 52*, 342-264.

Nobre, A. C., & McCarthy, G. (1994). Language-related ERPs: Scalp distributions and modulation by word type and semantic priming. *Journal of Cognitive Neuroscience, 6*, 233-255.

Nobre, A. C., & McCarthy, G. (1995). Language-related field potentials in the anterior-medial temporal lobe: II. Effects of word type and semantic priming. *Journal of Neuroscience, 15*, 1090-1099.

Novak, G. P., Ritter, W., Vaughan, H. G., & Wiznitzer, M. L. (1990). Differentiation of negative event-related potentials in an auditory discrimination task. *Electroencephalography and Clinical Neurophysiology, 75*, 255-275.

Novak, G. P., Ritter, W., Vaughan, H. G., & Wiznitzer, M. L. (1992). Differentiation of negative event-related potentials in an auditory discrimination task. *Electroencephalography and Clinical Neurophysiology, 75*, 255-275.

Oades, R. D., Dittmann-Balcar, A., & Zerbin, D. (1997). Development and topography of auditory event-related potentials (ERPs): Mismatch and processing negativity in individuals 8-22 years of age. *Psychophysiology, 34*, 677-693.

Oades, R. D., Zerbin, D., & Dittman-Balcar, A. (1995). The topography of event-related potentials in passive and active conditions of a 3-tone auditory oddball test. *International Journal of Neuroscience, 81*, 249-264.

Osterhout, L., & Hagoort, P. (1999). A superficial resemblance does not necessarily mean your are part of the family: Counterarguments to Coulson, King and Kutas (1998) in the P600/SPS-P300 debate. *Language and Cognitive Processes, 14*, 1-14.

Osterhout, L., & Holcomb, P. J. (1990). Event-related potentials elicited by grammatical anomalies. In C. H. M. Brunia, A. W. K. Gaillard, & A. Kok (Eds.), *Psychological brain research*. Tilburg: Tilburg University Press.

Osterhout, L. & Holcomb, P. J. (1994). The electrophysiology of language comprehension. In M. Rugg & M. C. H. Coles (Eds.), *Electrophysiological studies of human cognitive function*. Oxford: Oxford University Press.

Palmer, B., Nasman, V. T., & Wilson, G. F. (1994). Task detection difficulty: Effects on ERPs in a same-different letter classification task. *Biological Psychology, 38*(2-3), 199-214.

Pennington, B. F. (1995). Genetics of learning disabilities. *Journal of Child Neurology, 10*(Suppl 1): S69-S77.

Picton, T. W. (1988). The endogenous evoked potentials. In E. Baser (Ed.), *Dynamics of sensory and cognitive processes in the brain*. New York: Springer Verlag.

Picton, T. W. (1995). The neurophysiological calculation of auditory discrimination. *Ear and Hearing, 16*, 1-5.

Picton, T. W., Hillyard, S. A., Krausz, H. I., & Galambos, R. (1974). Human auditory evoked potentials: I. Evaluation of components. *Electroencephalography and Clinical Neurophysiology, 36*, 179-190.

Pinkerton. F., Watson, D. R., & McClelland, R. J. (1989). A neurophysiological study of children with reading, writing and spelling difficulties. *Developmental and Medical Child Neurolology, 31*, 569-81.

Plante, E., Van-Petten, C., & Senkfor, A. J. (2000). Electrophysiological dissociation between verbal and nonverbal semantic processing in learning disabled adults. *Neuropsychologia, 38*, 1669-1684.

Polich, J. M. (1985). Semantic categorization and event-related potentials. *Brain and Language, 26*, 304-321.

Polich, J. M. (1987). Task difficulty, probability, and inter-stimulus interval as determinants of P300 from auditory stimuli. *Electroencephalography and Clinical Neurophysiology: Evoked Potentials, 68*, 311-320.

Polich, J. M. (1989). Habituation of P300 from auditory stimuli. *Psychobiology, 17,* 19-28.

Polich, J., & Heine, M. R. D. (1996). P300 topography and modality effects from a single-stimulus paradigm. *Psychophysiology, 33*, 747-752.

Polich J. M., Howard L, Starr A. (1985). Effects of age on the P300 component of the event-related potential from auditory stimuli: peak definition, variation, and measurement. *Journal of Gerontology, 40*, 721-6.

Potts, G. F., Hirayasu, Y., O'Donnell, B. F., Shenton, M. E., & McCarley, R. W. (1998). High-density recording and topographic analysis of the auditory oddball event-related potential in patients with schizophrenia. *Biological-Psychiatry, 44*, 982-989.

Pratarelli, M. E. (1994). Semantic processing of pictures and spoken words: Evidence from event-related potentials. *Brain and Cognition, 24*, 137-157.

Proverbio, A. M., & Zani, A. (2004). Time course of brain activation during graphemic/ phonologic processing in reading: An ERP study. *Brain & Language, 87*(3): 412-420.

Raney, G. E. (1993). Monitoring changes in cognitive load during reading: An event-related brain potential and reaction time analysis. *Journal of Experimental Psychology: Learning, Memory, and Cognition, 19*, 51-69.

Rispens, J. E., Been, P. H., & Zwarts, F. (2006). Brain Responses to Subject-Verb Agreement Violations in Spoken Language in Developmental Dyslexia: An ERP Study. *Dyslexia, 12*, 134-149.

Ritter, W., Simson, R., Vaughan, H. G., & Macht, M. (1982). Manipulation of event-related potential manifestations of information processing stages. *Science, 218*(4575), 909-911.

Robichon, F., Besson, M., & Habib, M. (2002). An electrophysiological study of dyslexic and control adults in a sentence reading task. *Biological Psychology, 59*, 29-53.

Ruchkin, D. S., Sutton, S., & Stega, M. (1980). Emitted P300 and slow wave event-related potentials in guessing and detection tasks. *Electroencephalography and Clinical Neurophysiology, 49*(1-2):1-14.

Rugg, M. D. (1985). Event-related potentials and the phonological processing of words and non-words. *Neuropsychologia, 22*, 435-443.

Rugg, M. D. (1987). Dissociation of semantic priming, word and word repetition effects by event-related potentials. *Quarterly Journal of Experimental Psychology, 39A*, 123-147.

Rugg, M. D., & Doyle, M. C. (1992). Event-related potentials and recognition memory for low and high frequency words. *Journal of Cognitive Neuroscience, 4*, 69-79.

Rugg, M. D., & Nagy, M. E. (1987). Lexical contribution to nonword-repetition effects: Evidence from event-related potentials. *Memory and Cognition, 15*, 473-481.

Russeler, J., Probst, S., Johannes, S., & Münte, T. (2003). Recognition memory for high- and low-frequency words in adult normal and dyslexic readers: an event-related brain potential study. *Journal of Clinical and Experimental Neuropsychology, 25*, 815-829.

Schulte-Koerne, G., Deimel, W., Bartling, J. & Remschmidt, H. (1998). Auditory processing and dyslexia: Evidence for a specific speech processing deficit. *Neuroreport, 9*(2), 337-340.

Schulte-Koerne. G., Bartling, J., Deimel, W. & Remschmidt, H. (1999). Attenuated hemispheric lateralization in dyslexia: Evidence of a visual processing deficit. *Neuroreport, 10*(17), 3697-3701.

Schulte-Koerne, G., Deimel, W., Bartling, J. & Remschmidt, H. (2001). Speech perception deficit in dyslexic adults as measured by mismatch negativity (MMN). *International Journal of Psychophysiology, 40,* 77-87.

Shaul, S. (2005). The Characteristics of Young and Adult Dyslexics Readers on Reading and Reading Related Cognitive Tasks as Compared to Normal Readers. *Dyslexia, 11,* 132-151.

Silva-Pereyra, J., Fernandez, T., Harmony, T., Bernal, J., Galan, L., Diaz-Comas, L., et al. (2001). Delayed P300 during Sternberg and color discrimination tasks in poor readers. *International Journal of Psychophysiology, 40*, 17-32.

Smith, M. E. (1993). Neurophysiological manifestations of recollective experience during recognition memory judgments. *Journal of Cognitive Neuroscience, 5,* 1-13.

Solan, H. A., Sutiji, V. G., Ficcara, A. P., & Wurst, S. A. (1990). Binocular advantage and visual processing in dyslexic and control children as measured by visual evoked potentials. *Optometry and Vision Science, 67*, 105-110.

Squires, N. K., Squires, K. C., & Hillyard, S. A. (1975). Two varieties of long-latency positive waves evoked by unpredictable auditory stimuli in man. *Electroencephalography and Clinical Neurophysiology, 38*, 387-410.

Stein, J. (2001). The neurobiology of reading difficulties. In M. Wolf (Ed.), *Dyslexia, fluency and the brain* (pp. 3-21). Cambridge, MA: York press.

Stelmack, R. M., & Miles, J. (1990). The effect of picture priming on event-related potentials of normal and disabled readers during a word recognition memory task. *Journal of Clinical and Experimental Neuropsychology, 6*, 857-873.

Stelmack, R. M., Saxe, B. J., Noldy-Cullum, N., Campbell, K. B., & Armitage, R. (1988). Recognition memory for words and event related potentials: A comparison of normal and disabled readers. *Journal of Experimental Neuropsychology, 10*, 185-200.

Stuss, D. T., Picton, T. W., & Cerri, A. N. (1986). Searching for the names of pictures: An event-related potential study. *Psychophysiology, 23*, 215-223.

Taylor, M. J., & Keenan, N. K. (1990). Event related potentials to visual and language stimuli in normal and dyslexic children. *Psychophysiology, 27*, 318-327.

Taylor, M. J., & Keenan, N. K. (1999). ERPs to orthographic, phonological, and semantic tasks in dyslexic children with auditory processing impairment. *Developmental Neuropsychology, 15*, 307-326.

Taylor, M. J., Smith, M. L., & Iron, K. S. (1990). Event-related potential evidence of sex differences in verbal and nonverbal memory. *Neuropsychologia, 28*, 691-705.

Tiitinen, H., Sinkkonen, J., May, P., & Näätänen, R. (1994). The auditory transient 40-Hz response is insensitive to changes in stimulus features. *Neuroreport, 6*, 190-192.

Tonnquist-Uhlen, I. (1996). Topography of auditory evoked long-latency potentials in children with severe language impairment: The P2 and N2 components. *Ear and Hearing, 17*, 314-326.

Tonnquist-Uhlen, I., Borg, E., Persson, H. E., & Spens, K. E. (1996). Topography of auditory evoked cortical potentials in children with severe language impairment: The N1 component. *Electroencephalography and Clinical Neurophysiology: Evoked Potentials, 100*(3), 250-260.

Tremblay, K., Kraus, N., & McGee, T. (1998). The time course of auditory perceptual learning: Neurophysiological changes during speech-sound training. *Neuroreport, 9,* 3557-3560.

Van Herten, M., Kolk, H. H. J., & Chwilla, D. J. (2005). An ERP study of P600 effects elicited by semantic anomalies. *Cognitive Brain Research, 22*, 241-255.

Van Petten, C., & Kutas, M. (1987). Ambiguous words in context: An event-related potential analysis of the time course of meaning activation. *Journal of Memory and Language, 26,* 188-208.

Van Petten, C., & Kutas, M. (1991). Influences of semantic and syntactic context on open and closed-class words. *Memory and Cognition, 19*, 95-112.

Vaughan, H. G., Jr., & Kurtzberg, D. (1992). Electrophysiologic indices of human brain maturation and cognitive development. In M. R. Gunnar & C. Nelson (Eds.), *Minnesota Symposia on Child Psychology: Vol. 24* (pp. 1-36). Hillsdale, NJ: Lawrence Erlbaum Associates.

Verbaten, M. N., Huyben, M. A., & Kemner, C. (1997). Processing capacity and the frontal P3. *International Journal of Psychophysiology, 25,* 237-248.

Wijers, A. A., Mulder, G., Van-Hooff, H., & Lange, J. (1993). Topography and source analysis of brain activity associated with selective spatial attention and memory search. *Brain Topography, 5,* 383-388.

Wijers, A. A., Lange, J. J., Mulder, G., & Mulder, L. J. (1997). An ERP study of visual spatial attention and letter target detection for isoluminant and nonisoluminant stimuli. *Psychophysiology, 34*, 553-565.

Wijker, W., Molenaar, P. C., & Van-der Molen, M. W. (1989). Age changes in scalp distribution of cognitive event-related potentials elicited in odd-ball task. *Journal of Psychophysiology, 3,* 179-189.

Wilding, E. L., & Rugg, M. D. (1996). An event-related potential study of recognition memory with and without retrieval of source. *Brain, 119*, 889-905.

Wilding, E. L., & Rugg, M. D. (1997).An event-related potential study of recognition memory for words spoken aloud or heard. *Neuropsychologia, 35,* 1185-1195.

Wilson, G. F., Swain, C. R., & Ullsperger, P. (1998). ERP components elicited in response to warning stimuli: The influence of task difficulty. *Biological Psychology, 47*, 137-158.

Winkler, I., Paavilainen, P., & Näätänen, R. (1992). Can echoic memory store two traces simultaneously? A study of event-related brain potentials. *Psychophysiology, 29,* 337-349.

Wong, C. A. N., Gauthier, I., Woroch, B., DeBuse, C., & Curran, T. (2005). An early electrophysiological response associated with expertise in letter perception. *Cognitive, Affective and Behavioral Neuroscience, 5,* 306-318.

Yingling, C. D., Galin, D., Fein, G., Peltzman, D., & Davenport, L. (1986). Neurometrics does not detect "pure" dyslexics. *Electroencephalography and Clinical Neurophysiology, 63*, 426-430.

3

AUDITORY P2 IS REDUCED IN 5 MONTH OLD INFANTS FROM DYSLEXIC FAMILIES

Pieter H. Been[1,2], Theo H. van Leeuwen[3,4], Marieke van Herten[5], Ben Maassen[5], Aryan van der Leij[3] and Frans Zwarts[1]

[1]School for Behavioral and Cognitive Neuroscience, University of Groningen, [2]Neuroimaging Center, University of Groningen, [3]Faculty of Behavioral and Social Sciences, University of Amsterdam, [4]Department of Clinical Neurophysiology, Municipal Hospital Slotervaart, Amsterdam, [5]Medical Psychology, Radboud University Nijmegen Medical Centre, The Netherlands

Abstract: In this ERP study we examined the auditory processing of 5-month-old infants from dyslexic families (n=121) and controls (n=73) as part of a national longitudinal research program in The Netherlands on developmental dyslexia. A natural manipulated speech stimulus /bak/ was presented to these infants as the standard stimulus (about 400 repetitive presentations) in an oddball paradigm. Infants were either awake, watching a silent video, or asleep during the repetitive presentation of the stimulus. In this study we tested the prediction from a dynamic neuronal model study that the P2 should be reduced in infants from dyslexic families. The data indicates that infants from dyslexic families have a reduced P2 in the frontal-central-parietal regions in both hemispheres. During sleep the P2 amplitude was reduced compared with the awake state, but there was no difference between sleeping stages. Somewhat unexpectedly we did not find gender differences in this study. Cortical generators of the P2 were found in the auditory cortex and in Wernicke's and Broca's area. P2 amplitude explains 18% of the variance in verb production of the same infants at the age of 17 months. A discriminant analysis shows that infants are classified as deficient in auditory processing in 10% of the controls and 35% of the infants from dyslexic families. These numbers are well in line with the normal population risk and the elevated risk in infants from dyslexic families.

Key words: auditory processing, developmental dyslexia, ERP, P2, infants, family risk, sleeping stage, gender

1. INTRODUCTION

Developmental dyslexia is usually defined as a reading disability which is unexpected relative to intelligence and which is not attributable to instruction, the social environment or acquired sensory or neurological deficits (Critchley, 1964). Converging evidence indicates that developmental dyslexia is a language disorder which often critically affects the phonological domain of language (Olson, 1994). The phonological deficit may arise from a deficit in speech perception as reported in a number of studies showing deviant patterns of identification and discrimination among poor readers.

The origin of the disorder is biological (Paulesu et al., 2001) and affects boys at least twice as often as girls (Rutter et al., 2003). Regarding gender differences in brain development and activation patterns during reading tasks, separation of males and females in dyslexia research has been proposed to detect possible functional differences (Lambe, 1999).

Dyslexia runs in families (Pennington, 1990), is for a substantial part hereditary (DeFries, Fulker, & Labuda, 1987) and is probably of heterogeneous genetic origin (Grigorenko, 2001).

Post mortem studies show among others that dyslexia is accompanied by fundamental changes in the anatomy and physiology of the brain, which involves an anomalous balance in cerebral hemisphere development. Galaburda and his colleagues (Galaburda, Sherman, Rosen, Aboitiz, & Geschwind, 1985; Humphreys, Kaufmann, & Galaburda, 1990) have found alterations in the pattern of cortical asymmetry which may point to left hemisphere brain dysfunction. Specifically, the ordinary pattern of leftward asymmetry of the planum temporale is absent, and the perisylvian cortex displays minor cytoarchitectonic malformations, including foci of ectopic neurons in the molecular layer and focal microgyria (Galaburda, Rosen, & Sherman, 1989; Galaburda, 1994) and an excessive number of neurons in the deeper layers of the neocortex but relatively few in the upper layers (Galaburda, 1983; Galaburda & Kemper, 1979; Kemper, 1984).

Regarding the early maturation of the auditory processes related to reading problems, delayed or deviant maturational processes during the first year of life could be used for the early diagnosis of risk at dyslexia.

We adopted such an approach in a Dutch prospective study (NWO, 1996) starting assessments from the age of 2 months onwards.

In the study infants from dyslexic families and control families are enrolled, and speech perception by very young infants as a precursor and potential predictor of later language skills is one of the target variables. Employing an oddball paradigm in ERP assessments, eliciting mismatch negativity (MMN), auditory discrimination during quiet sleep at the age of 2 months has been addressed, showing that MMN is absent in infants from dyslexic families (van Leeuwen et al., 2006). The stimuli used in the oddball paradigm are from a /bak/-/dak/ continuum (van Beinum et al., 2005). Based on a dynamic neuronal model simulation study tailored to this specific continuum we generated and tested a number of predictions in the behavioral and the ERP domain (Been & Zwarts, 2003, 2004). Assuming a reduced neuronal density, reflecting ectopies in the upper parts of the cortical layers, one of the predictions was that in the case of dyslexia a reduced P2 component in the ERP during auditory processing should occur. It is this prediction that we address here in the full sample of 5 month-old infants, both from dyslexic and control families, using the standard stimulus of the oddball paradigm. Regarding the number of repetitive presentations of the standard stimulus (more than 400 to each infant) an averaged evoked potential with a large signal to noise ratio results, making it a potential reliable predictor for dyslexia suitable for individual diagnosis. This possibility shall be explored in a preliminary fashion. As the data were obtained when the infants were either awake or asleep during the assessments, state e.g., awake or sleeping stage, should be taken into account in the analysis of the data.

1.1 Familial dyslexia: prevalence rates

The observation that common forms of dyslexia are hereditary has recently been the focus of renewed interest. Familial transmission of dyslexia and the significant genetic risk to first-degree relatives have both been known for almost a century (Pennington, 1990). Recent evidence from large data sets, such as the Iowa Family Study of Reading Disabilities (Gilger, Pennington, & DeFries, 1991), indicates that both dyslexic boys and girls often have an affected parent. The odds are five- to seven-fold increased for boys and ten- to twelve-fold for girls. Bayesian estimates of the posterior probability that a child will be dyslexic given a dyslexic parent vary from 0.38 to 0.53 (median rate: 0.43) for male offspring of dyslexic men (Gilger et al., 1991). These estimates are in line with results from prospective studies.

Scarborough (1991) reported that 65% of a sample of children from families with a history of dyslexia could be classified as reading-disabled at the age of eight years. Gallagher, Frith, and Snowling (2000) found that 57% of a sample of 63 children with familial risk at dyslexia were delayed in literacy development at 6 years compared to 12% of a control group of 34 children. Pennington and Lefly (2001) report that 34% (15 males, 7 females) of a group of 67 children with familial risk became reading-disabled as assessed at the end of second grade compared with 6% of a control group of 57 children. So, retrospective and prospective studies show an elevated risk for children from dyslexic families in the range of about 35 to 65% to become reading-disabled.

1.2 Phonology

Phonological processing entails the segmental analysis of words for ordinary speaking and listening, as well as the metaphonological skills required for analyzing the sound structure of speech into the phonemic components represented by the alphabet. Many studies have shown dyslexic children to be "inferior to same-age normal readers in their perceptual discrimination of phonemes, phonological awareness measured by tasks requiring the isolation and manipulation of phonemes within words, speed and accuracy in lexical access for picture names, verbal short-term and working memory, syntactic awareness, and semantic processing in tasks such as listening comprehension" (Olson, 1994). A number of studies have provided ample evidence that differences in spoken language skills - especially awareness of phonemic segments - lead to difficulties in the phonological coding of written language, which is a key prerequisite for word recognition and spelling ability. The processing problems manifested by dyslexics give rise to the most diagnostic symptom of reading impairment: difficulty in pronouncing pseudo-words (Bruck 1988, 1990, 1992; Felton & Wood, 1992; Liberman & Shankweiler, 1985; Mann, 1984; Siegel & Ryan, 1988; Snowling, 1981, 1991; Stanovich, 1986). Although reading skills contribute reciprocally to the development of phonological skills as well (Wagner & Torgesen, 1987), indications are that a phonological deficit is causal to reading disability (Bradley & Bryant, 1978, 1983; Stanovich, 1988; Wagner, 1986).

The phonological deficit may arise from a deficit in speech perception as reported in a number of studies showing deviant patterns of identification and discrimination among poor readers. Godfrey, Syrdal-Lasky, Millay, and Knox (1981), comparing performances on two synthetic continua, [ba]-[da] and [da]-[ga], found that dyslexic children were significantly less consistent in identification, even at the extremes of the continua. Other studies have reported similar results for [ba]-[da] (Reed, 1989; Werker & Tees, 1987) and for [sa]-[sta] (Steffens, Eilers, Gross-Glen, & Jallad, 1992). In several of these studies, inconsistent identification also gave rise to deviant patterns of discrimination along synthetic continua. Impaired readers performed significantly worse than normal controls between phoneme categories but not within, indicating that they could not easily exploit the phonological contrast which normally enhances discrimination across a phoneme boundary (De Weirdt, 1988; Godfrey et al., 1981; Pallay, 1986; Werker & Tees, 1987). Their difficulties were primarily in identifying and discriminating phonetically similar, though phonologically contrastive, synthetic syllables. Such results suggest that speech categories may be broader and less sharply separated in reading-disabled compared to normal readers (Mody, Studdert-Kennedy, & Brady, 1996; Reed, 1989; Studdert-Kennedy & Mody, 1995).

1.3 Phoneme processing: ERP's, development, neural substrates and sleep

The auditory system matures during the first year of life. The cortical processing of the phonetical features of speech in adults is mainly handled by the left hemisphere (Zatorre, Evans, Meyer & Gjedde, 1992). Left hemisphere cortical processing is tuned to the mother language. Listening to an unknown other language activates both hemispheres (Mazoyer, et al., 1993). This hemisphere specialization develops soon after birth. Four days old babies can differentiate the mother language from an unknown language, and two unknown languages from each other. At the age of two months the language specialization of the left hemisphere seems to be established. The mother language can be differentiated from an unknown language, but the ability to differentiate two unknown languages from each other has vanished (Mehler, Dupoux, Pallier, & Dehaene-Lambertz, 1995). For adults it is difficult to discriminate between vowels and consonants of other languages which are alien to the own language. Yet very young children are able to make these discriminations of alien vowels and consonants The ability to discriminate alien consonants vanishes between the age of eight and twelve months (Werker & Tees, 1984) and the ability to discriminate alien vowels at the age of about six months (Kuhl, Williams, Lacerda, Stevens, & Linblom, 1992).

Phoneme perception is crucial for language processing and behavioral studies show similar capacities in infants and adults sub-served by the same neural substrates. MMN-studies, addressing auditory discrimination in the ERP-domain, show the plausibility that representations in the brain computed from speech are immediately phonemic and not proceeded by an acoustic representation, although an acoustic representation can be computed in parallel (Dehaene-Lambertz, & Gliga, 2004). Dipole models of the phonemic MMN suggest that the phonemic representation in adults is in the planum temporale in both hemispheres but favors the left hemisphere (Tervaniemi et al., 1999) and that this asymmetry occurs both during attentive and pre-attentive levels of processing (Tervaniemi & Hugdahl, 2003). Also in infants dipole models show that consonant-vowel syllables elicit an ERP and a MMN that favors the left hemisphere (Dehaene et al., 2004). As in adults MMN can be observed in infants even when attention is not directed to the stimulus either because they are watching interesting visual stimuli to keep them quiet or during sleep (Dehaene-Lambertz & Pena, 2001). Several studies show a reduced lateralization of the MMN to the left hemisphere in dyslexics or infants at risk for dyslexia during phoneme processing (Lyytinen et al., 2005).

Auditory stimuli typically elicit a P1-N1-P2-N2 complex. The P2 is a positive deflection that is evoked at about 200 ms in adults and is assumed to represent at least partially an exogeneous response, related to sensory activity, and elicited by both attended and un-attended stimuli. P2 can be dissociated along several parameters from N1. Generators of the P2 are probably located in the vicinity of the auditory cortex, the planum temporale and Brodmann's area 22 (Wernicke's area) involved in auditory association. Developmental studies show that the P2 latency matures early to adult values at the age of about 2 to 3 years and that there is probably an age related-increase in amplitude at the anterior electrodes. Adults show an increase of P2 amplitude at sleep onset and the amplitude continues to increase into stage2 and slow wave sleep (Crowley & Colrain, 2004). However, in 6-week-old infants mean P2 amplitudes and latencies elicited by the standard stimulus in an oddball presentation are equal across quiet and active sleep states (Duclaux, Challamel, Collet, Roullet-Solignac, & Revol, 1991). This suggests that sleeping stage perhaps affects the P2 differently in adults and infants, but at least that in the analysis of the P2 sleep states need to be controlled for.

Until recently little attention has been paid to the auditory P2 in dyslexia research (e.g., Lyytinen et al., 2005 for an overview). Recently it has received interest within the context of the work on asynchrony in speed of processing between the auditory-phonological and the visual-orthographic modalities in the case of dyslexia (Breznitz, 2002). In the auditory-phonological modality adult male dyslexics show delayed P2 peak latencies (Breznitz & Meyler, 2003; Breznitz & Misra, 2003). In a study with mixed gender delayed P2 latencies and lower P2 amplitudes were found in response to phonological patterns among adult dyslexic readers (Meyler & Breznitz, 2005).

2. MATERIALS AND METHODS

2.1 Study participants

The participants were 121 5-month-old infants at genetic risk for dyslexia (51 girls, 69 boys) and 73 control infants (33 girls, 40 boys). These infants were recruited from the Dutch population and were included in the Dutch Prospective Dyslexia Study. Inclusion in the at-risk group was based on (1) a family history of the parents with respect to reading problems and dyslexia and (2) scores of the affected parents, and of an additional first- or second-degree relative of these parents, on a test battery including speed tests on real word reading, nonword decoding and verbal IQ (Kuijpers et al., 2003). Dyslexia did not occur in the control group families and both parents had to score above criterion on our dyslexia test. All participating families received oral and written information about the study and all gave informed consent. The study protocol was approved by a medical ethics committee.

2.2 Stimuli, paradigm and procedure

The stimulus used in this study was the second stimulus from a /bak/-/dak/ continuum which is perceived as the Dutch word /bak/

(=tray) containing transients in the second and third formant. The stimulus starts, after a silent period of 20 ms, with a silent vocal murmur (170 ms), followed by a burst (/b/, 10ms), the vowel /a/ (250 ms), a silent /k/ occlusion (55 ms) and the release of /k/ (110 ms) (Van Beinum, Schwippert, Been, van Leeuwen, & Kuijpers, 2005).

Stimulus onset asynchrony was 800 ms and stimuli (620 ms duration, 75 dB sound pressure level) were (binaurally) presented by speakers at 70 cm from the infant's head. The infants were lying in a child's safety seat while stimuli were presented and brain activity was recorded. The total duration was about 11 min. When the infants were awake they watched a silent video.

2.3 Electroencephalogram recording, processing and analysis

In all cases a 32-channel electroencephalogram was recorded with 500 Hz per channel and filter settings 0.01-100 Hz (Synamps model 5083, Neuroscan Inc., El Paso, Texas, USA). Infant caps (Easy Cap, FMS, Munich, Germany) with sintered Ag/AgCl electrodes included all 10-20 system locations (Oz, O1/2, Pz, P3/4, P7/8, CPz, CP3/4, TP7/8, Cz, C3/4, T7/8, FCz, FC3/4, FT7/8, Fz, F3/4, F7/8 and Fp1/2). Additional electrodes were used for recording the vertical electrooculogram (above and below the left eye) and the horizontal electrooculogram (at the outer canthus of each eye). Reference electrodes were attached to the mastoids. Impedance was kept below 20 kOhm. The electroencephalogram was digitally band-pass filtered (1-30 Hz, 48 dB/octave), and artefacts exceeding 175 μV in any channel were rejected from analysis (Brain Vision Analyzer, Brain Products, GmbH, Munich, Germany). Individual grand average ERPs were determined for the standards after baseline correction in the 200 ms pre-stimulus interval. Ocular artefacts were corrected by the Gratton and Coles algorithm (Gratton, Coles & Dorchin, 1983). Sources of responses to the standard stimulus were estimated by low-resolution electromagnetic tomography analysis (LORETA), which computes the smoothest possible current source density solution (in grey matter) without a priori assumptions about the number of generators (Pascual-Marqui, Michel, & Lehmann, 1994). For the LORETA analysis the ERP's were transformed to the average reference and the baseline correction was removed. Each individual unfiltered raw EEG (about 11 min recording time) was inspected in stretches of 1 min for state (awake, sleep) classification. Predominant states (at least lasting 90% of the time) were observed for 174 of the 194 infants: 73 deep quiet sleep, 46 high voltage sleep and 55 awake (Guilleminault & Souquet, 1979). The remaining 20 infants showed mixed states, e.g., partly awake and partly asleep, or REM-sleep and were omitted from the present analysis. All individual grand averages showed a P2 peak at the left and or right central electrodes in the 350 to 550 ms interval after stimulus onset. The mean number of valid trials after artefact rejection was 345 (SD=98) with a lower bound of 100 valid trials.

3. RESULTS

For the purpose of illustration in Figure 1 the grand mean of the P2 of control boys during deep sleep is shown. Activity is gravitating at the left and right central electrodes (C3-C4). The peak latency is 410 ms after stimulus onset (220 ms after the start of the vocal burst).

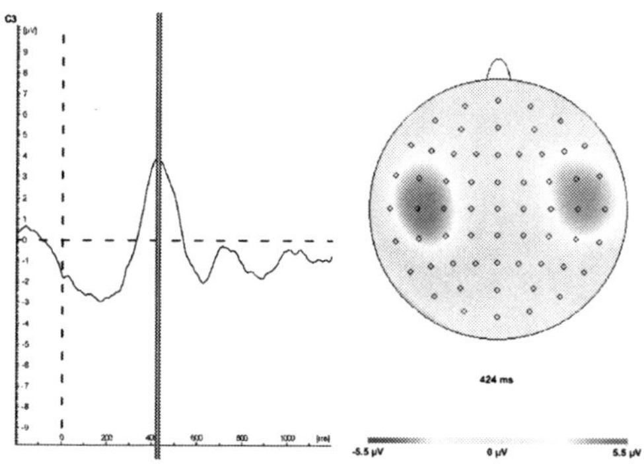

Figure 1. P2 of control boys during deep sleep (grand average). The left and right hemispheres are active.

A repeated measures MANOVA was conducted with the factors group (at risk vs control), gender (boys, girls) and state (deep sleep, high voltage sleep, awake) on the individual P2-peaks in the 350 to 550 ms interval after stimulus onset at the left frontal-central-parietal electrodes (FC3,FT7,C3,T7,CP3,TP7) and right frontal-central-parietal electrodes (FC4,FT8,C4,T8,CP4,TP8). Where appropriate the Greenhouse-Geisser correction was applied. The analysis yielded main effects for group [F(1,161)=8.10,p=.005] and for state [F(1,161)= 3.80,p=.025]. The state effect (Figure 2b) reflects the difference of the lower amplitudes during sleep, both deep and high voltage, and the awake state. An analysis with the same factors on the latencies of the P2 did not yield any significant results. There was no effect for gender [F(1,161)=.18,p=.83].

At the bivariate level only midline electrode pairs showed significant effects for group: FC3/FC4 [F(1,161)=7.72,p=.006], C3/C4[F(1,161)=7.68,p=.006] and CP3/CP4[F(1.161)=5.89,p=.016]. The repeated measures MANOVA for the left and right midline electrode pairs simultaneously (FC3,FC4,C3,C4,CP3,CP4) showed in addition to the expected group effect [F(1,161)=4.91,p=.03] an hemisphere effect [F(1,161)=23.4,p<.001]. As can be seen in Figure 2a the P2 amplitude is larger for the control group at the right and left electrodes explaining the main effect and both groups show a left hemisphere advantage reflecting the hemisphere effect.

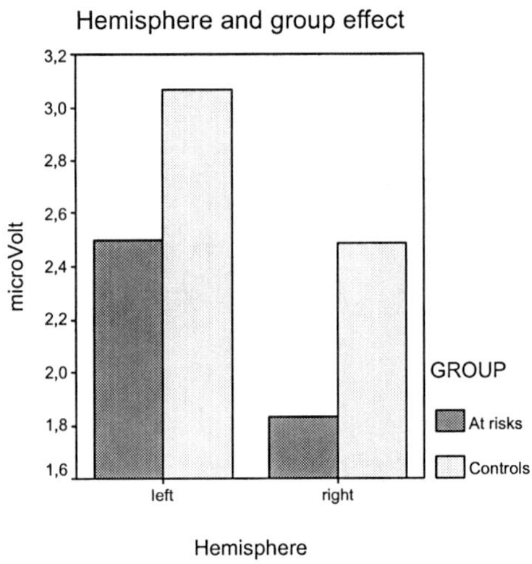

Figure 2a. P2 amplitudes for both groups on the left and right frontal-central-parietal electrodes yielding a main effect for group, at risks having diminished P2 amplitudes and yielding a left hemisphere advantage in both groups.

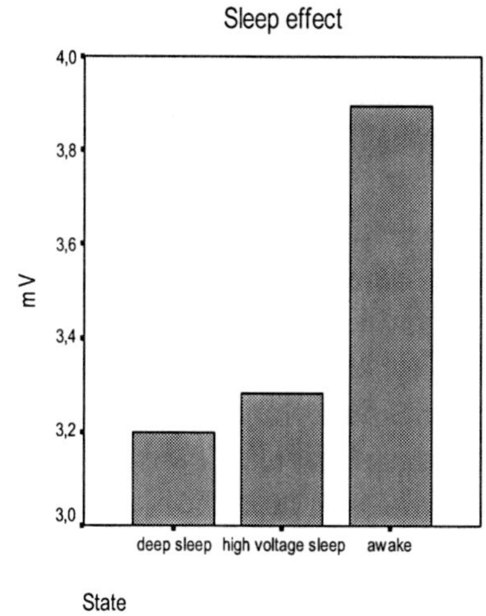

Figure 2b. There is an overall global effect of sleep, reflected in reduced P2 amplitudes compared with the P2 amplitude when the infants are awake.

To elucidate these results we conducted low resolution electromagnetic tomography analyses (LORETA) at the time of the P2 peaks at C3. Illustrative are the results obtained on the group grand means of the boys during deep sleep as depicted in Figure 3. In the left panel we see activation of both Broca's and Wernicke's area in both hemispheres, but more wide spread in the left hemisphere. In the right panel we see bilateral activation of the (secondary) auditory cortex.

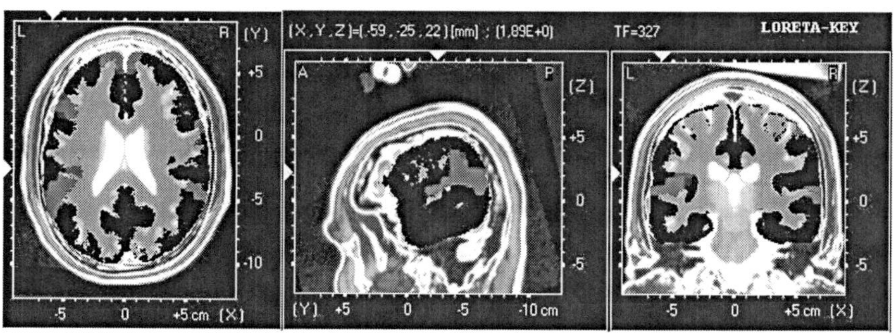

Figure 3. Low resolution electromagnetic tomography analysis (LORETA) of the P2 peak of the control boys during deep sleep.

Left panel: left and right central-parietal activation in the superior temporal gyrus (BA 22, Wernicke's area) at -59,-43,22 and 60,39,22 (Talairach coordinates); left and right frontal-central activation activation in the inferior frontal gyrus (BA 45, Broca's area) at -49,24,22 and 59,9,22.

Right panel: left and right central activation in the superior temporal gyrus of the temporal lobe (BA 42, secondary auditory cortex) at -63,-25,10 and 64,-25,9.

To explore the discriminating power of the P2 we performed a discriminant analysis with individual averaged P2-peak voltages at the left and right frontal-central-parietal electrodes and state (quiet sleep, high voltage sleep, awake) as predictors and group as criterion. The discriminatory power of the function was significant (Wilk's Lambda (df13)=.87,p=.03) and explained 14% of the variance (canonical correlation: 0.37). Taking prior group sizes reflecting the assumption that ultimately 40% of the at risk infants will become dyslexic we obtained the classification results in Table 1. About 10% of the controls are predicted to become dyslexic, well in line with the normal population risk, and about 35% of the at risk infants, in line with the lower bound of prospective studies.

Table 1. Classification summary table of the discriminant analysis. 10% of the controls are classified as dyslexic in line with the normal population risk and 35% of the at risk infants are classified as dyslexic in line with the lower bound of prospective studies.

		Group	Predicted Group Membership		Total
			Dyslexic	Normal reader	
Original	Count	At risk	37	70	107
		Control	6	61	67

The predictive validity of the P2-peak voltages was tested on language developmental data of the infants at the age of 17 months. At this age there is no difference between both groups in the overall production of words, but the groups differ in the number of verbs and grammatical words that are used, the at risks infants being lower producers (Koster et al., 2005). Using the same predictors as in the discriminant analysis the regression analysis between the predictors and the production of verbs at 17 months explained 18% of the variance ($r=.43$, $F(16,143)=1.8, p=.03$). We did not find a significant relation with overall word production or the production of grammatical words.

4. DISCUSSION

The main objective of this study was to test the prediction from a neuronal dynamic model study, tailored to the auditory stimulus used in this experiment that the presumed reduced neuronal density in the case of dyslexia will show in a reduced P2-amplitude during processing of the stimulus in the neural substrates involved. As noted in §1.3 the P2 evoked by auditory stimuli is representing at least a partially exogeneous response related to auditory sensory activity. As such it is not suited to address the process of auditory discrimination in phoneme processing as a potential underlying cause of a phonological deficit, but only auditory sensory activity as involved in phoneme processing. Assuming that there is an elevated risk in infants from dyslexic families in the range from about 35% to 65% to become reading disabled, a reduced P2-amplitude should show up in the averaged mean of this group compared to a control group. In general, our results indicate a consistent significant P2-amplitude difference between both groups at the left and right electrodes in the frontal-central-parietal area covering the areas involved in phoneme processing. This P2-amplitude is a robust measure with a high signal to noise ratio at the individual level, on the average based on the grand mean of 345 repetitive presentations. Somewhat contrary to our expectations we did not find gender differences in this analysis. As expected from phoneme processing studies in infants and adults (§1.3) we found a left hemisphere advantage. As far as sleeping state is concerned our results are in line with the results from a 6-week-old infant study (§1.3), also using the background stimulus in an oddball paradigm, showing no P2 amplitude and latency differences across sleeping stages. In addition we found here that there is a difference in P2-amplitude between the awake state and the sleep states (high voltage sleep, deep quiet sleep) addressed in this study. One should hesitate to compare the results of this study with the P2-studies in the context of the work on asynchrony in speed of processing between the auditory-phonological and the visual-orthographic modalities in the case of dyslexia (§1.3), as the tasks involved are attended phonemic decision tasks carried out by adult dyslexics and controls. We did not find differences in P2-latencies as were consistently found in these studies, although our P2 amplitude differences fit one study (Meyler & Breznitz, 2005).

As expected we found cortical generators of the P2 in the auditory cortex and Wernicke's area involved in auditory association (§1.3) in our LORETA analysis. In addition we found activation in Broca's area normally involved in the generation of speech code. The selective involvement of these language processing areas corroborates the validity of our results. So does the predictive validity significantly relating our electrophysiological results to verb production at the age of 17 months in the same groups of infants and specifically so because this difference in a specific language production category differentiates between at risk infants and controls at this age. Finally we observe that the classification results, based on our electrophysiological data, fit the normal population risk of the controls and the lower bound of the elevated risk of the infants from dyslexic families. As we observed at the beginning of our discussion this classification is based on robust electrophysiological measures with a high signal to noise ratio. Once the final diagnosis of dyslexia of our infants is available when they have reached the age of 9 or 10 years, the results of a discriminant analysis, differentiating between dyslexia and normal reading, can be used - if still significant - for computing individual probabilities of group membership for new cases based on the same electrophysiological measures as used in our prospective study. Regarding our sample sizes and number of variables used for prediction the shrinkage of predictive validity in new samples will be very reduced (Stevens, 1996). As such this study can potentially contribute to diagnostic systems applicable at the very young age of 5 months, making very early intervention feasible.

5. ACKNOWLEDGEMENTS

Our gratitude goes to all participating children and their parents and to the Netherlands Organization for Scientific Research for funding.

REFERENCES

Been, P. H., & Zwarts, F. (2003). Developmental dyslexia and discrimination in speech perception: a dynamic model study. *Brain and Language, 86,* 395-412.

Been, P. H., & Zwarts, F. (2004). Language disorders across modalities: the case of developmental dyslexia. In L. Verhoeven & H. van Balkom (Eds.), *Classification of developmental language disorders. Theoretical issues and clinical implications.* Mahwah, NJ: Lawrence Erlbaum.

Bradley, L., & Bryant, P. E. (1978). Difficulties in auditory organisation as a possible cause of reading backwardness. *Nature, 271*, 746-747.

Bradley, L., & Bryant, P. E. (1983). Categorizing sounds and learning to read - a causal connection. *Nature, 301*, 419-421.

Breznitz, Z. (2002). Asynchrony of visual-orthographic and auditory-phonological word recognition processes. An underlying factor in dyslexia. *Reading and Writing, 15,* 15-42.

Breznitz, Z., & Meyler, A. (2003). Speed of lower-level auditory and visual processing as a basic factor in dyslexia: electrophysiological evidence. *Brain and Language, 85,* 166-184.

Breznitz, Z., & Misra, M. (2003). Speed of processing of the visual-orthographic and auditory-phonological systems in adult dyslexics: the contribution of asynchrony to word recognition deficits. *Brain and Language, 85,* 486-502.

Bruck, M. (1988). The word recognition and spelling of dyslexic children. *Reading Research Quarterly, 23*, 51-69.

Bruck, M. (1990). Word-recognition skills of adults with childhood diagnoses of dyslexia. *Developmental Psychology, 26*, 439-454.

Bruck, M. (1992). Persistence of dyslexics' phonological awareness deficits. *Developmental Psychology, 28*, 874-886.

Critchley, M. (1964). *Developmental Dyslexia.* London: William Heineman Medical Books Limited.

Crowley, K. E., & Colrain, I. M. (2004). A review of the evidence for P2 being an independent component process: age, sleep and modality. *Clinical Neurophysiology, 115,* 732-744.

DeFries, J. C., Fulker, D. W., & LaBuda, M. C. (1987). Evidence for a genetic aetiology in reading disability of twins. *Nature, 329,* 537-539.

Dehaene-Lambertz, G. & Gliga, T. (2004). Common neural basis for phoneme processing in infants and adults. *Journal of Cognitive Neuroscience, 168,* 1375-1378.

Dehaene-Lambertz, G., & Pena, M. (2001). Electrophysiological evidence for automatic phonetic processing in neonates. *Neurorport, 12,* 3155-3158.

De Weirdt, W. (1988). Speech perception and frequency discrimination in good and poor readers. *Applied Psycholinguistics*, *16*, 163-183.

Duclaux, R., Callamel, M. J., Collet, L., Roullet-Solignac, I., & Revol, M. (1991). Hemispheric asymmetry of late auditory evoked response induced by pitch change in infants: influence of sleep stages. *Brain Research, 566(1-2),* 152-158.

Felton, R. H., & Wood, F. R. (1992). A reading level match study of nonword reading skills in poor readers with varying IQs. *Journal of Learning Disabilities*, 25, 318-326.

Galaburda, A. (1983). Developmental dyslexia: Current anatomical research. *Annals of Dyslexia, 33,* 41-53.

Galaburda, A. M. (1994). Developmental dyslexia and animal studies: At the interface between cognition and neurology. *Cognition, 50,* 133-149.

Galaburda, A. M., & Kemper, T. L. (1979). Cytoarchitectonic abnormalities in developmental dyslexia: A case study. *Annals of Neurology, 6,* 94-100.

Galaburda, A. M., Rosen, G. D. & Sherman, G. F. (1989). The neural origin of developmental dyslexia: Implications for medicine, neurology, and cognition. In A. M. Galaburda (Ed.), *From reading to neurons.* Cambridge, MA: MIT Press.

Galaburda, A. M., Sherman, G. F., Rosen, G. D., Aboitiz, F., & Geschwind, N. (1985). Developmental dyslexia: Four consecutive cases with cortical anomalies. *Annals of Neurology, 18,* 222-233.

Gallagher, A., Frith, U., & Snowling, M. J. (2000). Precursors of literacy delay among children at genetic risk for dyslexia. *Journal of Child Psychology and Psychiatry, 41(2),* 203-213.

Gilger, J. W., Pennington, B. F., & DeFries, J. C. (1991). Risk for reading disability as a function of parental history in three family studies. *Reading and Writing: An Interdisciplinary Journal, 3,* 205-217.

Godfrey, J. J., Syrdal-Lasky, A. K., Millay, K. K., & Knox, C. M. (1981). Performance of dyslexic children on speech perception tests. *Journal of Experimental Child Psychology, 32,* 401-424.

Guilleminault, C., & Souquet, M. (1979). Sleep states and related pathology. In R. Korobkin and C. Guilleminault (Eds.), *Advances in perinatal neurology, (Vol. 1).* New York: Spectrum.

Gratton, G., Coles, M. G. H., & Donchin, E. (1983). A new method for off-line removal of ocular artifact. *Electroencephalography and Clinical Neurophysiology,* 55, 468-484.

Grigorenko, E. L. (2001). Developmental dyslexia: an update on genes, brains and environments. *Journal of Child Psychology and Psychiatry, 42,* 91-125.

Humphreys, P., Kaufmann, W. E., & Galaburda, A. M. (1990). Developmental dyslexia in women: Neuropathological findings in three cases. *Annals of Neurology, 28,* 727-738.

Kemper, T. L. (1984). Asymmetrical lesions in dyslexia. In N. Geschwind & A. M. Galaburda (Eds.), *Cerebral dominance: the biological foundations* (pp. 75-89). Cambridge, MA: Harvard University Press.

Koster, C., Been, P. H., Krikhaar, E. M., Zwarts, F., Diepstra, H. D. & Van Leeuwen, T. H. (2005). Differences at 17 months: productive language patterns in infants at familial risk for dyslexia and typically developing infants. *Journal of Speech, Language & Hearing Research, 48(2),* 426-438.

Kuhl, P., Williams, K., Lacerda, F., Stevens, K., & Lindblom, B. (1992). Linguistic experience alters phonetic perception in infants by 6 months of age. *Science, 255,* 606-608.

Kuijpers, C., Been, P. H., van Leeuwen, T., ter Keurs, M., van der Leij, A., & van den Bos, K. (2003). Leesproblemen op het voortgezet onderwijs: normering van een aantal tests. *Pedagogische Studieën, 241,* 272-287.

Lambe, E. K. (1999). Dyslexia, gender, and brain imaging. *Neuropsychologia, 37,* 521-536.

Liberman, I. Y. & Shankweiler, D. (1985). Phonology and the problems of learning to read and to write. *Remedial & Special Education,* 6, 8-17.

Lyytinen, H., Guttorm, T. K., Huttunen, T., Hämäläinen, J., Lappänen, P. H. T., & Vesterinen, M. (2005) Psychophysiology of developmental dyslexia: a review of findings including studies of children at risk for dyslexia. *Journal of Neurolinguistics, 18,* 167-195.

Mann, V. A. (1984). Longitudinal prediction and prevention of early reading difficulty. *Annals of Dyslexia, 34,* 117-136.

Mazoyer, B. M., Tzourio, N., Frak, V. et al. (1993). The cortical representation of speech. *Journal of Cognitive Neuroscience, 5,* 467-479.

Mehler, J., Dupoux, E., Pallier, C., & Dehaene-Lambertz (1995). Cross-linguistic approaches to speech processing. *Current Opinion in Neurobiology: Cognitive Neuroscience, 5,* 171-176.

Meyler, A., & Breznitz, Z. (2005). Impaired phonological and orthographic word representations among adult dyslexic readers: evidence from event-related potentials. *The Journal of Genetic Psychology, 166(2),* 215-238.

Mody, M., Studdert-Kennedy, M., & Brady, S. (1996). Speech perception deficits in poor readers: Auditory processing or phonological coding? *Journal of Experimental Child Psychology, 64,* 199-231.

NWO Netherlands Organization for Scientific Research (1996). Identifying the core features of developmental dyslexia: A multidisciplinary approach. NWO Nota Kennis verrijkt programma.

Olson, R. K. (1994). Language deficits in "specific" reading disability. In M. A. Gernsbacher (Ed.), *Handbook of psycholinguistics*. San Diego: Academic Press.

Pallay, S. L. (1986). *Speech perception in dyslexic children*. Unpublished doctoral dissertation, City University of New York.

Pascual-Marqui R. D., Michel, C. M., & Lehmann, D. Low resolution electromagnetic tomography: a new method for localizing electrical activity in the brain. *International Journal of Psychophysiology, 18,* 49-65.

Paulesu, E., Demonet, J. F., Fazio, F., McCrory, E., Chanoine, V., Brunswick, N. et al. (2001). Dyslexia: cultural diversity and biological unity. *Science, 291,* 2165-2167.

Pennington, B. F. (1990). The genetics of dyslexia. *Journal of Child Psychology and Psychiatry, 31*, 193-201.

Pennington, B., & Lefty, D. L. (2001). Early reading development in children at familial risk for dyslexia. *Child development, 72,* 816-833.

Reed, M. A. (1989). Speech perception and the discrimination of brief auditory cues in reading disabled children. *Journal of Experimental Child Psychology, 48*, 270-292.

Rutter, M., Avshalom, C., Fergusson, D., Horwood, L. J., Goodman, R., et al. (2004). Sex differences in developmental reading disability. New findings from 4 epidemiological studies. *Journal of the American Medical Association, 291,* 2007-2012.

Scarborough, H. (1991). Antecedents to reading disability: Preschool language development and literacy experiences of children from dyslexic families. *Reading and Writing: An Interdisciplinary Journal, 3,* 219-233.

Siegel, L. S., & Ryan, E. B. (1988). Development of grammatical-sensitivity, phonological, and short-term memory skills in normally achieving and learning disabled children. *Developmental Psychology, 24*, 28-37.

Snowling, M. (1981). Phonemic deficits in developmental dyslexia. *Psychological Research, 43,* 219-234.

Snowling, M. (1991). Developmental reading disorders. *Journal of Child Psychology and Psychiatry, 32*, 49-77.

Stanovich, K. E. (1988). Explaining the differences between the dyslexic and the garden-variety poor reader: The phonological-core variable-difference model. *Journal of Learning Disabilities, 21*, 590-604.

Steffens, M. L., Eilers, R., Gross-Glen, K., & Jallad, B. (1992). Speech perception deficits in adult subjects with familial dyslexia. *Journal of Speech and Hearing Research,* 35, 192-200.

Stevens, J (1996). *Applied multivariate statistics for the social sciences.* Mahwah, NJ: Lawrence Erlbaum Asssociates.

Studdert-Kennedy, M., & Mody, M. (1995). Auditory temporal perception deficits in the reading-impaired: A critical review of the evidence. *Psychonomic Bulletin and Review, 2,* 508-514.

Tervaniemi, M., Kujala, A., Alho, K., Virtanen, J., Ilmoniemi, R.J., & Naatanen, R. (1999). Functional specialization of the human auditory cortex in processing phonetic and musical sounds: a magnetoencephalographic (MEG) study. *Neuroimage, 9,* 330-336.

Tervaniemi, M., & Hugdahl, K. (2003) Lateralization of auditory-cortex functions. *Brain Research Reviews, 43,* 231-246.

Van Beinum, F. J., Schwippert, C., Been, P. H., van Leeuwen, T. H., & Kuijpers, C. (2005). Development and application of a /bAk/-/dAk/ continuum for testing auditory perception within the Dutch longitudinal dyslexia study. *Speech Communication, 47(1,2),* 124-142.

Van Leeuwen, Th., Been, P., Kuijpers, C., Zwarts, F., Maassen, B., & van der Leij, A. (2006). Mismatch response is absent in 2-month-old infants at risk for dyslexia. *Neuroreport, 4(17),* 351-355.

Van der Leij A, Lyytinen H., & Zwarts F. (2001). The study of infant cognitive processes in dyslexia. In A. Fawcett (Ed.), *Dyslexia: Theory & Good Practice* (pp. 160-81). London; Philadelphia: Whurr Publishers.
Wagner, R. K. (1986). Phonological processing abilities and reading: Implications for disabled readers. *Journal of Learning Disabilities*, *19*, 623-630.
Wagner, R. K. & Torgesen, J. K. (1987). The nature of phonological processing and its causal role in the acquisition of reading skills. *Psychological Bulletin*, *101*, 192-212.
Werker, R. F., & Tees, R. C. (1984). Cross-language speech perception: Evidence for perceptual reorganization during the first year of life. *Infant Behavior Development, 7*, 49-63.
Werker, J., & Tees, R. (1987). Speech perception in severely disabled and average reading children. *Canadian Journal of Psychology, 41*, 48-61.
Reed, M. A. (1989). Speech perception and the discrimination of brief auditory cues in reading disabled children. *Journal of Experimental Child Psychology*, *48*, 270-292.
Zatorre, R. J., Myer, E., Gjedde, A., & Evans, A. C. (1996). PET studies of phonetic processes in speech perception: renew, replication and reanalysis. *Cerebral Cortex, 6,* 21-30.

4

ELECTROPHYSIOLOGICAL FUNCTIONAL IMAGING OF AUDITORY PROCESSING IN HUMANS

From Auditory Object Definition to Language

Hillel Pratt
Evoked Potentials Laboratory, Technion – Israel Institute of Technology, Haifa 3200, Israel

Abstract: Changes in the auditory scene include the formation of new objects from the acoustic background, change in the properties of existing objects, in addition to the appearance or disappearance of objects from the scene. This chapter summarizes results of imaging the processing of these attributes of auditory stimuli that takes place in parallel during a time period of about 100 msec (80-170 msec) after onset of a sound.

Electrophysiological functional imaging of auditory processing of sound onset, offset, it's detection as deviant and its formation from a cluster of acoustic features allowed reasonable spatial resolution coupled with unparalleled temporal resolution. Such imaging allowed following the time course of processing a variety of sounds attributes. The time courses that are thus revealed are sensitive to the nature of the stimulus and different aspects of the stimulus were found to be analyzed in parallel in different brain areas. Different modes of processing manifest in different time courses of brain activity as revealed by electrophysiological functional imaging of dyslexics vs. normal readers.

These results indicate that the brain is a parallel processor that simultaneously handles many aspects of the processed material and adapts this processing with experience.

Key words: Event Related Potentials, auditory, speech, source estimation, functional imaging

1. INTRODUCTION

The auditory system, like all sensory systems, is sensitive to changes in the environment that may be critical to survival. The auditory environment is rich in simultaneous sounds, emanating from different sources with a variety of spectral characteristics. Yet, we can take this acoustic mixture and cluster in it distinct "auditory objects" (Bregman, 1990) that are discriminated by their frequency characteristics, temporal distinctness and where they are coming from.

Changes in the auditory scene include the formation of new objects from the acoustic background, change in the properties of existing objects, in addition to the appearance or disappearance of objects from the scene. In the well-known example of the Cocktail Party, in which individual speakers in a background babble of a cocktail party can be distinguished and listened to at will, we can detect new persons, an unexpected voice and the appearance and departure of a person. In addition, speech sounds are discriminated from other, non-speech, background sounds.

The grouping of the frequency components of sounds emanating from the same source into coherent auditory objects is performed by the auditory cortex (Creutzfeldt, Hellweg, & Schreiner, 1980; Gehr, Komiya, & Eggermont, 2000; Leppelsack, 1978; Newman & Wollberg, 1973; Pantev, Hoke, Lehnertz, Lukenhoner, Anogianakis, & Wittkowski, 1995; Wang, Merzenicj, Beitel, & Schreiner, 1995). However, evidence on processing other attributes of auditory objects, particularly in humans, are still lacking. This chapter summarizes results on processing of a variety of auditory attributes that all take place in parallel during a time period of about100 msec (80-170 msec) after onset of a sound. These results will demonstrate that the brain is a parallel processor that simultaneously handles many aspects of the processed material and adapts this processing with experience.

Information on normal processing of sounds can be used for better understanding of altered modes of processing in special populations. We studied auditory processing in 'phonological' dyslexics whose reading difficulty is associated with a general auditory processing impairment compared to normal readers. Several stimulus types were presented and the brain activity during the critical early period around 100 msec was compared with that of normal readers.

In these studies brain processes were studied by recording the electrical activity evoked by the auditory stimuli (Event-Related Potentials – ERPs) and imaging the intracranial current densities that could account for the surface recorded potentials. Current density distributions were used to compare the brain's electrical activity in the detection of auditory change, the fusion of acoustic elements to form a new auditory object, the detection of deviance of a stimulus from the preceding series of auditory events, onset and offset of a stimulus, the initial distinction of speech from non-speech sounds and the processing of meaningful well-rehearsed words (first language) as compared to that of less familiar words (second language).

2. METHODS

In all these studies, ERPs were recorded from 21 electrodes, distributed on the scalp according to the 10-20 system, while subjects performed an auditory discrimination task or while they passively listened to sounds. All subjects were young, neurologically and audiometrically normal university students between the ages of 19 and 28. Each group of subjects, in each of the studies comprised of at least 13 subjects, and only statistically significant group results are presented.

In the studies of fusion and of deviance, stimuli that were only elements of speech but not perceived as defined speech sounds: /a~a/ (base) and /g/ and the /d/ (formant transitions) were fused to create the speech sounds /aga/ and /ada/ (Figure 1). The base was always presented in front of the subject, while the formants were presented at the same (good fusion), or different (worse fusion) locations, to fuse with the base and form the vowel-consonant-vowel. Subjects listened to Vowel-Consonant-Vowel strings of two types - /aga/ and /ada/, and had to press one button to /aga/ and another to /ada/. Probabilities of the two stimuli were not equal so that the effect of probability and deviance could also be studied. The response to the introduction of the formant (the C-Complex) is actually a composite of a number of temporally overlapping events: The response to transition onset, activity associated with the actual fusion of acoustic elements to form a new object and the detection of deviance in case of a rare consonant. In order to separate these different contributions and study each one separately, the other overlapping contributions had to be subtracted.

The activity specific to object definition, or fusion of elements, the net response to fusion (F-Complex), was isolated by subtracting the sum of the responses to base alone and formant transitions alone from the response to the fused stimulus (Laufer & Pratt, 2003). The activity specific to deviance detection, the MMN, was derived by subtracting the response to the standard fused consonant from the response to the deviant rare consonant. The resultant potentials to object definition and to deviance detection overlap in their time courses. To determine if they are generated in the same brain areas and when the formation of a new auditory object and the detection of deviance separate, we conducted current density source estimation during deviance detection and during object definition and compared these distributions statistically using non-parametric procedures (see below) that are also used in fMRI BOLD comparisons (Laufer & Pratt, 2005).

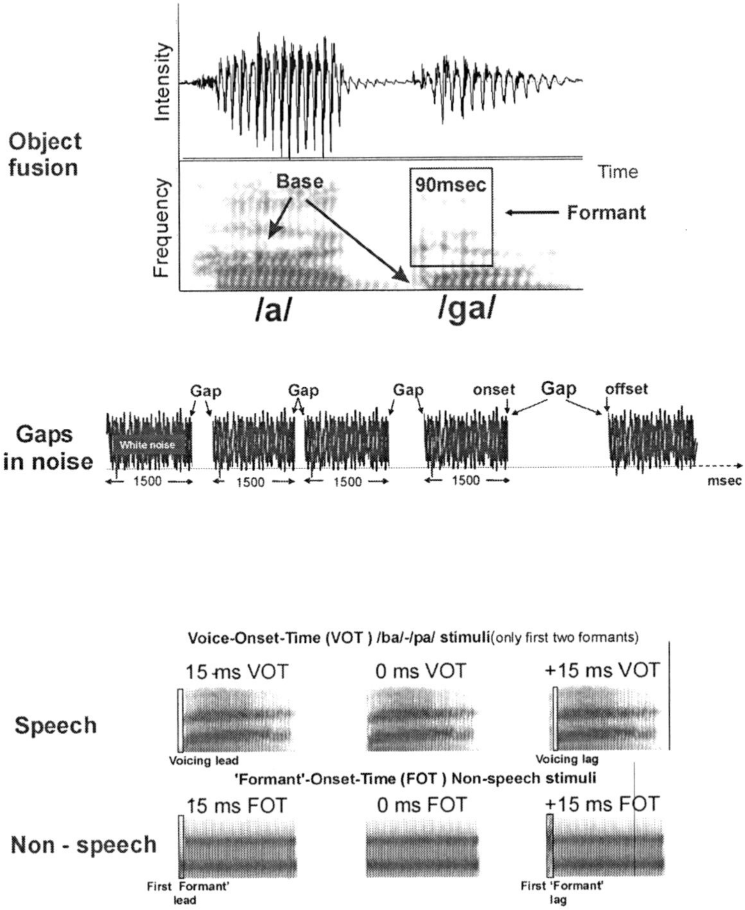

Figure 1. Stimuli used in the various studies (from top to bottom): To study acoustic fusion to form auditory objects, formant transitions and base were fused to result in V-C-V sequences /aga/ and /ada/. To study stimulus onsets and offsets, without the spectral changes associated with such transitions, gaps in white noise were used. Gap onsets were sound offsets while gap offsets were sound onsets. Speech and non-speech stimuli with the same spectro-temporal properties were compared using a Voice-Onset-Time (VOT) continuum, created by editing natural productions of /ba/ and /pa/ and an analogous non-speech continuum, comprised of two synthesized formants, varying in their onset time.

To study onsets and offsets of sounds without the concomitant spectral changes, gaps in continuous white noise were used. The gaps in noise stimuli consisted of randomly distributed gaps of different durations in a continuous white noise (Figure 1). With gaps in noise subjects had to press a button when they detected a gap in the continuous noise (Pratt, Bleich, & Mittelman, 2005).

Processing of speech, which is the primary and most often used mode of human communication, was compared to non-speech sounds while making sure that speech and non-speech sounds shared the very same physical attributes, such as spectral and temporal attributes, and differed only in their origin – natural speech vs synthesized sounds (Figure 1). The subjects' task was to discriminate /ba/ from /pa/ when speech stimuli were used, and between two synthesized sounds with the very same temporal and spectral properties, having almost the same spectrograms as the speech signals (Horev et al., 2006).

To study the effects of experience on auditory processing, the brain activity of processing first (well rehearsed) and second (less rehearsed) language was compared (Sinai and Pratt, 2003a,b). Subjects heard pairs of words to which they had to respond whether both were meaningful, only one was meaningful (and the other a pseudo-word) or whether both were meaningless pseudo-words, by pressing an appropriate button. The words were either Hebrew (first language) or English (second language) real words or pseudo-words, and subjects had to relate to their meaningfulness and not to the language they were in. The brain potentials to stimuli were sorted according to their language (first or second) and the accent they were in (Hebrew pseudo- and real words vs. English pseudo- and real words).

Intracranial brain activity was estimated from the scalp-recorded potentials using Low resolution electromagnetic tomography (LORETA; Pascual-Marqui, Esslen, Kochi, & Lehmann, 2002; Pascual-Marqui, Lehmann, Koeing, Kochi, Merlo, & Hell, 1999; Pascual-Marqui, Michel, & Lehmann, 1994; Vitacco, Brandeis, Pascual-Marqui, & Martin, 2002). LORETA is a functional brain imaging method that estimates the distribution of current density in the brain, displaying it in a 3D Talairach space. LORETA is a 3D distributed inverse solution which relies on the smoothness assumption (Pascual-Marqui et al., 1999) that neighboring neurons are simultaneously and synchronously active. The smoothness assumption results in low spatial resolution blurred beyond the 7 mm^3 voxels. The version of LORETA employed here used a three-shell spherical head model registered to the digitized Talairach and Tournoux (1988) atlas (Brain Imaging Centre, Montreal Neurological Institute).

LORETA was used in this study because of its minimal set of assumptions, its relative accuracy in localizing deep sources (Pasqual-Maqui, 1999) and low localization error (Menendez, Andino, Lantz, & Michel, 2001; Yao & He, 2001; Pascual-Marqui et al., 2002; Phillips, Rugg, & Friston, 2002a, 2002b). Pascual-Marqui et al. (2002) reviewed the experimental validation of LORETA based on the correct localization of primary sensory cortices, epileptic foci, language processing areas, and face processing areas. Other publications validated the method by providing experimental data (e.g., Anderer, Saletu, Semlitsch, & Pascual-Marqui, 2002; Maurer, Bucher, Brem, & Brandeis, 2003; Park et al., 2002; Pizzagalli et al., 2002; Vitacco, Brandeis, Pascual-Marqui, & Martin, 2002). Recently, in the context of a study to determine the time-course of emotional processing using LORETA (Esslen et al., 2004), a good correspondence was found with other brain imaging studies (PET/fMRI), with the added value of superior temporal resolution.

In our studies, Statistical non-Parametric Mapping (SnPM) was used to determine the time course of differences in current density distributions between experimental conditions or subject groups. The SnPM method estimates the probability distribution by using a randomization procedure, corrects for multiple comparisons and has the highest possible statistical power (Nichols & Holmes, 2002). The SnPM method was validated in our previous studies by comparing its results with more conventional ANOVA results (Laufer & Pratt, 2003b; Sinai & Pratt, 2003).

Specifically, we used the 'pseudo-t' statistic which reduced noise in the data by averaging over adjacent voxels (Nichols and Holmes, 2002). In order to trace time segments of significant differences between responses we compared them on a time-frame-by-time-frame voxel-by-voxel basis for a period of 256 time-frames (1sec.) from stimulus onset. A time-segment was designated significant only if it contained at least 5 contiguous significant ($P<0.01$) time-frames. We employed this procedure to reduce the probability that time-frames assigned with significance by chance alone due to alpha inflation would be included in the analysis. The second step was to compare average current density values obtained across the significant time-frames comprising each significant time-segment. Thus, a single

LORETA solution consisting of 2394 voxels representing the entire time segment was obtained. The two-step procedure outlined above was employed in order to trace significant time segments, utilizing the high temporal resolution of LORETA, while adhering to the method originally used by Nichols and Holmes (2002), of averaging significant t-values over space only.

We presented LORETA images of specific significant time segments using the 'fiducial cortical surface' (boundary midway through cortical thickness, Dickson, Drury, & Van Essen, 2001) and assigned it to the region in which the voxel with the maximal difference (local maxima) was found. However, some caveats associated with the LORETA method should be mentioned. Because the localization error of LORETA is at worst in the order of two voxels (Pascual-Marqui, 1999), which serves as an upper limit for correct localization, activation may only reside *in the vicinity* of the brain structures indicated by such maximal difference single voxel computations.

In addition, LORETA uses a fitting procedure (described in Pascual-Marqui et al., 1999) by which individually measured 3D electrode positions are fitted to the standardized Talairach scalp surface. We used this procedure, and did not rely on the individual MRI of each subject. Thus, the fitting procedure itself adds to the localization error of LORETA. In addition, since data have been pooled over subjects, individual differences should be taken into account in the pattern and location of gyral convolutions, and thus, activity may reside only in approximate regions to those specified in the text and plotted in the LORETA images.

3. RESULTS AND DISCUSSION

The current density distributions associated with acoustic fusion and with deviance detection did not differ significantly in the first 180 msec, and were both localized to the area of the auditory cortex. However, between 187 and 219 msec after stimulus onset their sources diverged and current density distributions were significantly different: Both were temporal, but Deviance Detection was bilateral in the posterior temporal lobe, while Object Definition was lateralized to the left, with a tendency to be slightly more anterior in the anterior and middle left temporal lobe (Figure 2).

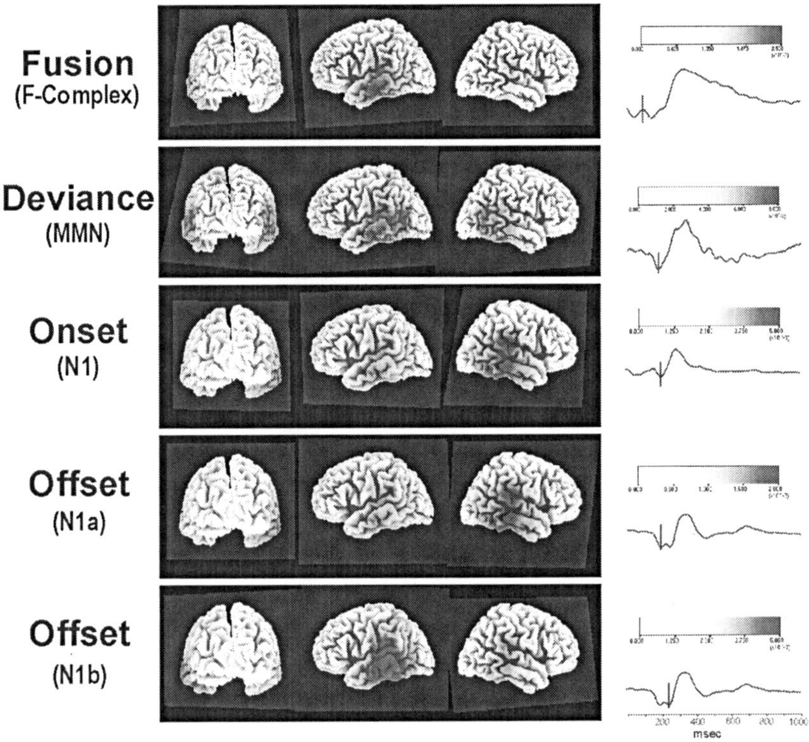

Figure 2. Source current density distributions of early brain processing of (from top to bottom): Fusion of acoustic features to form an auditory object (F-Complex), detection of a deviant stimulus in a string of frequent stimuli (MMN), detection of stimulus onset (N_1) and detection of stimulus offset (two sub-peaks of activity: N_{1a} and N_{1b}). The scalp derived waveforms and the points in time for which source estimation was conducted are displayed to the right of each image.

At the time period of object definition and deviance detection, activity specific to object appearance and disappearance (gap offset and onset) can be recorded as well. The current density distributions associated with object appearance and disappearance are distinct in time course and location in the brain This is best demonstrated by the potentials to gaps in noise. The potentials to gaps in noise appeared when subjects detected the gaps and consisted of a double-peaked N_1 complex (N_{1a} and N_{1b}) which was not affected by attention. In response to long gaps, the double-peaked N_1 was observed only in response to noise offset (gap onset) and not to its onset (gap offset).

Noise onset potentials were similar to those evoked by clicks, while the bifid N-Complex to noise offset included two distinct constituents, one earlier and one later than the click and gap offset N_1 (Figure 2).

In terms of source current density distributions, N_{1a} was prominent on the left while N_1 to clicks was more prominent on the right, and N_{1b} was also more prominent on the right. N_1 to the onset of a sound (gap offset) was lateralized to the right central and posterior temporal lobe. Noise offset N_{1a} was lateralized to the left central and posterior temporal lobe, while N_{1b} was lateralized to the right central and posterior temporal lobe (Figure 2).

In summary, formation, deviance, appearance and cessation of sounds evoke physiologically distinct processes, reflecting different aspects of changes in the auditory scene. They all take place between 80 and 170 msec after event onset or offset, they are all unaffected by attention allocation and they all locate to the vicinity of auditory cortex and adjacent temporal lobe regions. However, their distributions in the brain are different: Formation lateralizes to the left, deviance is bilateral, appearance is lateralized to the right and cessation detection – to the left and then to the right. These change-detection processes are therefore simultaneous but distinctly represented in the brain.

The distinction of speech from non-speech sounds takes place from the very early stages of cortical processing. During the very same time period that sounds are grouped to objects, and are differentiated to expected vs deviant, etc., they are also differentiated according to whether they are speech or non-speech sounds, and all this happens in the same general area of the auditory cortex in the temporal lobe. This manifests, among others, in hemispheric prominence alternating at different times, in a different manner for speech and non-speech sounds (Figure 3).

The experience in processing auditory material affects the time course of activity in the brain. Comparing brain processing of first and seconds language revealed early and late differences in the associated brain activity. In general, the differences in brain activity around the N_1 component were related to the acoustics (accent) of the speech signal, whereas in later time frames (hundreds of msec from word onset) the differences related to the language and meaning, with more right hemisphere activity to second language (Figure 4), rather than the acoustics (Sinai & Pratt, 2003b).

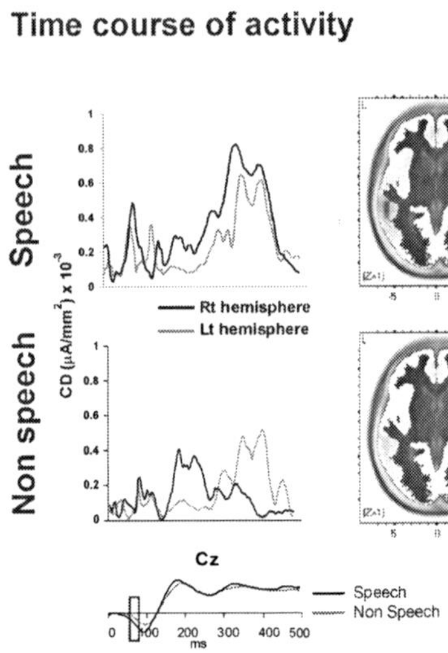

Figure 3. Time course of activation of the left and right hemispheres in response to speech and non-speech stimuli (left) and the source current density distribution around 100 msec, in response to speech and non-speech sounds (right). Hemispheric activation is expressed as the average current density across all voxels of the plotted hemisphere. The time course of scalp-recorded activity at the vertex (C_z) is plotted at the bottom, with the square showing the time frame for which current density distribution is displayed on the right.

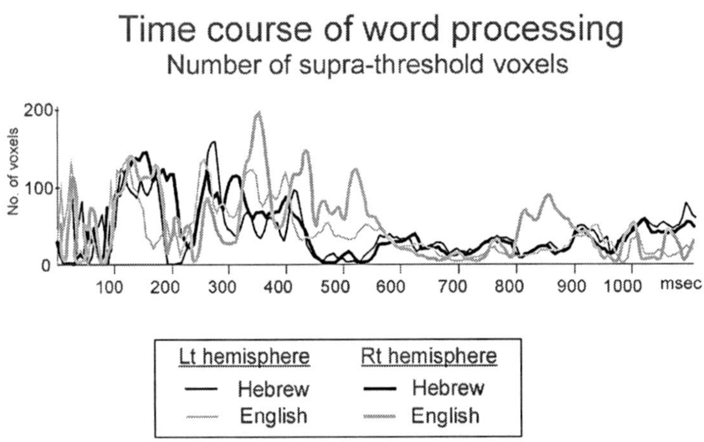

Figure 4. Time course of activation of the left and right hemispheres in response to first and second language words. Note the substantially larger activation of the right hemisphere in response to English (second language). Note in particular the latyeralization of activity to the left hemisphere with Hebrew words (second language) and to the right with English (second language) in the 80-100 msec time period after word onset.

When the processing of sounds in normals was compared to subjects with altered processing, the time course of processing was found to be different (Moisescu-Yiflach & Pratt, 2005). Following the time course of brain activation in this period: Controls showed activity beginning on the right, shifting to bilateral and ending on the left. In response to linguistic temporal cues (discriminating /ba/ from /pa/), Controls also showed activity beginning on the right, shifting to bilateral and ending on the left, to both non-linguistic and linguistic temporal cues. In contrast, dyslexics showed activity that was lateralized to the left throughout the time period.

4. CONCLUSIONS

The results outlined in this report show a variety of brain activities associated with the formation of an auditory object, a change in an ongoing sound, appearance of a sound, disappearance of a sound, distinction between speech and non-speech material and even differentiation of accent, all taking place between 80 and 170 msec after the change in the auditory environment, and each involving a unique set of brain structures.

From clinical observations on the effects of brain lesions, and from reaction-time studies in normal subjects, there are indications that the left hemisphere of the brain specializes in processing speech, while non-speech is processed mostly in the right hemisphere. Electrophysiological imaging of processing speech and non-speech sounds and following the time course of hemispheric lateralization in processing these sounds allowed a more detailed account of hemispheric lateralization. Lateralization of processing any sound alternates between right and left and the time course of this lateralization is different in speech and in non-speech material. Moreover, lateralization time course is even different between processing first and second language. Therefore, rather than describing the left hemisphere as the speech hemisphere and the right hemisphere as the non-speech hemisphere, the left appears to process well-rehearsed and more familiar material, while the right hemisphere specializes in material that is less familiar and requires more scrutiny in processing.

The results of comparing the time course of early processing of auditory speech and non-speech material by dyslexics with processing in normal readers indicate that compared to the changing lateralization of activity in normals, lateralization of activity in the Dyslexic subjects remains static. Thus, abnormal modes of processing during the critical period around N_1 manifest in impaired performance that may manifest in skills such as reading.

In summary, electrophysiological functional imaging of auditory processing allows reasonable spatial resolution coupled with unparalleled temporal resolution which allows following the time course of processing sounds. The time courses that are thus revealed are sensitive to the nature of the stimulus. Different aspects of the stimulus are analyzed in parallel in different brain areas. Different modes of processing manifest in different time courses of brain activity as revealed by electrophysiological functional imaging.

5. ACKNOWLEDGEMENTS

The results reported in this chapter were compiled and analyzed by the staff and graduate students of the Technion Evoked Potentials Laboratory without whom these studies could not have been conducted. All credits therefore belong to Naomi Bleich, Nitza Horev, Ilan Laufer, Naomi Mittelman, Tsuf Moisesko-Yiflach and Alon Sinai, and any faults are the sole responsibility of HP.

REFERENCES

Anderer, P., Saletu, B., Semlitsch, H. V., & Pascual-Marqui, R. D. (2002). Non-invasive localization of P300 sources in normal aging and age-associated memory impairment. *Neurobiological Aging*, *24*, 463-479.

Bregman, A. S. (1990). Auditory scene analysis, Cambridge, MA: MIT Press.

Creutzfeldt, O., Hellweg, F. C., & Schreiner, C. (1980). Thalamocortical transformation of responses to complex auditory stimuli. *Experimental Brain Research*, *39*, 87-104.

Dickson, J., Drury, H., & Van Essen, D.C. (2001). Surface management system (SuMS): a surface-based database to aid cortical surface reconstruction, visualization and analysis. *Philosophical Transactions of the Royal Society of London. Series B, Biological Sciiences*, *356*, 1277-1292.

Esslen, M., Pascual-Marqui, R. D, Hell, D., Kochi, K., & Lehmann, D. (2000). Brain areas and time course of emotional processing. *Neuroimage*, *21*, 1189-1203.

Gehr, D. D., Komiya, H., Eggermont, J. J. (2000). Neuronal responses in cat primary auditory cortex to natural and altered species-specific calls. *Ear & Hear*, *150*, 27-42.

Horev, N., Most, T., & Pratt, H., in press, Categorical Perception of Speech (VOT) and Analogous Non-Speech (FOT) Signals: Behavioral and Electrophysiological Correlates. *Ear & Hear*.

Laufer, I., & Pratt, H. (2003). The Electrophysiological Net Response (F-complex) to Spatial Fusion of Speech Elements Forming an Auditory Object. *Clinical Neurophysiology, 114*, 818-834.

Laufer, I., & Pratt, H. (2005). The 'F-complex' and MMN tap different aspects of deviance, *Clinical Neurophysiol*ogy, *116*, 336-352.

Leppelsack, H. J. (1978). Unit responses to species-specific sounds in the auditory forebrain center of birds. *Federation Proceedings, 137*, 2336-2341.

Maurer, U., Bucher, K., Brem, S., & Brandeis, D. (2003). Development of the automatic mismatch response: from frontal positivity in kindergarten children to the mismatch negativity. *Clinical Neurophysiology, 114*, 808-817.

Menendez, R. G. D, Andino, S. G., Lantz, G., Michel, C. M., & Landis, T. (2001). Noninvasive localization of electromagnetic epileptic activity. I. Method descriptions and simulations. *Brain Topography, 14*, 131-137.

Moisescu-Yiflach, T., & Pratt, H. (2005). Auditory Event Related Potentials and Source Current Density Estimation in Phonologic/Auditory Dyslexics. *Clinical Neurophysiol*ogy, *116*, 2632-2647.

Newman, J. D., & Wollberg, Z. (1973). Multiple coding of species-specific vocalizations in the auditory cortex of squirrel monkeys. *Brain Research, 54*, 287-304.

Nichols, T. E., Holmes, A. P. (2002). Nonparametric permutation tests for functional neuroimaging: a primer with examples. *Human Brain Mapping, 15*, 1-25.

Pantev, C., Hoke, M., Lehnertz, K., Lukenhoner, B., Anogianakis, G., & Wittkowski, W. (1995). Tonotopic organization of different areas of the human auditory cortex revealed by simultaneous magnetic and electric recordings. *Electroencephalography and Clinical* Neurophysiology, *94*, 26-40.

Park, H. J., Kwon, J. S., Youn, T., Pae, J. S., Kim, J. J., Kim, M. S., & Ha, K. S. (2002). Statistical parametric mapping of LORETA using high density EEG and individual MRI: application to mismatch negativities in schizophrenia. *Human Brain Mapping, 17*, 168-178.

Pascual-Marqui, R. D., Esslen, M., Kochi, K., & Lehmann, D. (2002). Functional imaging with low-resolution brain electromagnetic tomography (LORETA): a review. *Methods & Findings in Experimental & Clinical Pharmacology, 24* Suppl C, 91-95.

Pascual-Marqui, R. D., Lehmann, D., Koeing, T., Kochi, K., Merlo, M. C. G., Hell, D., & Koukkou, M. (1999). Low resolution brain electromagnetic tomography (LORETA) functional imaging in acute, neuroleptic-naïve, first-episode, productive schizophrenia. *Psychiatry Research: Neuroimaging, 90*, 169-179.

Pascual-Marqui, R. D., Michel, C. M., & Lehmann, D. (1994). Low resolution electromagnetic tomography: a new method for localizing electrical activity in the brain. *International Journal of Psychophysiology, 18*, 49-65.

Pascual-Marqui, R. D. (1999). Review of methods for solving the EEG inverse problem. *International Journal of Bioelectromagnetism, 1*, 75-86.

Phillips, C., Rugg, M. D., & Friston, K. J. (2002a). Anatomically informed basis functions for EEG source localization: combining functional and anatomical constraints. *Neuroimage, 16,* 678-95.

Phillips, C., Rugg, M. D., & Friston, K. J. (2002b). Systematic regularization of linear inverse solutions of the EEG source localization problem. *Neuroimage, 17*, 287-301.

Pizzagalli, D. A., Lehmann, D., Hendrick, A. M., Regard, M., Pascual-Marqui, R. D., & Davidson, R. J. (2002). Affective judgments of faces modulate early activity (approximately 160 ms) within the fusiform gyri. *Neuroimage, 16*, 663-677.

Pratt, H., Bleich, N., & Mittelman, N. (2005). The composite N_1 component to gaps in noise. *Clinical Neurophysiology, 116*, 2648-2663.

Sinai, A., & Pratt, H. (2003a). High Resolution Time Course of Hemispheric Dominance Revealed by Low-Resolution Electromagnetic Tomography (LORETA). *Clinical Neurophysiol*ogy, 1181-1188.

Sinai, A., & Pratt, H. (2003b). Semantic Processing of Unattended Words and Pseudowords in First and Second Language: An ERP Study. *Journal of Basic and Clinical Physiology and* Pharmacology, *14*, 177-190.

Talairach, J., & Tournoux. P. (1988). Co-planar stereotaxic atlas of the human brain, in: *3-dimensional proportional system: an approach to cerebral imaging*. Stuttgart, George Thiem Verlag.

Vitacco, D., Brandeis, D., Pascual-Marqui, R., & Martin, E. (2002). Correspondence of event-related potential tomography and functional magnetic resonance imaging during language processing. *Human Brain Mapping*, *17,* 4-12.

Wang, X., Merzenich, M. M., Beitel, R., & Schreiner, C. E. (1995). Representation of a species-specific vocalization in the primary auditory cortex of the common marmoset: temporal and spectral characteristics. *Journal of Neurophysiology*, *74*, 2685-2706.

Yao, D., & He, B. (2001). A self-coherence enhancement algorithm and its application to enhancing three-dimensional source estimation from EEGs. *Annals Biomedical Engineering*, *29*, 1019-1027.

5

OVERLAPPING TASKS METHODOLOGY AS A TOOL FOR INVESTIGATING LANGUAGE PERCEPTION

Werner Sommer[1] and Annette Hohlfeld[2]
[1]Humboldt-University Berlin; [2]Center for Human Evolution, Madrid

Abstract: A series of studies is reviewed that investigated the effects of additional tasks on the N400 component of the event-related brain potential (ERP) within the framework of an overlapping tasks paradigm. In all studies the N400 component was elicited by words that could be either synonymous or non-synonymous to a preceding word and by subtracting the ERP to synonymous from those to non-synonymous words. Additional task stimuli were visual and could be presented at high to low temporal overlap with the words. The N400 was delayed in time when there was high temporal overlap with the additional task stimulus. The delay was more pronounced when the additional task was more difficult and more language-like. Second-language speakers showed very similar interference effects albeit at a globally slower level. Somewhat different interference effects were obtained when the meaning of the eliciting words were irrelevant to the task. In contrast, eye movements and visuo-spatial attention shifts had no effects on N400 latency. Together, the results indicate that the N400-eliciting processes – presumably the access to semantic knowledge – belong to a group of central processes that form a bottleneck in the cognitive system because they can handle only one process at a time. On the basis of these findings dual-task methodology is suggested to be a valuable tool not only for investigating the processes supporting language perception and, more generally, the retrieval of semantic knowledge but also for other language perception processes.

Key words: Event Related Potentials, N400 component, dual-task

1. INTRODUCTION

Judicious combination of two tasks that have to be performed concurrently is a time-honoured method for investigating the nature of psychological processes and, in particular, of language processing. Whereas traditional dual task research suffers from the lack of control over the timing of the processes involved, this is not the case for overlapping tasks where the critical stimuli are presented at specified onset asynchronies. As yet, only few studies have applied these methods to language processing. Even fewer studies have combined overlapping tasks with the recording of language-sensitive event-related brain potentials (ERPs). This has been done in a recent series of experiments conducted by the authors and their co-workers. These experiments indicate that the semantic processing of words is delayed by concurrent, overlapping tasks. This delay depends on the amount of temporal overlap between tasks, on the difficulty of the decisions to be made on the concurrent stimulus, and – possibly – on the linguistic content of the decision. In order to explain these effects we suggest a model where the access to the semantic content of a word – or semantic knowledge in general – is part of those central cognitive processes that act like a bottleneck because they can deal with only one piece of information at a time. We further discuss other findings which are better explained in a graded resource sharing account.

2. DUAL TASKS AS A TRADITIONAL METHOD IN LANGUAGE RESEARCH

Studying the effects of combing two or more tasks is of interest from at least two broadly defined perspectives, enhancing basic knowledge about human cognition and its application to every day situations. From a basic research perspective, dual and multiple tasks are of interest because such situations very often lead to slower or degraded performance in at least one of the tasks as compared to the corresponding single task conditions. This holds true for many task combinations even when there is no obvious interference on a sensory or motor level. However, some tasks can be combined without costs and in other combinations, the presence and degree of inter-task interference may depend on the nature of the cognitive processes involved and on the level of expertise. Therefore, it seems that in principle, dual-task methodology appears to be a fruitful way to study the structure of the human mind. This certainly also holds true for language processing.

Dual task methodology in language research has in many cases applied complex tasks where many subprocesses have to be performed in an unspecified temporal order. In such condition there have been reports of skilled and seemingly cost-free multi-tasking processes[i]. Thus Spelke, Hirst, and Neisser (1976) successfully trained two persons over 85 one-hour sessions to read short stories for comprehension and take dictation of single words, discover relations among dictated words, and categorize words for meaning. These results were replicated and extended by Hirst, Spelke, Caharack, and Neisser (1980) and were taken as evidence that with increasing levels of skills capacity limits for multiple task performance vanish. There sometimes seem to be virtually no limits of how much a skilled human mind can accomplish at a given time.

Others have used the dual task methodology in order to investigate the relationship between different kinds of processes with the idea that when processes depend on similar or different mechanisms, there should be high or low interference, respectively, when these processes are simultaneously active. This tradition is especially prominent in research on working memory. For example, as reviewed by Caplan and Waters (1999) the degree to which sentence comprehension depends on verbal working memory has been studied by presenting sentences of varying syntactic complexity to participants while they had to keep a verbal load in short term memory. In experiments that required first to memorize a random sequence of digits and then to read a sentence, which had to be assigned to a picture, Caplan and Waters reported main effects of load in the error rates, but never an interaction of load and syntactic complexity. In contrast, if the task required reading a sentence, which had to be assessed for acceptability, and to memorize a sequence of digits that was presented together with the sentence, an interaction of load and syntactic complexity was observed. Based on these findings Caplan and Waters concluded that concurrent digit load only interferes with syntactic processing when the sentence task as well as the digit recall task are processed in an interrupted fashion. They further argued that retaining digits and structuring a sentence do not compete for the same resource pool, but that the ability to structure a sentence is affected by attention shifts induced by the additional task.

In the context of non-linguistic research, often a visuo-manual tracking procedure (cf. Heuer, 1991, for a review) has been combined with a second task such as a choice response or a memory task. Whereas early reports supported the view that tracking only interferes with manual primary tasks (McLeod, 1977), Jäncke (1994) showed that verbal rehearsal and speaking also disturbs tracking performance. In addition, he found speaking to disturb rightward movements in particular, possibly indicating neural overlap of left-hemispheric brain structures.

Experiments which involve complex tasks with many different pieces of information being delivered or processed at undefined time points – often termed as continuous tasks – have been criticised as being inconclusive with respect to the kind of interaction between tasks. In principle such continuous tasks can not exclude the possibility that participants rapidly alternate between tasks and therefore actually perform one task after the other (e.g., Pashler & Johnston, 1998). Therefore, in non-linguistic research there has been a recent shift towards using designs where the relevant stimuli for the tasks are presented at precisely specified time points. The most prevalent design is the overlapping tasks or psychological refractory period (PRP) paradigm[ii].

2.1 Overlapping tasks

In the PRP-paradigm two stimuli (S1 and S2) are presented at specified stimulus-onset asynchronies (SOAs), ranging typically between 50 ms and 1 s. Each of these stimuli is related to a task and requires a corresponding response (R1 and R2). Usually the first stimulus is given priority and has to be responded to first and as fast and accurate as possible, whereas the response to the second stimulus has to come next but also at maximal speed and accuracy. In many cases both speed and accuracy for S1 are independent of SOA. In contrast, RT2 is usually much prolonged when SOA gets shorter (cf. Fig. 1). The two most important explanations for this phenomenon are the single channel bottleneck account and the resource sharing account.

The first and probably most widely accepted account was first proposed by Welford (1952) and was elaborated upon in recent models (e.g., Pashler, 1994; cf. Fig. 1, Panel C). It ascribes dual task interference to limitations of certain processing stages. Welford

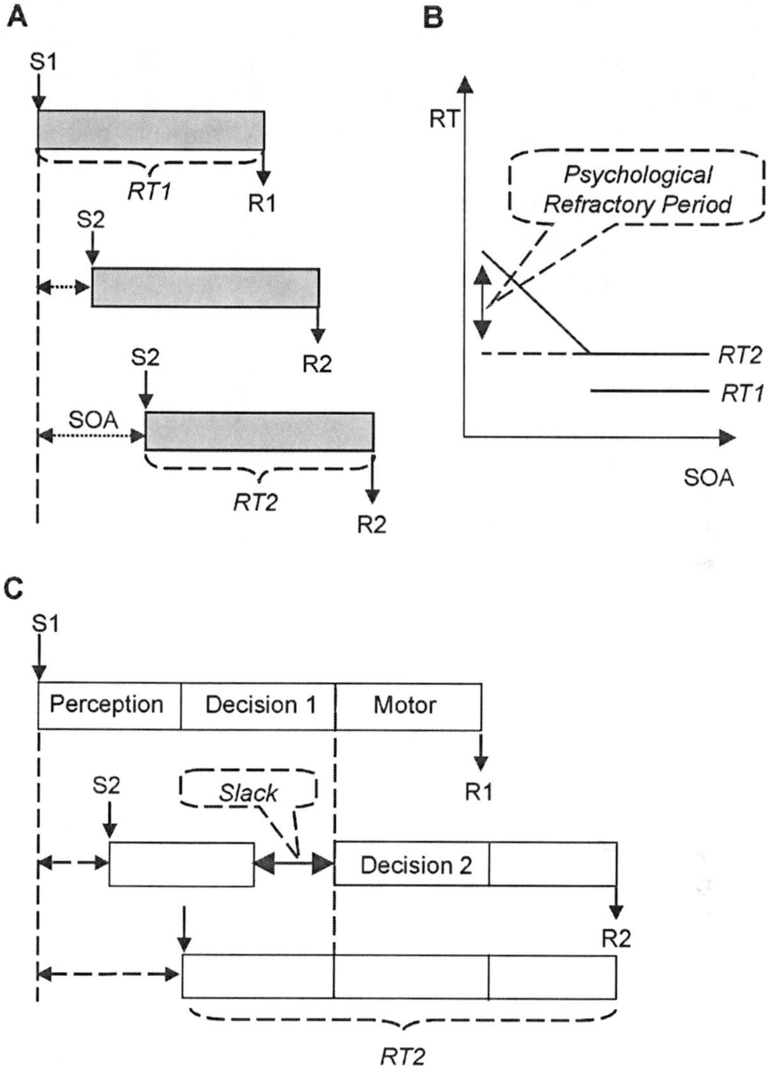

Figure 1. Panel A shows the basic Design for Overlapping Tasks. Stimuli S1 and S2 require two independent responses, R1 and R2. The stimulus onset asynchrony (SOA) between S1 and S2 is varied across several levels and the reaction times for both responses (RT1 and RT2) are recorded. Panel B represents a typical pattern of findings from this paradigm. While RT1 is often unaffected by SOA, RT2 is longest at short SOAs and decreases as SOA increases. The delay of RT2 at short SOAs is termed psychological refractory period (PRP). Panel C represents a theoretical model for PRP effects. There is a central bottleneck during the processing of S2, consisting, e.g. of a decision to be made. Processing of S2 can proceed in parallel with S1 processing until the bottleneck stage during which processing comes to a halt, is reached. The ensuing slack period increases RT2 as an inverse function of SOA.

suggested that the delay in reaction time (RT) to a stimulus that immediately follows another stimulus occurs because there is only a single processing channel, forming a bottleneck. While this channel is occupied with Task 1, the processing of other tasks is halted. Clearly, this halt is more pronounced at short SOAs were the bottleneck is occupied with processing S1 for a longer time after S2 presentation. When SOA is long enough, there is no halt and RT2 can be as short as in single tasks. However, at a certain point RT2 increases by the same amount of time as SOA becomes shorter, causing the typical negative slope of RT2 depicted in panel B of Figure 1.

More recently, it has been suggested that not all processing stages produce such kinds of bottlenecks while being occupied with S1 (Pashler & Johnston, 1989). Especially sensory, simple perceptual, and late motor processes may be exempt from this limitation. However, it is not quite clear which kinds of stages or subprocesses induce such bottlenecks. The most widely accepted bottleneck inducing processes are decision or response selection processes. When these processes are manipulated in their time demands, for example, by making the stimulus-response assignment for S2/R2 more complex, RT2 increases independently of SOA (additive effects – McCann & Johnston, 1992). In contrast, when sensory processes are manipulated, for example, by varying S2 intensity, effects in RT2 are only observed at long SOAs; at short SOAs the variations in processing time are absorbed into the slack period during which S2-processing is halted (underadditive effects).

More generally speaking, the contrast between experimental effects of S2-related manipulations that are either additive or under-additive with SOA has become a widely used gauge for testing whether the manipulated stage is subject to the central bottleneck or not. The locus-of-slack-logic (Schweickert, 1978) suggests that if the effect of the manipulation required for S2 is underadditive with the factor SOA – being smaller at short as compared to long SOAs – the manipulated stage can be absorbed into the slack and therefore can run in parallel with the central processes taking place for S1. If the effect of the manipulation is additive with the factor SOA, the stage is postponed by the bottleneck because it cannot be carried out in parallel with central processes, indicating that the postponed process itself is a central one (cf. Lien et al., 2006). Apart from response selection also other bottleneck-inducing – and therefore central – stages have been suggested, such as difficult perceptual identification, memory retrieval, action planning, and response initiation (De Jong, 1993; Pashler & Johnston, 1989).

A second class of explanations for dual task interference argues with the distribution of processing resources. Early resource concepts (e.g., Kahneman, 1973), proposed a general limited pool of unitary processing resources that had to be shared between the tasks at hand. Later, this model had to be revised because the observed task interference appeared to depend on the type or modality of the involved tasks. Therefore, multiple resources were proposed, claiming separate resource pools for different task modalities, processing stages or types of information (Navon & Gopher, 1979; Wickens, 1984). Since resources are thought to be allocated from limited resource pools, improvement of one task may be associated with performance decrements in a concurrent second task, if (and only if) they draw on the same resource pool. Thus, multiple task performance should primarily depend on the resource overlap of the involved tasks and, in addition, on the dynamic allocation of the available resources (Gopher, 1986). The multiple resource approach has been criticized primarily because of its lack of theoretical constraints. Thus, the model could easily be adapted to account for any given pattern of interference.

Although bottleneck or time-sharing models seem to be more popular at present, it is not easy to demonstrate their superiority over resource sharing accounts. Thus, Navon and Miller (2002) have shown that typical results from psychological refractory period experiments can also be explained by resource sharing. Accordingly, recent attempts to explain dual task conflicts incorporate both time and resource sharing views. For example, Meyer and Kieras (1997) assumed executive processes such as task priority management to account for asymmetric interference effects in the PRP paradigm. Here, the relative processing priority of the involved tasks changes over time, e.g., as a function of task demands. Meyer and Kieras (1997) suggested that dual task interference might be a kind of task artifact due to participant's strategies or lack of practice. In some cases it has indeed been shown that after extensive practice dual task costs can become very small or even nonexistent (e.g., Sangals, Wilwer, & Sommer, in press; Schumacher et al., 2001).

2.2 Language research with PRP-paradigms

Despite the multitude of studies about dual-task processing, demonstrating their fruitfulness (for a review see Pashler, Johnston & Ruthruff, 2001), in the linguistic domain this approach has mainly been used with continuous performance tasks. However, there is a growing body of research that applies the PRP paradigm to the investigation of language perception or production processes. Of common interest is the question whether certain subprocesses interfere with other central processes and can thus be considered to be central and non-automatic in nature. Furthermore, the PRP paradigm has been shown to be useful for investigating the modularity of linguistic processes. As discussed by Ferrreira and Pashler (2002) interferences with other non-linguistic processes are not to be expected if linguistic processes are specialized and based on cognitively, anatomically and genetically distinct substrates as suggested for example by Pinker (1994).

Which are the subprocesses that are being investigated within this context? With respect to auditory word perception the following processing stages are distinguished (Dietrich, 2002; Hagoort & Brown, 2000; Van Petten, Coulson, Rubin, Plante, & Parks, 1999): In a first step the sensory word form is accessed (sensory decoding of acoustic-phonetic input) and selected (word identification). In a second step the auditory word form needs to be mapped onto the appropriate concept. In this process the mental lexicon serves as an interface between language form and language content, which are considered as two fundamentally distinct knowledge domains (Jackendoff, 2002; Wiese, 2004). Mapping the input signal onto word form representations in the mental lexicon results in the retrieval of information associated with this word form including syntactic properties (such as gender or word class) as well as meaning. If more complex linguistic items, i.e., complete sentences have to be perceived the syntactic structure has to be analysed and assigned to the single lexical items (parsing). During word production the activation of conceptual features, access to the mental lexicon comprising lemma (syntactic properties) as well as word-form information and finally the selection of corresponding phonemes are distinguished as separate processing stages (Levelt, Roelofs, & Meyer, 1999). There is much debate in how far processing is serial, parallel or incremental.

Several studies with PRP designs have investigated the effects of lexical processing by means of registering performance measures. These will be reviewed next, followed by a singular report on phonological recoding and by the only report about word production. Our own studies have focussed on word meaning and combined behavioural measures with the recording of event-related brain potentials and will therefore be reported after explaining ERPs.

McCann, Remington, and Van Selst (2000) combined a pitch discrimination Task 1 with either lexical decisions or word naming as Task 2. In each case, the frequency of the words was manipulated. Word frequency affected reaction time (shorter RTs to high than low frequency words) but it never interacted with SOA. These findings were taken to indicate that word processing is not as automatic as activation models suggest and that lexical processing may tap central stages of processing. However, the findings of McCann et al. (2000) were challenged by several later studies. Allen et al. (2002) combined a lexical decision task for written words with a visual shape discrimination task. The shapes (triangle vs. rectangle) surrounded the words in order to preclude competition of spatial attention between tasks. Allen et al. (2002) found underadditive interactions between word frequency and SOA, indicating that lexical processes can run in parallel with central bottleneck-processes. Interestingly, in older adults the underadditivity was even more pronounced than in younger adults. Lien et al. (2006) confirmed the superiority of older adults in parallel lexical processing and attributed it to the greater cumulative experience of older adults with these processes. In a nonlexical experiment however, there was no evidence for greater parallel processing for older adults, indicating the specificity of this finding.

Cleland, Gaskell, Quinlan, and Tamminen (2006) combined a simple perceptual choice as Task 1 with lexical decisions for written or spoken words of different frequency as Task 2. In both visual and auditory conditions the frequency effect was underadditive with SOA implying parallel processing. The discrepancy to the findings of McCann et al. (2000) was explained by a lack of statistical power. In fact, the frequency effect of Cleland was much larger than that of McCann et al. and in some of the experiments a tantalizing, albeit insignificant trend toward a reduction of the frequency effect with decreasing SOA was to be seen. Although these studies leave open the question under which condition younger adults show parallel processing, they demonstrate that the dual task approach may be a powerful tool to functionally localize linguistic processes and determine their delimiting conditions.

Other dual task approaches to language processing have looked at phonological recoding (Reynolds & Besner, 2006) and on language production (Ferreira & Pashler, 2002). To investigate the nature of the underlying processes during the generation of phonological codes from print Reynolds and Besner asked their participants to discriminate tones in a primary task and to read aloud in a secondary task. In a series of seven experiments the locus-of slack-logic was applied by manipulating, for instance, grapheme-phoneme complexity or orthographic neighbourhood density that are assumed to affect the duration of different processing stages during reading aloud. As a result of these manipulations these authors were able to distinguish between processes that do or do not require central attention during reading. Whereas the activation of representations in the orthographic lexicon does not require central attention, the assignment of a phonological code to print uses central attention or occurs after central processing. Also feed-forward activation from the orthographic to the phonological lexicon is assumed to depend on central attention.

The study of Ferreira and Pashler (2002) investigated in how far completion of a tone discrimination Task 2 is hindered by a picture naming Task 1. In more detail, they aimed at elucidating, which subprocesses of word production (lemma selection, word-form, and phoneme selection) delay tone discrimination responses and can thus be considered to cause a central processing bottleneck. Experiment 1 manipulated the duration of the lemma as well as of the word-form selection process by manipulating cloze probability and word frequency, respectively. Both manipulations lead to a delay of response times in the tone discrimination as well as in the picture naming task. In a second experiment phoneme selection was manipulated by presenting pictures with phonologically related distractor words. This manipulation, however, did not yield any effects. In sum, these findings were interpreted as indicating that lemma as well as word-form selection belong to the central processes causing processing bottlenecks, whereas phoneme selection does not.

A very fruitful approach in recent language research has been the recording of event-related brain potentials in response to specific linguistic events (for a review, see Kutas, van Petten, & Kluender, 2006). In our own research we have combined ERP recordings with the PRP design. Before reviewing our results, we will therefore describe ERP methodology, some basic ERP findings from language research, and how ERP recordings can be combined with the PRP design.

3. LANGUAGE RESEARCH WITH EVENT-RELATED POTENTIALS

ERPs is just one of many available techniques that allows insight into (neuro)physiological concomitants of cognitive and emotional processes (Rugg & Coles, 1995). Alongside with magnetoencephalic recordings the ERP technique excels in its temporal resolution. In addition, the amplitude of the ERP or, more specifically, of the various components of the ERP, is indicative of the amount of neuronal activity involved in a given process. The voltage distribution across the scalp is one of the parameters that allow distinguishing between ERP components and – within limits – to localize their neural sources.

In the present context, ERPs were mainly used in order to study the temporal dynamics of specific processing stages (ERP component latency) and the intensity of cognitive processes under different types of overlapping tasks (ERP component amplitude). Such markers are especially valuable when combined with behavioral observations. Performance data, such as reaction times or error rates, are only directly informative about the end products of processing, and inferences about the mediating processing stages are by necessity indirect. In contrast, ERPs allow a more direct observation of cognitive processes.

ERPs are extracted from the continuous electroencephalogram (EEG) by averaging the EEG time-point by time-point and in synchrony with a specific type of event (e.g., a certain kind of stimulus or response) over a number of trials. This procedure isolates the characteristic wave-shape in relationship to the ERP-eliciting event by reducing (averaging out) the background EEG. Numerous components, which can in many cases be considered as peaks and troughs within the complex wave-shape of the averaged ERP, can be identified that have been related to specific cognitive processing stages.

With respect to the studies reported below the N400 potential is of central interest here. The N400 is an electrically negative-going ERP component with a maximal deflection at around 400 milliseconds elicited by spoken, written or signed words. The N400 is especially clear when the eliciting word does not fit the semantic context provided by a preceding sentence fragment or even by a single word. In the experimental paradigm of our own studies a semantic context was established by a prime word, which was always a noun. This was followed by a second noun (target) that was either synonymous to the prime, such as *physician – doctor, quarrel – dispute*, or non-synonymous, for example *physician – dispute.* The N400 is best visualized by calculating the voltage difference between the ERP to context-incongruent and -congruent words. Figure 2 gives an illustration of the brain response to spoken words that are either synonymous (strong semantic context) or non-synonymous in meaning (no context) to a preceding spoken noun. The difference wave between these ERPs is a pure measure of the N400 component.

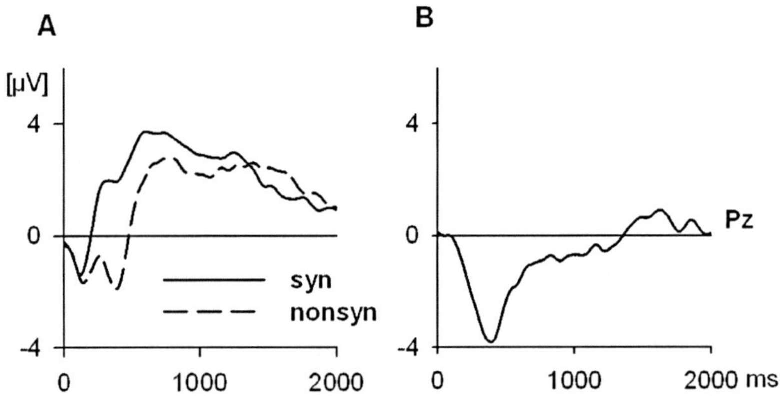

Figure 2. Event-related Brain Responses (ERPs): ERPs to spoken words at a single electrode Pz, which is located parieto-centrally, i.e. just behind the vertex of the head. The abscissae show the first 2 seconds after the onset of the spoken word, whereas the ordinates show the voltage of the brain's response to those words (in microvolt). Each curve represents the grand average across 16 subjects and about forty responses per condition elicited in each subject. Panel A distinguishes between words that are synonymous or unrelated in meaning to a word that was presented about two seconds before (continuous vs. broken line, respectively). Evidently, there is a large difference between these ERPs, which consists of a more negative-going response to non-synonymous words with the greatest difference around 400 ms after word onset. This is highlighted in Panel B, which shows the difference wave between nonsynonymous and synonymous words, calculated time point by time point; this difference wave constitutes the so-called N400 component (for further explanations see text).

There is good evidence that the N400 can be used as an index of language comprehension (Kutas et al., 2006). The time course of the N400 indicates the temporal dynamics of integrating a word into a given context, with onset and peak latency as convenient time markers of the beginning and maximal activity of that process, respectively. The N400 amplitude reflects the neuronal activation involved in this process.

ERP components typically reported for syntactic processing are the so-called LAN (left anterior negativity) as well as the P600. The LAN was initially reported by Kluender and Kutas (1993). In a number of studies the LAN was found between 200 and 500 ms from word onset (Coulson, King, & Kutas, 1998; Osterhout & Holcomb, 1992), thus it occurs in the same latency range as the N400. In other studies it was found even earlier, between 100 and 300 ms (Hahne & Friederici, 1999). Due to this temporal variation, the early negative shift was labeled early left anterior negativity (ELAN). LAN effects refer to an amplitude difference between two conditions and have been reported to violations of word-category constraints, number, case, gender, and tense. Furthermore the LAN and the P600 (see below) have been shown to coexist, which seems to support the idea that the LAN reflects syntactic processing (Friederici, Pfeifer, Hahne, 1993; Neville, Nicol, Barss, Forster, & Garrett, 1991). Other authors suggest that this component reflects an early detection of an error in the syntactic structure (Kluender & Kutas, 1993). It is also argued by these authors that LAN indexes the use of verbal working memory during sentence comprehension (Coulson, King, & Kutas, 1998; Kluender & Kutas, 1993). According to this idea, LAN is related to general resource requirements for language comprehension rather than to syntactic processing.

The P600 is a well-established phenomenon – a positivity that occurs about 600 ms after stimulus onset and that is associated with syntactic analysis during language comprehension (Osterhout & Holcomb, 1992). It can be induced by violations of syntactic constraint, such as subject-verb agreement in number. The positive shift starts at about 500 ms after the onset of violation. It has been found with both written and acoustic input in different languages.

4. USING ERPS IN OVERLAPPING TASK PARADIGMS

In order to obtain more fine grained information about interference patterns in PRP paradigms, obviously one might measure ERPs. However, there is an intrinsic methodological problem. Because each stimulus (and response) is related to a series of ERP components spanning several hundred milliseconds, the ERPs to the Task 1 stimulus will still be going on when the Task 2 stimulus is presented. Therefore Task 1 and Task 2 ERPs will overlap and the degree of overlap will differ as a function of SOA, making ERP comparisons across SOAs problematic. However, it is possible to isolate ERP components to specific events even in this situation if the overlapping part of the ERP can be eliminated by a suitable subtraction procedure. Osman and Moore (1993) were the first to use this subtraction procedure in a PRP design. They demonstrated that ERP components that indicate movement preparation (the lateralized readiness potential, LRP) can be isolated in a PRP paradigm for each response (R1 and R2) by (1) manipulating the two responses independently of each other and (2) performing the LRP calculation which includes a subtraction procedure for each condition. Thus, one can isolate the effect of a given manipulation – in Osman and Moore's case preparing left vs. right response hand and foot, respectively – by making the subtraction between the conditions of interest at each SOA.

This logic has been applied in other LRP studies (e.g., Sommer, Leuthold, & Schubert, 2001; Sangals, Ross & Sommer, 2004; Sangals et al. in press) and has also been extended to other ERP components. Thus Luck (1998) isolated the P300 component in a PRP paradigm by using rare and frequent stimuli – rareness increases P300 amplitude – and by studying the effects of SOA and stimulus discriminability (brightness). SOA had a much stronger effect on reaction time than on P300 latency. Stimulus discriminability interacted underadditively with SOA in RTs and additively in P3 latency. These findings were taken as converging evidence that the locus of interference in PRP paradigms follows stimulus identification and categorization. Two further observations of Luck (1998) are of interest here. Although in his Experiment 1, SOA had very little effect on P300 latency, it strongly reduced P300 amplitude. This finding was interpreted as indicating a reduction of available resources for stimulus identification and categorization. A further ERP component, the P2, which is also sensitive to stimulus probability and precedes P300, was not affected by SOA – neither in amplitude nor in latency. Together these findings from the non-linguistic domain indicate that ERPs can be fruitfully applied to investigate interference effects at various levels of processing and to distinguish effects of resource competition and temporal postponement. In the following we will review our studies that have applied the combination of PRP designs and ERP recording to questions of language processing.

5. EFFECTS OF ADDITIONAL TASKS ON SEMANTIC PROCESSING

The initial objective of our studies was to investigate effects of an additional task on semantic processing during word perception. They were motivated within an applied context, namely how the ability of an operator team, such as airplane crews or surgery teams to verbally communicate, would be affected by high task load, such as demands on manoeuvring during landing. These applied aspects of our research have been reported elsewhere (Hohlfeld et al., 2004c). Here we will focus on the basic research aspects of our investigations.

Our studies focussed on the N400 component, which is elicited when a word does not have an appropriate semantic context (see above). The N400 was elicited by spoken German noun pairs that were either semantically unrelated in meaning or synonymous. That is, in the former case, an N400 was expected (Rösler, Streb, & Haan, 2001) whereas in the latter case it should be small or absent. This was indeed the case as confirmed in a single task experiment that involved the same stimulus procedure as the dual experiments except that responses were only required to the word stimuli (Hohlfeld, Sangals & Sommer, 2004b, Exp. 1; cf. Fig. 2).

In a first dual task study (Hohlfeld et al., 2004b, Exp. 2) the additional task (Task 1) required foot responses to visual stimuli (the letters L or R), which had to be processed with priority. The language task (Task 2) demanded hand responses to the nouns. The second word of the noun pair (target) required decisions about its synonymy with the first word (prime). Target words were presented at one of three possible intervals after the prime (see Fig. 3). The letter was presented as the stimulus for the additional task at a fixed interval after the prime and before the target word was presented. Task load was manipulated in two ways. First, the degree of overlap between the additional task and the language task was manipulated by varying the time between the onset of the letter and the target word in three steps (SOA 100, 400, and 700 ms). Second, the compatibility of stimulus to response mapping in the additional task was manipulated. The visual stimulus had to be responded to with right and left foot reactions when the mappings were compatible. In the incompatible condition, R had to be responded to with the left foot and L with the right foot.

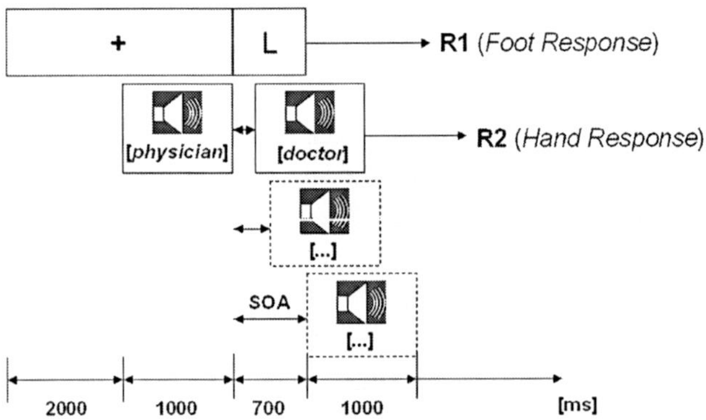

Figure 3. Chronometric description of an experimental trial. For explanation see text.

In order to eliminate the overlap effects of the S1- and R1-elicited ERPs, the N400 was calculated as difference wave between ERPs to incongruent and congruent target words at each SOA and compatibility condition. The single task control of Experiment 1 had shown that the N400 was not noticeably affected by SOA as such when the letter stimulus was irrelevant. Now, when the letter stimulus had to be responded to, the N400 was similiar as in the single task experiment, provided that temporal overlap between the tasks was low (long SOA). However, when overlap was high (short SOA) N400 was strongly delayed by up to 270 ms. When subjects had to give incompatible foot responses in the additional task, for example, respond with the left foot to the letter R, N400 was delayed even more and this was more pronounced at short than at long SOA (see Fig. 4 A). Interestingly, when the mean amplitude for all three SOAs within a set time range was compared, no effects on the total amplitude of the N400 component over the whole recording epoch were observed, indicating that the total amount of neural activity related to semantic integration had not been altered by the additional task.

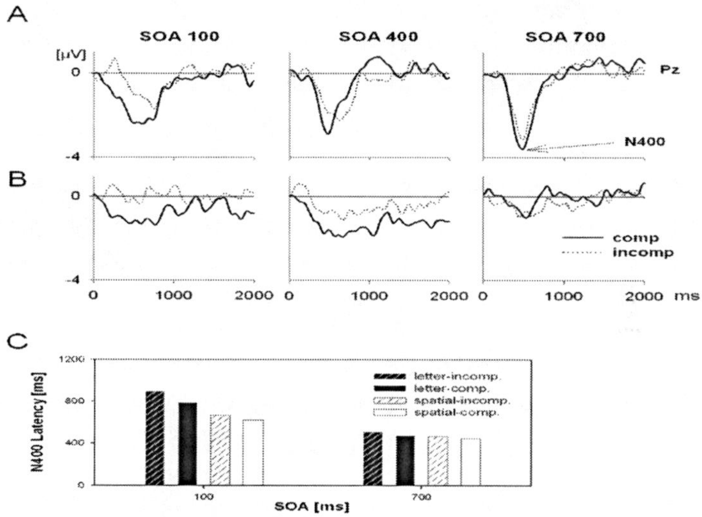

Figure 4. Difference Waves between Event-related Potentials Elicited by Non-synonymous and Synonymous Target Words (N400 component). This figure shows the difference waves in two dual task experiments as a function of stimulus onset asynchrony (SOA) with a letter (L or R) that had to be responded to with compatible or incompatible (comp vs. incomp) left and right pedal presses. Panels A and B show the N400 component when words had to be judged for meaning (synonymity) and for acoustic properties (voice pitch), respectively. When nouns were judged for meaning, task load delayed the N400 component (see panel A, SOA 100 incompatible). N400 was abolished when nouns had to be processed for acoustic properties under task load (see panel B, SOA 100 incompatible). The abscissae show the first 2 seconds after the onset of the spoken target word. The ordinates show the voltage of the brain's response to those words (in microvolt). Panel C. Latency of N400 Maximum as a Function of SOA: depending on whether the additional task stimulus was a letter (language-related) or a spatial location of a small square (spatial), as well as of the compatibility of response assignment to this stimulus (comp. vs. incomp.). Due to task overlap the peak latency of the N400 is more strongly delayed when letters had to be processed in an additional task than when squares had to be processed.

These results suggest that limitations in the availability of central processing stages postpone semantic integration, but do not necessarily compromise it. This is supported by reaction times and error rates. Although there was an increase in reaction times with decreasing SOA, there was no increase in error rates. This implies that in the incompatible dual task condition, participants eventually perceived the nouns and gave correct responses. The experimental effects on N400 activity indicate that concurrent task load genuinely affects the integration of a verbal message into the semantic context and not merely its conversion into a motoric response.

To obtain a better understanding of the causes of interference between the overlapping tasks, a further experiment investigated the effect of different types of stimuli in the additional task (Hohlfeld et al., 2004b, Exp. 3). The previous experiment used letters as stimuli in the additional task, which also require a degree of language processing. Therefore, the hypothesis was that semantic integration might be less affected when the demands on language processing in the additional task are reduced. To minimize the amount of language processing, spatial positions of simple squares were chosen as one type of stimuli. In addition, the language-related type of stimuli (the letters L and R), which were used in the previous experiment, were also applied here. Again, task load was manipulated by SOA (100 vs. 700 ms) and compatibility. Letters were presented in the centre of the computer screen, and the squares appeared to the right or left of a central fixation point. When trials were compatible, foot responses had to be given on the same side where the square appeared. Incompatible trials demanded foot responses opposite to the presentation side. The same language task was used as before (synonymity decisions).

The type of stimulus in the additional task had large effects on the time course of language perception. The latency of the N400 component was postponed more strongly in the case of language-related stimuli (letters) compared to spatial stimuli, particularly when tasks strongly overlapped (Fig. 4 C). For both types of stimuli, the manipulation of compatibility affected N400 latency, i.e., semantic integration. These effects are supported by reaction time data. Judgement of nouns' synonymity required more time when letters than when spatial stimuli had to be processed in the additional task. This also applies to the effect of stimulus-response compatibility: incompatible stimulus-response assignments led to a larger increase in reaction times in the case of letters than in the case of spatial stimuli. These findings imply that task interference increases when both tasks involve processing language-related items.

The reported findings about task load effects on N400 can be explained if we consider the processes underlying the N400 component as belonging to those processes that require the central bottleneck. Thus, if the N400-eliciting processes are central ones, they should be delayed by shortening SOA under all conditions. In addition, N400 should be further delayed by all processes that increase the duration of the bottleneck (Fig. 5). Thus, in more time consuming conditions for the additional task (Task 1), the central bottleneck is occupied for a longer period than in less time-consuming conditions, causing a corresponding delay also for the central processes in the language task.

The findings of Hohlfeld et al. (2004b) demonstrate that language processing at the semantic level can be postponed by additional tasks. But obviously the study leaves open many questions. One of which is the range of possible processes in the additional task that can cause such postponement. A potential source of interference that is also of considerable practical relevance are spatial attention shifts. In Experiment 3, reported above, the spatial stimuli had required small

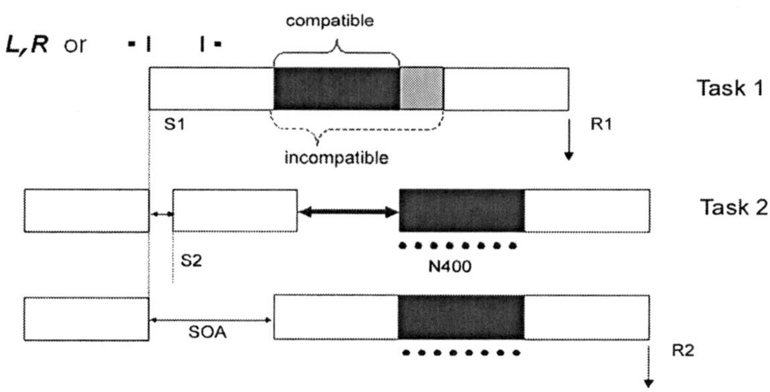

Figure 5. A possible account of the observed interference effects between two tasks.The central bottleneck is depicted in black, the prolongation of this stage in case of incompatible stimulus-response assignments is indicated by grey shading. This stage is preceded by the perceptual and succeeded by the motor stage (in white). If one believes the N400 eliciting processes in Task 2 to be central ones (indicated by the black dotted line), they are necessarily halted as long as central processes in Task 1 are unfinished.

attention shifts to the left or right. Although spatial attention shifts are unlikely sources for the interference found from the letter stimuli, it is conceivable that such attention shifts might have contributed to the interference observed for the non-linguistic spatial stimuli. As myriads of spatial attention shifts occur in everyday life as saccades are performed while observing our visual environment, it seemed to be of interest to study this question in some detail (Dimigen, Schild, Hohlfeld, Berg & Sommer, submitted). To this end, the paradigm used by Hohlfeld et al. (2004b) was modified. Now the words had to be responded to with the left or right foot and the additional task required index finger responses. More importantly, the additional task consisted of two small signs that could only be discriminated when visually fixated. These signs were presented at the fixation point or ten degrees to the left or right of fixation such that the participants had to make a saccade and shift their visuo-spatial attention in order to perform the task of discriminating the signs.

A first experiment replicated the additional task effects on reaction time and N400 latency for central presentation of the additional task stimuli. Importantly, it seemed that these interference effects were enhanced when these stimuli were presented at the eccentric locations. However, in order to conclude from these findings to a genuine interference effect on language processing one has to take into account that in the eccentric condition processing of the additional task stimulus cannot start before the end of the saccade, which requires about 200 ms on average. In a second experiment this delay of processing initiation was compensated by equating the effective SOAs in the central and eccentric conditions. Following these adjustments there were no significant differences anymore between the central and eccentric conditions, neither in reaction times nor in the N400 to the word stimuli. Therefore it appears that reflexive saccades of the type required here and visuo-spatial attention shifts do not directly interfere with auditory language perception. The study of Dimigen et al. also contained a condition with an effective negative SOA, that is, the word stimulus was presented prior to the visual signal. In this case a decoupling of N400 latency and reaction time occurred. Whereas N400 occured around the usual 400-ms peak latency, reaction time was strongly delayed, probably because participants hat to withhold their responses in this condition. This observation demonstrates that the shift of N400 latency is not a consequence or even artefact of RT delays.

Up to this point the evidence can be summarized as demonstrating that additional task load, that is, high temporal overlap between language perception and an important other task, can have strong effects on language processing at the semantic level. These effects consist in a delay in reaction time, which would be expected on the basis on many existing studies with the PRP paradigm. Analyses of the N400 component of the ERP demonstrate that the postponement takes place for integrating the message into the context of the preceding word. Because neither error rates nor N400 amplitude were substantially influenced by task overlap, these conform to an interpretation in the framework of single channel processing models. Interestingly, a further experiment demonstrated that there can also be result patterns that are difficult to integrate into a single channel model but rather seem to indicate some kind of resource sharing or depletion elicited by additional tasks.

In order to assess whether the findings of semantic integration postponement depend on explicit processing of semantic meaning, Hohlfeld and Sommer (2005) performed an experiment where participants did not have to process the language stimuli (nouns pairs) for meaning but for their acoustic properties. As before, the additional task required the discrimination of the letters L and R with compatible and incompatible stimulus-response assignments. The task for the language stimuli consisted in discriminating the pitch of the target noun relative to that of the prime noun. To this end the basic frequency of each of the target nouns was lowered or raised by a fifth relative to the natural frequency, with which the speaker had articulated the word. Figure 4 B depicts the N400 component, super-imposed for the compatible and incompatible conditions. The difference waves for these conditions are similar at the long SOA (no task overlap) but diverge at the intermediate and short SOAs (medium and high overlap). The difference wave, indicating semantic integration, is essentially zero in the incompatible condition at SOA 100. In contrast, the brain activation that signals semantic integration is merely delayed rather than diminished when meaning is explicitly processed (see Fig. 4 A). In fact, in the study of Hohlfeld and Sommer (2005) N400 was abolished when overlap and difficulty was combined. This finding implies that when a message is not explicitly processed for meaning but rather at a more shallow level, its meaning may be accessible to the system only when task load is relatively low (low overlap as in the case of SOA 700 and compatible stimulus-response mappings). This is confirmed by results from a single task experiment (Hohlfeld & Sommer, 2005, Exp. 1) that had applied identical stimulation but only required responses to acoustic properties of the nouns. In this single task condition not only a clear – albeit small – N400 component had been observed; there had also been a synonymity effect in response times in the pitch discrimination task, demonstrating the availability of semantic meaning, although this was not required, when additional task load is absent.

The finding of an amplitude reduction rather than a latency shift in the N400 component in the dual task condition is hard to integrate into a model based on the timing or postponement of processing stages as suggested above. Thus, in this case it is more appropriate to interpret interference effects in terms of a resource model. Attention can be viewed as a resource that has to be allocated to the two tasks, letter processing and pitch processing. Attention to semantic aspects of the words is not required although the words as such have to be attended in order to discriminate their pitch. Because N400 is present in the single task and at least to some extend in the easier conditions of the dual task (medium SOA) and is absent in the most difficult condition (short SOA, incompatible letter-to-foot mapping) it seems that attentional resources can be withdrawn from the semantic properties of words that are attended to for the sake of extracting task-relevant non-semantic properties. A similar interpretation based on the deletion of processing resources was used to explain the amplitude reduction of the P300 component by Luck (1998). In case of the processes underlying N400 it seems that, depending on the circumstances, they may be subject to both resource depletion and postponement.

As a final point in this review of additional task effects on semantic processes we will describe a study that was motivated even more directly by an applied context but does shed light an basic issues as well. A potentially critical aspect in many work places is that communication does not take place in the native language. Although team members are proficient in the second language (L2) when formal tests are applied, evidence suggests that under stress, there is a tendency to return to the native language and that the likelihood for mistakes in processing the second language may increase (Cushing, 1994). Therefore, it seemed to be conceivable that language perception in second language speakers is more susceptible to task load than in native speakers. This question was addressed by Hohlfeld, Mierke, and Sommer (2004a). The design of the experiment was identical to Experiment 2 of Hohlfeld et al. (2004b) reported above, using German language stimuli. However, the subjects' native language was Russian. German, as their L2 has been acquired after puberty but to a high degree of competence. In an offline multiple choice test, which assessed second language speakers' understanding of the presented German nouns, they performed relatively well. They had 91 per cent correct responses while native speakers achieved 98 per cent.

In this experiment, the N400 component in second language speakers was delayed in peak latency by more than 200 milliseconds when compared to first language speakers. In addition, the duration of semantic processing in second language speakers was longer than in first language speakers, indicated by a wider spread of the N400 component over time. Importantly, the delay of language perception in second language speakers occurred on top of the additional task load effects but were additive with them. That is, the disadvantage of second language speakers in processing word meaning is not aggravated by additional task load. With respect to underlying mechanisms these results indicate that in second language processing the temporal duration of semantic access may be increased. Some evidence for a higher susceptibility for additional task load in second language speakers was provided by the error rates, that were higher than in native speakers for all conditions but especially at short SOAs.

6. EXTENSIONS OF THE PARADIGM AND OUTLOOK

Our studies reviewed in the previous section had all used a single-word context in order to study semantic processing. Obviously it is of interest to consider more natural contexts at least at the sentence level in order to assess, whether our previous findings can be extended to this level. This has recently been done by Hohlfeld, Martín-Loeches, and Sommer (in prep.) in a study with Spanish sentences. Spanish has the advantage that in one and the same word semantic and syntactic congruence can be manipulated with respect to the same reference word (Martín-Loeches, Nigbur, Casado, Hohlfeld, & Sommer, 2006). This property of the Spanish language was exploited in order to investigate under otherwise identical conditions the effects of additional task load on both semantic and lexical processes. Thus, Spanish sentences of the type determiner-noun-adjective-verb were presented. The adjective could be consistent and inconsistent with noun meaning or congruent and incongruent with respect to the noun's grammatical gender. Additional task stimuli (high or low pitched tones) were presented 100, 400, or 700 ms before the adjective.

The N400, elicited by the adjectives inconsistent in meaning was largest at long SOA and decreased in amplitude with SOA. Effects of SOA on N400 latency were very slight. These results are accounted for best by resource sharing, possibly in working memory. In case of adjectives incongruent in gender with the preceding noun a LAN as well as a P600 were elicited; the degree of temporal overlap affected only the P600 which was delayed at the short SOA. From these findings it may be concluded that early syntactic processes as reflected in the LAN do not belong to central processes, whereas those reflected in the P600 underlie a processing bottleneck. According to these results the findings derived from the earlier studies and explicit meaning processing of spoken German word pairs cannot be directly transferred to written Spanish sentences. Clearly, it remains to be determined why exactly, these differences occur. Elucidation of these reasons may shed light on important properties of language processing.

Where can we go from here? The combined application of dual tasks with ERP recordings could be carried on to study language processing in greater depths. Thus, it is of interest under which conditions semantic processing undergoes resource depletion or post-ponement. Also of interest would be to compare different languages and to study second language processing in more depths, for example as a function of graded expertise level (e.g., McLaughlin, Osterhout, & Kim, 2004). The approach could be extended to other language processes, such as syntactic and phonological processes. Such work is underway; as described above, Hohlfeld et al. (in preparation) studied syntactic processes under additional task load and Rabovsky, Alvarez, Hohlfeld, and Sommer (in preparation) have recently extended the overlapping task approach to phonological and lexical processes by manipulating syllable frequency in a lexical decision task.

There is also a more principled perspective for this line of research. The N400 component may not merely reflect the integration process of a word into a semantic context. Kutas and Federmeier (2000) have proposed that the N400 reflects the access to semantic memory in general. On that assumption, the combined approach of dual tasks with N400 recording may be applied to study processes in semantic memory and to resolve pertinent questions. For example, as pointed out by Fischer (2006) there is contradictory evidence whether retrieval from long-term memory can proceed in parallel with central bottleneck processes or not. Thus, Carrier und Pashler (1995) found additivity of SOA and the difficulty of retrieving pair associations. According to locus-of-slack logic this indicates that retrieval of verbally coded knowledge from long term memory is part of central bottleneck processes. In contrast, Logan und Schulkind (2000) found evidence for parallel retrieval by using the so-called cross-talk logic. Cross-talk between the two tasks occurred when similar but not when different stimulus response translations (task sets) were required. The employment of the N400 as an ERP component that indicates retrieval from semantic memory might be most valuable in order to help resolve such controversial issues.

In conclusion, the well-controlled and well-studied PRP design appears to be a valuable tool in order to investigate the microstructure of language processing. We believe that the power of this research tool can be enhanced by combining it with the recording of ERPs. A review of our own work with this approach shows that the access to semantic properties of words can be described in many cases as limited by a central bottleneck. However, in other conditions, a resource sharing account appears to be more appropriate. The delineation of the conditions under which these accounts hold may shed important light on elementary boundary conditions of this process. Also very promising appears to be the extension of this approach to other specific aspects of language processing and to semantic memory in general.

REFERENCES

Allen, P. A., Lien, M. C., Murphy, M. D., Sanders, R. E., Judge, K. S., & McCann, R. S. (2002). Age differences in overlapping-task performance: Evidence for efficient parallel processing in older adults. *Psychology and Aging, 17*, 505-519.

Caplan, D., & Waters, G. S. (1999). Verbal working memory and sentence comprehension. *Behavioral and Brain Sciences, 22*, 77-126.

Carrier, L. M., & Pashler, H. (1995). Attentional limits in memory retrieval. *Journal of Experimental Psychology-Learning Memory and Cognition, 21*, 1339-1348.

Cleland, A. A., Gaskell, M. G., Quinlan, P. T., & Tamminen, J. (2006). Frequency effects in spoken and visual word recognition: Evidence from dual-task methodologies. *Journal of Experimental Psychology-Human Perception and Performance, 32*, 104-119.

Coulson, S., King, J., & Kutas, M. (1998). Expect the unexpected: Event-related brain response to morphosyntactic violations. *Language and Cognitive Processes, 13*, 21-58.

Cushing, S. (1994), *Fatal Words: Communication clashes and aircraft crashes*, Chicago: University of Chicago Press.

De Jong, R. (1993). Multiple bottlenecks in overlapping task performance. *Journal of Experimental Psychology-Human Perception and Performance, 19*, 965-980.

Dietrich, R. (2002). *Psycholinguistik*. 1. Stuttgart, Germany: Metzler.

Dimigen, O., Schild, U., Hohlfeld, A., Berg, P. & Sommer, W. (submitted). Auditory language comprehension during saccadic eye movements: An investigation with event-related brain potentials.

Ferreira, V. S., & Pashler, H. (2002). Central bottleneck influences on the processing stages of word production. *Journal of Experimental Psychology-Learning Memory and Cognition, 28*, 1187-1199.

Fischer, R. (2005). *Parallel memory retrieval in dual task situations*? Unpublished Dissertation. Berlin: Humboldt-University.

Friederici, A. D., Pfeifer, E., & Hahne, A. (1993). Event-related brain potentials during natural speech processing: Effects of semantic morphological and syntactic violations. *Cognitive Brain Research, 1*, 183-192.

Gopher, D. (1986), Energetics and Resources. In G. R. J., Hockey, A. W. K., Gaillard, & M. G. H., Coles, (Eds.), *Adaptation to stress and task demands. NATO Advanced Research Workshop*, New York: Plenum Press.

Hagoort, P., & Brown, C. M. (2000). ERP effects of listening to speech: semantic ERP effects. *Neuropsychologia, 38*, 1518-1530.

Hahne, A., & Friederici, A. D. (1999). Electrophysiological evidence for two steps in syntactic analysis: Early automatic and late controlled processes. *Journal of Cognitive Neuroscience, 11*, 193-204.

Heuer, H. (1991). Motor Constraints in Dual-Task Performance. In D. L. Damos, (Ed), *Multiple-Task Performance* (pp. 173-204). London: Taylor & Francis.

Hirst, W., Spelke, E. S., Caharack, G., & Neisser, U. (1980). Dividing attention without alternation or automaticity. *Journal of Experimental Psychology-General, 109*, 98-117.

Hohlfeld, A., Fukuda, R., Neuper, S., Sangals, J., Sommer, W., & Straeter, O. (2004c). Task load effects on language processing: experimental approaches. In R. Dietrich & T. M. Childress (Eds.), *Group interaction in high risk environments* (pp. 209-240). Aldershot, England: Ashgate.

Hohlfeld, A., Martín-Loeches, M., & Sommer, W. (in preparation). Semantic and syntactic processing in Spanish sentences and additional task load.

Hohlfeld, A., Mierke, K. & Sommer, W. (2004a). Is word perception in a second-language more vulnerable than in one's native language? Evidence from brain potentials in a dual task setting. *Brain & Language, 89*, 569-579.

Hohlfeld, A., Sangals, J., & Sommer, W. (2004b). Effects of additional tasks on language perception: An ERP investigation. *Journal of Experimental Psychology: Learning, Memory, & Cognition, 30*, 1012-1025.

Hohlfeld, A., & Sommer, W. (2005). Semantic Processing of Unattended Meaning is Modulated by Additional Task Load: Evidence from Electrophysiology. *Cognitive Brain Research, 24*, 500-512.

Jackendoff, R. (2002). *Foundations of language. Brain, meaning, grammar, evolution.* Oxford, England: Oxford University Press.

Jäncke, L. (1994). Horizontal pursuit right-arm movements and dual-tasks interferences: A replication and extension, *Cortex, 30*, 695-700.

Kahneman, D. (1973), *Attention and effort*. Englewood Cliffs, NJ: Prentice Hall.

Kluender, R., & Kutas, M. (1993). Bridging the gap: evidence from ERPs on the processing of unbounded dependencies. *Journal of Cognitive Neuroscience, 5*, 196-214.

Kutas, M., & Federmeier, K. D. (2000). Electrophysiology reveals semantic memory use in language comprehension. *Trends in Cognitive Sciences, 4*, 463-470.

Kutas, M., Van Petten, C., & Kluender, R. (2006). Psycholinguistics electrified II. In M. A. Gernsbacher & M. Traxler (Eds.), *Handbook of Psycholinguistics* (2nd ed.). New York: Elsevier Press.

Levelt, W. J. M., Roelofs, A., & Meyer, A. S. (1999). A theory of lexical access in speech production. *Behavioral and Brain Sciences, 22,* 1-75.

Lien, M. C., Allen, P. A., Ruthruff, E., Grabbe, J., McCann, R. S., & Remington, R. W. (2006). Visual word recognition without central attention: Evidence for greater automaticity with advancing age. *Psychology and Aging, 21*, 431-447.

Logan, G. D., & Schulkind, M. D. (2000). Parallel memory retrieval in dual-task situations: I. Semantic memory. *Journal of Experimental Psychology-Human Perception and Performance, 26*, 1072-1090.

Luck, S. J. (1998). Sources of dual-task interference - Evidence from human electrophysiology. *Psychological Science, 9,* 223-227.

Martín-Loeches, M., Nigbur, R., Casado, P., Hohlfeld, A., & Sommer, W. (2006). Semantics prevalence over syntax during sentence processing: A brain potential study of noun-adjective agreement in Spanish. *Brain Research, 1093*, 178-189.

McCann, R. S., & Johnston, J. C. (1992). Locus of the single-channel bottleneck in dual-task interference. *Journal of Experimental Psychology-Human Perception and Performance, 18,* 471-484.

McCann, R. S., Remington, R. W., & Van Selst, M. (2000). A dual-task investigation of automaticity in visual word processing. *Journal of Experimental Psychology-Human Perception and Performance, 26*, 1352-1370.

McLaughlin, J., Osterhout, L., & Kim, A. (2004). Neural correlates of second-language word learning: minimal instruction produces rapid change. *Nature Neuroscience, 7,* 703-704.

McLeod, P. (1977). A dual task response modality effect: Support for multiprocessor models of attention. *Quarterly Journal of Experimental Psychology*, 29, 651-667.

Meyer, D. E., & Kieras, D. E. (1997). A computational theory of executive cognitive processes and multiple-task performance: Part 2. Accounts of psychological refractory-period phenomena. *Psychological Review, 104*, 749-91.

Navon, D., & Gopher, D. (1979), On the economy of the human-processing system. *Psychological Reveiw, 86*, 214-255.

Navon, D. A. and Miller, J. (2002). Queuing or sharing? A critical evaluation of the single-bottleneck notion. *Cognitive Psychology, 44*, 193-251.

Neville, H. J., Nicol, J., Barss, A., Forster, K. I., & Garrett, M. F. (1991). Syntactically based processing classes: evidence from event-related brain potentials. *Journal of Cognitive Neuroscience, 3,* 151-165.

Osman, A. & Moore, C. M. (1993). The locus of dual-task interference: Psychological refractory effects on movement-related brain potentials. *Journal of Experimental Psychology: Human Perception and Performance, 19*, 1292-1312.

Osterhout, L. & Holcomb, P. J. (1992). Event-related brain potentials elicited by syntactic anomaly. *Journal of Memory and Language, 31*, 785-806.

Pashler, H. (1994). Dual-task interference in simple tasks: Data and theory. *Psychological Bulletin, 116*, 220-44.

Pashler, H., & Johnston, J. C. (1989). Chronometric evidence for central postponement in temporally overlapping tasks. *Quarterly Journal of Experimental Psychology, 41A*, 19-45.

Pashler, H., & Johnston, J. C. (1998). Attentional limitations in dual task performance. In H. Pashler (Ed.), Attention (pp. 155-189). Hove: Psychology Press.

Pashler, H., Johnston, J. C., & Ruthruff, E. (2001). Attention and performance. *Annual Review of Psychology, 52,* 629-651.

Pinker, S. (1994). *The language instinct.* New York: Morrow.

Rabovsky, M., Alvarez, C., Hohlfeld, A., & Sommer, W., (in preparation). Effects of an additional task on visual word recognition: An ERP study.

Reynolds, M., & Besner, D. (2006). Reading aloud is not automatic: Processing capacity is required to generate a phonological code from print. *Journal of Experimental Psychology-Human Perception and Performance, 32,* 1303-1323.

Rösler, F., Streb, J., & Haan, H. (2001). Event-related brain potentials evoked by verbs and nouns in a primed lexical decision task. *Psychophysiology*, 38, 694-703.

Rugg, M. D., & Coles, M. G. H. (1995). Electrophysiology of mind. Event-related potentials and cognition. -220. Oxford, England: Oxford University Press.

Sangals, J., Ross, L., & Sommer, W. (2004). Time pressure effects on information processing in overlapping tasks: Evidence from the lateralized readiness potential. *Acta Psychologica, 117,* 275-294.

Sangals, J., Wilwer, M., & Sommer, W. (in press). Localising practice effects in dual-task performance. *Quarterly Journal of Experimental Psychology.*

Schumacher, E. H., Seymour, T. L., Glass, J. M., Fencsik, D. E., Lauber, E. J. & Kieras, D. E. (2001). Virtually perfect time sharing in dual-task performance: Uncorking the central cognitive bottleneck. *Psychological Science, 12*, 101-8.

Schweickert, R. (1978). A critical path generalization of the additive factor method: Analysis of a Stroop task. *Journal of Mathematical Psychology, 18,* 105-139.

Sommer, W., Leuthold, H. & Schubert, T. (2001). Multiple bottlenecks in information processing? An electrophysiological examination. *Psychonomic Bulletin & Review, 8,* 81-8.

Spelke, E. S., Hirst, W., & Neisser, U. (1976). Skills of divided attention. *Cognition, 4*, 215-230.

Van Petten, C., Coulson, S., Rubin, S., Plante, E., & Parks, M. (1999). Time course of word identification and semantic integration in spoken language. *Journal of Experimental Psychology: Learning, Memory, and Cognition, 25*, 394-417.

Welford, A. T. (1952). The "Psychological refractory period" and the timing of high speed performance - A review and a theory. *British Journal of Psychology, 43,* 2-19.

Wickens, C. D. (1984). Processing resources in attention. In R. Parasuraman, R. Davies & J. Beatty (Eds.), *Varieties of attention* (pp. 63-102*).* New York: Academic Press.

Wiese, H. (2004). Semantics as a gateway to language. In H. Härtl & H. Tappe (Eds.), *Mediating between concepts and language* (Trends in linguistics 152, pp. 197-222). Berlin, New York: de Gruyter.

---

[i] Some anecdotal evidence about astonishing multi-task performance may be of interest here. In a letter to his sister from April 20, 1782 Mozart mentioned having composed a praeludium while at the same time writing the corresponding fugue and the Japanese Prince Shotoku (574-622) was said to have been able to listen to ten people at once and decide all their suits without error. We thank Werner Felber, Dresden, and Hiroaki Masaki, Tokyo, for communicating these clues.

[ii] The PRP paradigm is named because it was assumed that the reaction times delay that is often observed when a stimulus is presented shortly after a preceding stimulus has been likened to the refractory period in the action potential of nerve cells. Although this analogy has turned out to be misleading, the name has stuck.

6

A SAMPLER OF EVENT-RELATED BRAIN POTENTIAL (ERP) ANALYSES OF LANGUAGE PROCESSING

Marta Kutas[1,2,3] and Katherine A. Delong[1]

[1]Department of Cognitive Science, University of California San Diego, La Jolla, California, 92093, USA. [2]Depatment of Neurosciences, University of California San Diego, La Jolla, California, 92093, USA. [3]Center for Research in Language, University of California San Diego, La Jolla, California, 92093, USA.

Abstract: In large part, language comprehension and production occur quickly and unavailable to conscious reflection. Electrophysiological methods – event-related brain potentials (ERPs) and other measures of electrical brain activity – afford a view of the brain in action as it supports these language processes as they unfold in real time. Moreover, ERPs can be utilized even when a comprehender's only task is to understand a word, phrase or sentence or to produce names or more elaborate utterances. Recording electrical brain activity in response to written and spoken words (as well as smaller and larger linguistic units) thus provides a means of tracking the brain's sensitivity to various linguistic inputs, revealing which factors are important to processing and the time course of their influence. As a continuous measure of processing, ERPs allow simultaneous looks at brain activity at the multiple time scales at which language processing transpires, from the first milliseconds of processing a word to the seconds required to comprehend a sentence, or even longer for a discourse. One of the greatest advantages to using ERPs, then, is that this combination of methodological features allows for investigations of aspects of language processing that are otherwise difficult if not impossible to detect via other measures. In this chapter, we will examine such instances, outlining five very different groups of ERP studies which exemplify some of the unique insights made possible by use of the methodology in the study of language-related neural processes. In particular, we will discuss the paradigms and the kinds of information that can be gathered from using ERPs to look at language processing outside the focus of attention, during language learning (before explicit knowing), for individuals in unconscious states, in determining the nature of predictive processing, and for testing how specific contextual cues may activate information in semantic memory. Our examination of these specific experimental examples makes clear the important role that ERPs have to play in studying language processing, both traditionally and as the number of neuroimaging techniques continues to grow.

Key words: Event Related Potentials, N400, MMN, P600, language processing, minimally conscious state, sleep, lexico-semantic processing, attention, spatial selective attention, attentional blink, event location, masking, second language acquisition, speech segmentation, verb aspect, prediction

1. INTRODUCTION

In the 1960's the idea of investigating the psychology of language by recording electrical activity from the human scalp seemed as fantastical as putting a man on the moon. One could perhaps look at differential engagement of the two cerebral hemispheres by measuring the language-specific suppression of alpha activity, but that was a far cry from what psycholinguists wanted to know about language processing. By the 1980's, however, Armstrong's moon walk was part of history, and the idea of using electrophysiology to study linguistic phenomena was becoming a respectable enterprise. Different types of electrical brain responses were being observed at the scalp to words that were incongruent with prior contexts at semantic, syntactic, and phonological levels. Even more interestingly, it had been shown that event-related brain potentials (ERPs) were sensitive to psycholinguistic variables of all sorts in perfectly normal sentences, even when all of the experimental sentences were grammatically well formed and meaningful. Such findings paved the way for the virtual explosion of ERP and magnetoencephalographic (MEG) investigations of language processing over the past quarter century. With a diversity of studies running the gamut from phoneme categorization to discourse processing, with groups ranging from healthy to brain damaged individuals, with measures recorded from populations spanning infancy through old age, virtually no area remained untouched by cognitive ERP researchers.

A major advantage of the ERP technique in the study of cognition is that it affords a continuous but time-stamped look at ongoing neural activity as individuals make sense of the barrage of sensory and internal stimulation they encounter while sensing, perceiving, encoding, recoding, retrieving, and sometimes responding to real or imagined events. ERPs provide a series of snapshots of the synaptic potentials generated primarily by pyramidal cells in the neocortex, which are thought to perform the computations critical for comprehension and cognition. In many cases, ERP effects are highly correlated with overt behaviors and lead to inferences that could just as easily be made from external performance measures such as various speed and accuracy judgments, or the scanning patterns of eye movements across either scenes as people listen to sentences or across printed words as they read text. Such converging measures are important for amassing databases of psycholinguistic phenomena and for constructing comprehensive theories. However, ERP and performance measures are at times dissociable and can occasionally offer different pictures of the same cognitive acts; thus, for thorough understanding of a particular area of interest, the different perspectives afforded by the varying methods must be integrated. Perhaps most importantly though, and in response to those who might advocate the use of only more basic behavioral methods for reasons of time and expense, there are also cases in which ERPs provide a unique view into moment-by-moment cognitive processing, with no parallel in other measures. While the limitations of various performance measures are sometimes clear at the point when the experimental design is conceived, in other instances it is not possible to tell whether more basic methods will provide sufficient power to reveal potential differences between conditions. As experimental design does not come with a crystal ball, it is often only with subsequent testing using more neurally-informed and informative methodologies, such as ERPs, that differences between conditions are revealed where none were originally detected.

In this chapter we will outline five different examples of areas in which ERPs afford insights into language processing that are not readily, if at all, available through other existing methodologies. Specifically, we will review studies in which ERPs are used to: (1) localize the processing source when linguistic content is presented outside of focused attention, (2) monitor lexico-semantic processes during learning, (3) assess cognitive and language competence during alternate states of arousal and awareness (e.g., coma, vegetative state and sleep), (4) capture predictive processes during language comprehension, and (5) test a specific hypothesis about one type of information (event location) that context words (specifically verb aspect) activate in semantic memory. These examples rely on the ERP as an instantaneous detector of current flow across membranes with a temporal resolution on the order of milliseconds. They also take advantage of the fact that ERP measures can be elicited by stimuli regardless of whether they require an immediate overt response. In other words, no additional task is necessary above and beyond the natural behaviors of viewing, reading or listening.

2. LINGUISTIC PROCESSING OUTSIDE THE FOCUS OF ATTENTION

One of the greatest advantages of ERPs is that they allow researchers to investigate aspects of language processing that are inaccessible to conscious reflection, and consequently are difficult, if not impossible, to detect via other measures. They can reveal activity that does not reach overt awareness, cannot be talked about, or might not have immediate behavioral consequences. In this respect, some longstanding and controversial questions about semantic language processing have been examined within the context of selective attention and attentional blink paradigms. Specifically, these paradigms have been used to assess the degree to which language processing is automatic, fast-acting, and largely unconscious versus more slow-acting, strategically controlled, and post-lexical, with the challenge being to tease apart these two classes of processes (assuming of course that these are true distinctions that the human brain honors). So doing would be difficult without a way of observing neural processes as they unfold in real time. Both ERP and MEG recordings afford us just such a view, albeit imperfect. Because ERPs provide continuous measures of neocortical processing between stimuli and responses we can better pinpoint the times at which processing is affected by certain experimental manipulations. The effects of early and later processes (for instance pre-attentive versus post-attentive) are at times not as conflated as they are in final output measures.

In particular, the N400 component has been at the heart of much of this testing. The N400 was first described by Kutas & Hillyard

(1980), who observed that relative to congruous words, semantically anomalous words in a given sentence context (e.g., the word *dog* in '*I take my coffee with cream and dog.*') were characterized by greater negativity between 250-500 ms or so after target word onset, peaking around 400 ms post-stimulus. The component has since been interpreted as the default neural response to any potentially meaningful item, be it a written or spoken word, a picture, or a sign, with an amplitude sensitive to a variety of factors. These factors include, but are not limited to word frequency, repetition, concreteness, number of orthographic neighbors, sentence position, semantic word association, and predictability within a sentence or discourse (see Kutas, Federmeier, Staab, & Kluender, in press, for a review). The N400 is especially large in response to items that do not semantically fit with their preceding context (whether at the word, sentence, or discourse level), but the modulation is also evident in responses to all but the most highly expected of items, even when they fit with the context. It has a peak latency around 400 ms that is relatively stable across experimental paradigms, and a centro-posterior scalp distribution that depends on several factors including whether eliciting stimuli are auditory or visual, pictorial, linguistic or nonlinguistic in nature, etc. In general then, the N400 is thought to reflect the degree of ease or difficulty in retrieving stored knowledge associated with a potentially meaningful item from semantic memory, contingent upon both the characteristics of the stored item itself, as well as the contextual cues available (Kutas & Federmeier, 2000).

Modulations in N400 amplitude and latency in controlled tasks are a good way to track semantic processing (as long as other factors to which N400 is sensitive are held constant) and have been used to probe a wide variety of linguistic phenomena. These range from word priming and message level processing to the role of attention and consciousness in language comprehension, to differences in hemispheric activation of semantic memory, to vocabulary building in language learning, just to name a few. The component has been used in a diverse assortment of experimental paradigms, including comparisons between conditions within experiments (e.g., expected sentence completion exemplars vs. less probable continuations or category violations; contextually sensible endings vs. violations of world knowledge), between different subject populations (e.g., young vs. elderly, healthy vs. schizophrenic patients), and less commonly, longitudinally (e.g., novice second language learners before vs. after learning has occurred). In sum, as a tool for investigating issues relating to the time course of language processing and the structure of semantic memory, the N400 has proven remarkably informative, even though it is not unique to language processing.

Although it is clear that N400 amplitude modulation indexes some aspect of semantic processing, it remains a point of contention precisely which process(es) the component reflect(s). One controversy centers around the degree to which the electrical activity during the N400 time window is elicited by more automatic versus more controlled processing. To this end, spatial selective attention and attentional blink ERP studies have been somewhat informative. Respectively, these studies have examined how semantic processing is influenced by manipulating the allocation of spatial attention to primes or probes and by having participants detect multiple target stimuli during rapid serial visual presentation (RSVP) conditions. We will review findings from examples of both of these types of experiments and describe how ERPs have been used with these paradigms to inform us about the temporal locus of the cognitive effects in question.

2.1 Spatial selective attention

McCarthy and Nobre (1993) investigated the role of spatial selective attention on semantic and repetition priming N400 effects. Their main goal was to adjudicate between early versus late selection theories of attention. Early selection theories posit that spatial attention acts to filter out unattended stimuli at an early (pre-semantic) stage of cognitive processing. By contrast, late selection theories propose that all stimuli, even unattended items, are processed automatically and fully, including access to their meaning, with a subsequent filtering stage determining whether or not the items gain access to consciousness. To discriminate between these two possibilities, participants were asked to maintain central eye fixation while ERPs were recorded to words presented lateralized to the left or right visual field. Within each field, the stimulus list consisted of words that were semantically related, semantically unrelated or repetitions. Participants were instructed to focus their attention alternately on one of the visual fields and to detect words that belonged to a specified semantic category (exemplars). If spatially unattended prime words modulated semantic priming and repetition effects as indexed by N400 amplitude modulation, then this would be taken as support for the hypothesis that the N400 reflects some aspect of automatic semantic processing, such as spreading activation; this outcome would correspond more closely to late selection models of attention. If however, there were no N400 amplitude modulations of semantically related or repeated words in the unattended channel, then this would be taken as support for the hypothesis that the N400 reflects more controlled processing; this outcome would correspond more closely to early selection models of attention.

In line with prior results, only exemplars presented to the attended visual field elicited large amplitude P300s compared to those exemplars presented to the unattended visual field. The absence of a reliable P300 effect between 400-800 ms to unattended stimuli suggests that the exemplars were not categorized and consolidated into working memory, and thus argues for selection some time prior to these processes. However, it does not settle the question of whether the unattended words are processed at some semantic level, as the N400 often precedes the P300. In this experiment, however, there were also no N400 effects to either semantically related or literally repeated target items in the unattended channel, in contrast to reliable semantic and repetition related modulation of N400 amplitudes for targets in the attended channel. From this pattern of results, McCarthy and Nobre (1993) concluded that the N400 did not reflect automatic, unconscious processing and that active suppression of processing in a spatial location can indeed influence the extent to which a word is processed at a semantic/conceptual level.

2.2 Attentional blink

As demonstrated by the McCarthy and Nobre (1993) study, an invaluable strength of the ERP technique is that it offers a means of teasing apart different stages and/or subprocesses of analysis. Under the appropriate experimental conditions, different aspects of the ERP waveform can be analyzed to determine whether and when certain neural/mental operations transpire. For example, (1) early sensory potentials such as the occipital P1 and the N1 indicate whether a stimulus is sensed and perceived, (2) potentials between 200 to 550 ms or so post stimulus (the time region of the N400) over posterior scalp sites indicate whether once perceived, a particular event reaches a semantic/conceptual level of analysis, and (3) late positivities between 400 to 600 ms over centro-parietal scalp sites (the P300 or more precisely the P3b) indicate whether the stimulus item was identified, categorized, and consolidated in working memory. ERP researchers have capitalized on this affordance of being able to look at qualitatively different mental processes to isolate the temporal locus of the attentional blink phenomenon. The attentional blink is a short refractory period after the detection of a target item in a stream of rapidly presented stimuli during which subsequent targets are missed (Raymond, Shapiro, & Arnell, 1992). For instance, when individuals are shown rapidly flashing characters (e.g., B T D A 3 N P **Z** F R K M) at a rate 10 per second or less, and are asked to report on two targets (e.g., a number and a letter in a contrasting color – in this example the number 3 and the letter **Z**), they can accurately report whether the first target (T1) is odd or even, but are less accurate at identifying whether the second target (T2, occurring at lag 3) is a vowel or a consonant. This impairment occurs when T2 falls within 300-600 ms after the first target (the attentional blink), but rather surprisingly not when T2 occurs immediately after T1 (at lag 1). Expectedly, T2 targets appearing much later (e.g., at lag 7) also are easily detected. But for a target falling within the period of the attentional blink, it could be that participants are neither sensing nor perceiving the second target, *or* perhaps that participants are detecting the second target, but are unable to identify and categorize it or to consolidate it into working memory.

To establish which of these subprocesses is implicated in the attentional blink (AB), Vogel, Luck, and Shapiro (1998) presented participants with a context word at the beginning of each trial (e.g., *shoe*), followed by a stream of consonant strings presented at a rate of one every 83 ms. Within this rapid stream there were two critical target items: the first (T1) was a string of numbers (e.g., *8888888*) and the second (T2) was a word that was either related to the context word (e.g., *foot*) or unrelated (e.g., *pickle*) to it (Figure 1a). T2 occurred at one of three lags: immediately after T1 (lag 1), at lag 3, or at lag 7. It was always followed by additional consonant strings plus a 1-second delay, after which participants were asked to report on the targets. Participants received both dual and single-target detection trials: in the dual-target condition instructions were to make forced choice responses at the end of each trial on both T1 (odd or even) and T2 (related or unrelated to the context word), and in the single-target condition they only had to perform the T2 task. For the single-target condition, there was no effect of lag in either reporting on T2 or in the ERPs. In the dual-target condition, participants were quite accurate at reporting the even/odd number categorization regardless of the lag. They were also accurate at reporting whether T2 was semantically related to the context word at lags 1 and 7. However, at lag 3 (the attentional blink) participants were not very accurate at making the relatedness judgment (Figure 1b).

A

Stimulus Type	Time (ms)	Related Trial	Unrelated Trial
Context Word	1000	SHOE	PICKLE
Blank	1000		
Distractor	83	PNVCSZP	KDSWPVZ
Distractor	83	GRSDPKN	VNMCPKL
Distractor	83	BVCPLMS	FDPMCNV
Distractor	83	DSPWTFR	VPMTDZM
Distractor	83	RLDJHGK	HJDLGFP
Distractor	83	SPLDJMF	DFPLJKH
T1	83	7777777	8888888
Distractor	83	WDPTBNF	GHJDMVT
Distractor	83	SCDPVBF	HDVCBNM
T2	83	XFOOTXX	XROPEXX
Distractor	83	FDLNLKB	NMCVPHJ
Distractor	83	DLJJCNW	DCVPBJM
Distractor	83	WPSCDSN	PCNBVLK
Distractor	83	DPWVCPB	NPMTVDK
Distractor	83	CBNDPNJ	BRTFPMF
Distractor	83	RTPMVBC	JLSDCDK
Distractor	83	TWSCLMN	LKSDVCP
Distractor	83	LJVBCMH	DKKHNVP
Distractor	83	RMVCPKL	WKLDMZP
Distractor	83	DPNMNVZ	CPNHVGB
Blank	1000		
Response Cue	2000	?	?
Blank	2000		

Figure 1a. Example stimuli.

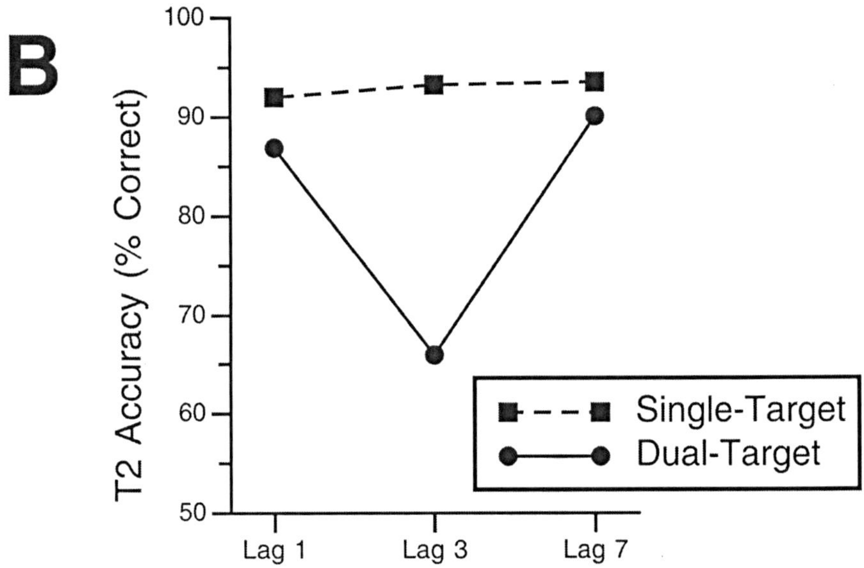

Figure 1b. Mean discrimination accuracy for the second target (T2) word as a function of lag for the single- and dual-target conditions[i].

In contrast, the relatedness effect in the ERP waveforms (the difference between the ERPs to related and unrelated words) at T2 was unaffected by lag: there was a large, similarly sized N400 semantic relatedness effect at all three lags (Figure 2). So although participants could neither identify nor classify words occurring during the attentional blink in terms of their relation to the meaning of the context word, these words nonetheless elicited an N400 semantic priming effect, indicating that they had been analyzed to a semantic/conceptual level. These waveforms were recorded at midline electrode sites and were averaged across participants. Negative is plotted upward. T2 = second target.

In other experiments of this type, Vogel and colleagues demonstrated that the stimuli presented during the attentional blink were perceived and analyzed for sensory characteristics (as evidenced by the normal early sensory components), but were not consolidated into working memory (as indicated by the totally suppressed P3 components). In this manner, ERP analyses were utilized to do what they do best – temporal localization. Specifically, ERPs implicated the synaptic computations involved in stimulus categorization and consolidation into working memory as the ones that were primarily

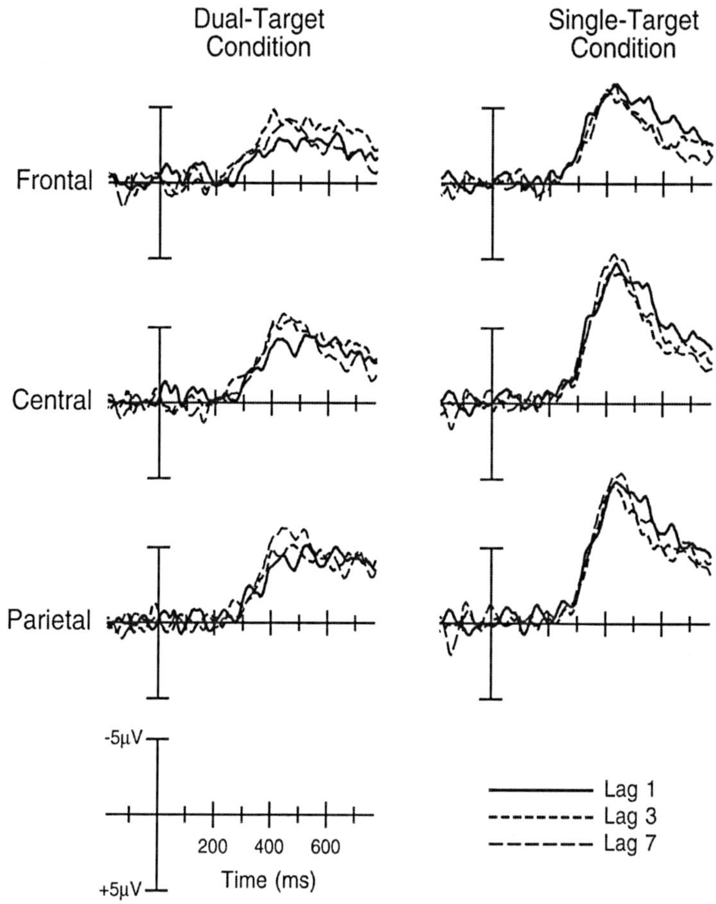

Figure 2. Grand average event-related potential difference waveforms, formed by subtracting related T2 trials from unrelated T2 trials[ii].

responsible for the attentional blink phenomenon. These results can be contrasted to the findings from the McCarthy and Nobre (1993) study, where those experimenters observed neither an N400 nor a P3 effect to spatially unattended stimuli. In that study, active suppression of items in a specific spatial location prevented words from being processed semantically/conceptually (as reflected by the absence of an N400 effect). In contrast, the attentional blink studies showed that if attention is paid to a stream of inputs, then a conceptual level of analysis can be attained, even if individuals report being unaware of the stimulus or certain aspects of the stimulus and are unable to later report on those items. These findings support the idea that perception, and some degree of attention, are needed to facilitate semantic processing, but that semantic processing is not contingent upon consoliation in working memory, as evidenced by the absence of a P3 effect.

The spatial selective attention and attentional blink experiments are clever examples of harnessing ERP components, including those sensitive to linguistic stimuli and semantic variables, to capture specific computational processes in action. In doing so, they help to delineate the time course of processing leading to particular behavioral phenomena. In general then, the effectiveness of ERPs rests on the finding that different effects are functionally specific indices of different neural, and hence presumably cognitive, computations. The methodology thus offers a powerful tool for the functional demarcation and dissection of cognitive architectures. More specifically, in the case of the attentional blink studies, there was an immediate effect of semantic relatedness in brain processing – the N400 priming effect – that was not manifest in the subsequent behavioral response, as evidenced by participants not being able to consistently report on the T2 targets. In this sense, the ERP data were essential to analyzing the informational flow leading to the attentional blink. This dissociation of the ERP and overt performance measures is not uncommon in the literature, with frequent examples of the two measures telling different stories about which factors impact processing at which stages. Such results should remind us of the utility of looking at the electroagnetic activity within the brain, especially in situations where behavioral outputs may not be sensitive enough, wholly accurate, or readily, if at all, available.

3. LANGUAGE LEARNING

Language learning is another area where ERPs have been useful in uncovering evidence of certain kinds of linguistic analysis, when more overt behavioral tests revealed no or only slight differences. We know that the dynamics of different language representations in the brain are modulated over the course of development, when individuals acquire first and second languages. In these cases, we also know that there may be delays between comprehenders' declarative knowledge (i.e., what they can talk about) and their implicit knowledge of specific language information. Accordingly, it is the combination of high temporal sensitivity in detecting fast, presumably automatic processing (which imaging techniques like fMRI or PET cannot easily provide) along with the fact that ERPs also allow some insights into the neural underpinnings of how learning affects processing that make it an effective technique for studying language learning. An added advantage of ERPs in studying processing related to language learning is that whereas it is often difficult to use the same behavioral task with different groups of subjects, for instance with infants, monolinguals, and bilingual speakers, with some ERP paradigms it is possible; ERPs thus can at times allow researchers to compare and contrast the time course and mechanisms of language processing across groups.

3.1 Second language acquisition

ERPs have proven particularly useful in studying the early phases of second language acquisition, when explicit testing may underestimate what language learners' brains know about their new language. McLaughlin, Osterhout, and Kim (2004), for example, used the known sensitivity of the N400 to semantic relationships and lexicality (or wordness – the property of a string of letters representing an actual word), to assess the degree to which college students learning French as a second language knew French words at different stages of learning. Specifically, participants were shown semantically related word pairs (e.g., *chien-chat*, Eng. *dog-cat*), semantically unrelated word pairs (e.g., *maison-soif*, Eng. *house-thirst*), and word-pseudoword pairs (e.g., mot-nasier, Eng. *word*-pseudoword), and asked to make a lexical decision. As expected, a control group of non-learners showed no differences in the ERPs to the second member of the word pair, indicating no sensitivity to either word/nonword status or to the semantic relationship between the words (Figure 3). By contrast, the group of French learners showed differences in N400 amplitude (larger for nonwords) after an average of only 14 hours of instruction, indicating an appreciation of wordness within the second language (Figure 4a); conversely, at this same stage of training, lexical decision performance (assessed by *d'* sensitivity measures) was on average at chance (Figure 4b). Moreover, for the French learners, an ERP pattern indicative of semantic processing – smaller N400s to the related than the unrelated words – was observed after an average of only 63 hours of instruction (and also after 138 hours), even though behavioral responses, although improving, were still relatively poor.

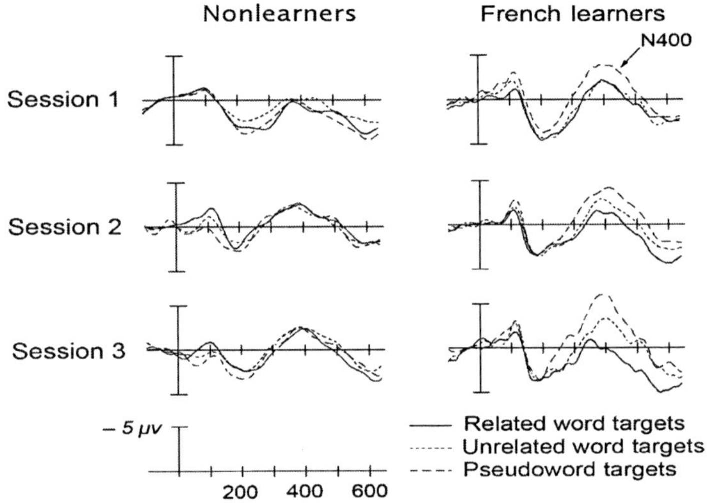

Figure 3. ERPs to word and pseudoword targets during the three testing sessions, for the nonlearners and French learners. Data acquired over the central midline site (Cz) are shown[iii].

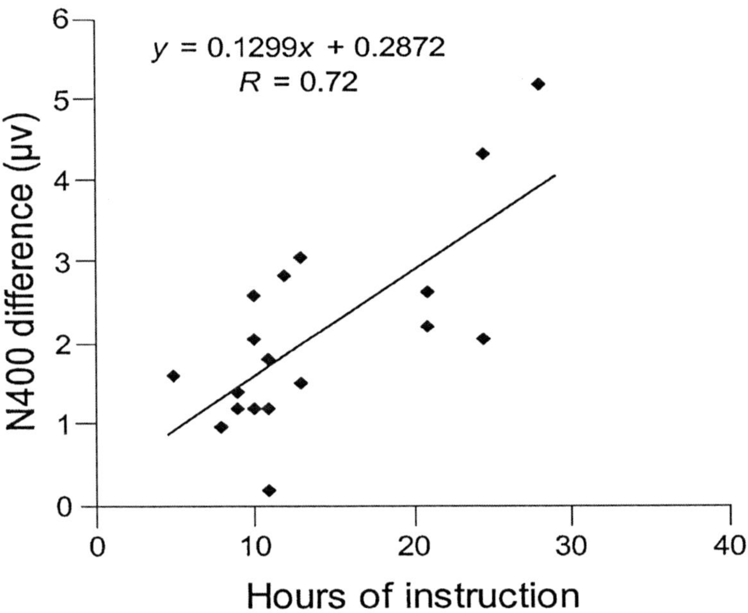

Figure 4a. Session 1 N400 amplitude difference between words and pseudowords. N400 differences were correlated with hours of instruction[iv].

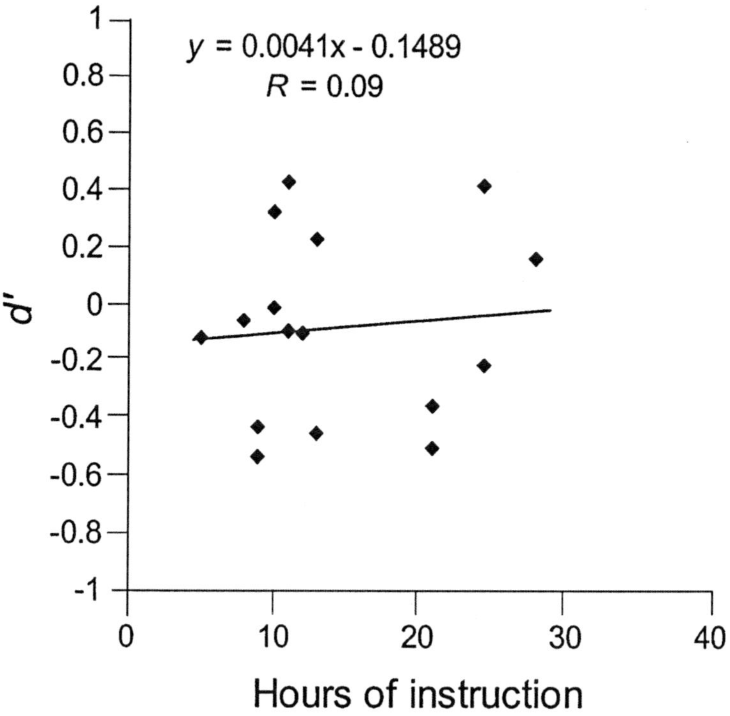

Figure 4b. d' scores regressed onto hours of instruction before session 1. d' scores were not correlated with hours of instruction.

3.2 Speech segmentation

The method of comparing ERPs before and after linguistic training also has been used to monitor speech segmentation processes (Sanders, Newport, & Neville, 2002). After establishing that the initial syllables of (actual) English words elicited larger sensory N100 components than medial syllables presented in continuous speech (Sanders & Neville, 2003), these researchers wanted to test whether the N1 indexed perceived word onsets. To that end, participants were trained to identify 3-syllable nonsense words like *babupu* or *bupada.* Learning was assessed behaviorally and monitored, with ERPs recorded to these "words" as they occurred in continuous speech streams both before and after training. Individuals' accuracy following training varied significantly, and was highly correlated with the change in N1 amplitudes before and after training: participants who learned more "words" showed larger N100 word-onset effects. These results suggest that N100 amplitude can serve as a marker for speech segmentation.

Moreover, as word onset effects occurred quite early, these data would seem to implicate predictive or very fast, automatic processes in speech segmentation. In this experiment, then, unlike the McLaughlin et al. (2004) second language learning study, the behavioral results and the ERPs went hand-in-hand, although in the latter, perhaps a different behavioral measure might have been more sensitive and/or correlated with the ERP data. Still, this ERP marker of speech segmentation has real utility in that it can be used to track speech continuously and not just at a few target test points. Critically, it can also be used in situations where even the most limited behavioral testing is not an option, as with infants or with various patient populations.

These language learning studies show us that ERPs are a good measure of synaptic plasticity. The changes in ERP indices of neural processing as a function of experience can be used to investigate, for instance, the effects of various instructional methods (e.g., temporally massed versus spaced, or immersion versus pictorial), similarities between first and second languages at multiple levels, or age of acquisition, to mention a few. For each of these contrasts, ERPs provide a tool for tapping into potential distinctions between language competence and performance.

4. UNCONSCIOUS STATES

4.1 ERPs to assess brain trauma patients

Arguably, the benefit ERPs afford in being able to observe cognitive and conceptual processing independent of behavioral or verbal output could be considered most advantageous in situations where individuals exhibit limited consciousness or behavioral responsivity. The methodology's value is particularly evident when assessing the integrity of the cognitive and language comprehension systems in patients who have survived severe brain trauma. These may include comatose individuals who show no indication of arousal or awareness, individuals in vegetative state who are awake but unaware of themselves or their environment, individuals in minimally conscious state (MCS) who are not in a vegetative state but are unable to communicate consistently (i.e., they can follow simple commands, make yes/no responses somehow, have intelligible speech, or exhibit purposeful behavior), and individuals with locked-in syndrome who show an awareness of their environment but are unable to move (for instance, quadriplegics). It is very difficult to assess the integrity of language comprehension in such individuals, and thus it is well worth an attempt to do so via electrical and hemodynamic neuroimaging methodologies, especially using auditory inputs. In these patient groups, there have been promising attempts to look for normal or delayed early sensory potentials (e.g., P1s and N1s), mismatch negativities (MMN), P3, N400, and P600 components, among others. The MMN, a frontal negativity recorded in response to infrequent, deviant stimuli embedded in a stream of auditory events has proven to be an especially good predictor of awakening in coma patients. For instance, Naccache, Puybasset, Gaillard, Serve, & Willer (2005) found that in 30 comatose patients, 10 showed a MMN, and 9 of these eventually awakened, whereas from the remaining 20 MMN-negative group, 13 died and 7 awakened. Although these findings are based on MMNs to tones, we can envision a MMN battery to different types of deviants – not just of frequency, intensity, duration, timbre, and phonetic content, but also of higher, more abstract linguistic and non-linguistic features which are known to elicit reliable MMNs (e.g., Paavilainen, 2001; Pulvermüller, Shtyrov, Kujala, & Näätänen, 2004; Saarinen, Paavilainen, Schöger, & Tervaniemi, 1992;). Testing of this sort would be relevant, because the MMN data imply the existence of a memory trace in which features of the frequent standard stimuli are represented.

A few researchers have examined semantic processing in such patients. Schoenle and Witkze (2004), for example, maintain that 38% of patients diagnosed as being in a vegetative state showed some evidence of N400 activity (although they specify that only 12% showed clear N400s), indicating some level of sensitivity to semantic or lexical processing. However, the data are rather poor quality and lacking in methodological controls. (N400s were assessed visually, not statistically, by three independent investigators. It is not specified whether these raters were blind to the patients' diagnoses or to the experimental conditions. It is also not clear from the description of the materials exactly what kind of sentence stimuli were used and which factors were or were not controlled for. The authors stated that they used 5-word sentences with either semantically correct or incorrect final words, yet the example they provide, "*The coffee is too hot to drink/fly*" is clearly longer than 5 words. Even assuming this was a misstatement, they do not indicate whether the stimuli were normed for semantic fit, nor whether the target words in the two conditions were matched on factors such as word frequency, length, or concreteness, to mention but a critical few. We believe these omissions are particularly relevant and potentially detrimental because if such studies are to be taken seriously as a means for diagnosing conditions as grave as vegetative state, then it is critical for these early investigations to be methodologically sound. Additionally, it was difficult for readers of this article to assess for themselves the ERP findings, as only a limited subset of single subject waveforms for selected vegetative state patients were shown, and even these were presented in a way not conducive to comparisons between conditions.) Kotchoubey (2005), using chord and vowel-sound P3 oddball paradigms as well as sentence and word pair N400 paradigms, have cleaner recordings and likewise claim that both the P3 and N400 occur in vegetative state patients with above chance frequency, suggesting that current methods for diagnosis may underestimate their remaining information processing abilities. Given the grave consequences to misdiagnosis in these cases, an ERP approach may be cost effective even for the occasional patient.

4.2 ERPs during sleep

ERPs also have been used to demonstrate the extent to which the human brain can process auditory information during sleep, when individuals cannot actively attend to or easily control their behavioral output. ERP studies have shown that sleeping brains are not completely isolated from the sensory environment and that at least some auditory information can be processed during sleep, sometimes in ways remarkably similar to wakefulness. For example, sleeping brains seem able to discriminate between different types of auditory stimuli by detecting deviant tone stimuli in oddball paradigms, exhibiting P300-like responses during rapid eye movement (REM) sleep, and various other ERP effects during other stages of sleep (see Bastuji, Perrin, & Garcia-Larrea, 2002, for a review). This indicates that at least some stimulus categorization is possible during this sleep stage, and that the responsible mechanism(s) overlap with those in the waking state.

But questions remain about whether these signs of auditory discrimination are related to higher-level semantic recognition, or whether they simply reflect the acoustic salience of the oddball. To test the sleeping brain's sensitivity to semantically relevant input, researchers have primarily used one of two different ERP experimental paradigms. The first examines the participant's own name, which during wakefulness elicits a large P300 compared to other names or words in a list, even without explicit instructions to attend or respond to one's own name. Participants' own names are used because their emotional content and high natural frequency in the individuals' everyday lives make them especially relevant stimuli that seem to be difficult to ignore consciously or unconsciously. Perrin, García-Larrea, Mauguière, and Bastuji (1999), for instance, recorded ERPs to the subject's own name presented equiprobably with 7 other names during waking and during REM (also known as paradoxical sleep or PS). In both cases participants' own names exhibited late positive waves between 400-600 ms, maximal over posterior scalp sites – in other words, a P300. Given that all the names were equiprobable, these results demonstrated that the sleeping ERP effect could not simply be due to the acoustic difference or physical rarity of the individual's own name. The authors concluded that the ERPs thus showed that some top-down processing remains functional during PS, since some sort of comparison of a deviant to a standard is necessary for detection. However, it is not clear whether these findings are due to the fact that as a pattern, one's own name is a more frequent stimulus relative to other environmental inputs, or whether the ERP response is more directly related to the name's inherent meaning. One potential way of addressing this question (which to our knowledge has not been done) might be to overtrain individuals over a period of days with some other name, not their own, and then determine whether the training influences the P3 during sleep to that particular name (relative to others that have not been so trained).

Because using the participant's own name might leave in question how "semantic" this processing is, due to the emotional content and higher natural occurrence baseline rate of individuals' own names, other ERP studies have instead employed word/word priming paradigms to argue for some degree of semantic analysis during sleep. In two separate studies, ERPs showed that related and unrelated words continued to elicit differential responses during sleep, and also indicated that differential responses to pseudowords were possible, depending on the stage of sleep. Perrin, Bastuji, and García-Larrea (2002) presented word primes followed by either congruous or incongruous target words, with pseudowords inserted between word pairs during waking, Stage 2 (S2) sleep, and PS. For both S2 and PS sleep, incongruous words showed larger N400-like waves than congruous words, with latencies and topographies similar to the waking N400. (Brualla, Romero, Serrano, & Valdizán, 1998 reported a similar finding, although with delayed N400 latencies during sleep.) Pseudowords, by contrast, elicited different ERPs depending on the vigilance state: during wakefulness they exhibited larger N400s than incongruous words, whereas during S2 sleep pseudowords and incongruous words elicited similarly greater amplitude N400s relative to congruous words. Less apparent is why during PS the ERPs to pseudowords, but not incongruous words, resembled those to congruous words. The authors suggest that these results are consistent with the finding by Stickgold, Scott, rittenhouse, & Hobson (1999) that linguistic absurdity is accepted in a different manner in dream-sleep than during waking, as reflected by an abnormal pattern of semantic behavioral priming (upon being awoken from PS) where weak primes show greater effects than strong primes. However, it is unclear why this pattern, for which the equivalent in the Perrin study would be reduced N400s to more weakly associated words, would not also hold for the incongruous words as well as for the pseudowords. Although the patterns observed for the pseudowords undoubtedly require deeper investigation, the finding of incongruous words continuing to elicit larger N400s relative to congruous words throughout S2 and PS sleep (as supported by two separate studies) is an intriguing one, and hints at a sleeping brain that is capable of processing language in a more semantically active way than perhaps previously would have been thought.

The sleeping brain reportedly is also sensitive to sentence level contextual priming. Ibáñez, López, and Cornejo (2006) examined both waking and sleeping participants using spoken Spanish sentence stems completed with endings of varying degrees of congruency, such as (translated from original Spanish) "*Something that flies and has a motor is a...*" followed by either a congruous ending (*airplane*), or one of three types of incongruous endings: 1) *bird* (incongruous with the second part of the sentence), 2) *car* (incongruous with the first part of the sentence), or 3) *television* (incongruous with both parts of the sentence). Waking individuals showed a significant differentiation in the N400 time window to the target types, with the largest negativities in response to the totally incongruous endings, the smallest negativities to congruous endings, and intermediate negativities to both Incongruous 1 and 2 endings which themselves were not discriminable. Sleeping participants were presented with the same stimuli during both Stage II and REM sleep, with ERP results showing no significant differences in relation to sleep stage, and overall a similar ERP congruency pattern to that of waking participants. The maximum negativity in both waking and sleep was in the left frontal regions, and was functionally similar regardless of sleep-wake status. Cognitive processing reflected by N400-like negativities it seems thus can be generated outside of conscious awareness.

The combination of superior temporal resolution, access to the neural activity generated by cortical networks, lack of necessity for an external response, and the added benefit of being able to collect data in bedside settings make ERPs an optimal methodology for monitoring the cognitive processes of brains in various states of consciousness. Using ERPs to examine unconscious states provides an important tool not just for gaining a better understanding of functions such as language comprehension (i.e., research in a more fundamental scientific sense), but also may turn out to have more practical applications as a critical component in establishing diagnostic criteria for patients who have suffered various degrees of brain trauma. The relatively untapped possibilities and potential knowledge to be gained in both areas represent an exciting new direction for ERP research, but one that calls for very careful experimental design.

5. PREDICTIVE LANGUAGE PROCESSING

Because so much of language processing occurs quickly and is unavailable to conscious reflection, ERPs have arguably made their greatest contributions in probing natural language processing in healthy, intact brains. One especially contentious issue in the language comprehension literature has been whether or not individuals might predict upcoming items at various linguistic levels (syntactic, semantic, phonological, etc.) Traditionally, a majority of psycholinguists have believed that language is too unpredictable and too ambiguous to allow for prediction except in very rare cases where contextual constraint is unusually high (e.g., Stanovich & West, 1979). More recently though, a few researchers have begun to propose that prediction (or perhaps better said, preactivation) may occur routinely (DeLong, Urbach, & Kutas, 2005; Federmeier & Kutas, 1999; Kamide, Altmann, & Haywood, 2003; van Berkum, Brown, Zwitserlood, Kooijman, &

Hogoort, 2005; Wicha, Moreno, & Kutas, 2004). Preactivation, however, is not so easy to capture, the difficulty being in how to observe the consequences of an event that has not yet occurred. ERPs are well suited for prediction research, though, because they can provide a continuous monitor of brain responses throughout the course of a sentence or discourse, i.e., prior to target events that might be subject to prediction. They also can provide a measure of the quantitative and qualitative changes that may distinguish two conditions, including sensitivity to semantic and syntactic variables and processing. In these ways, ERPs can be used to explore research questions that behavioral or in some cases even eye-tracking studies cannot as easily resolve.

In a precursor to electrophysiological studies designed specifically to track prediction, Van Petten, Coulson, Rubin, Plante, and Parks (1999) used ERPs to investigate whether or not semantic integration could begin to operate prior to the complete identification of a spoken word. Participants listened to sentences (e.g., "*It was a pleasant surprise to find that the car repair bill was only seventeen...*") that were completed by a word that was either a high cloze probability semantically congruous word (*dollars*) or one of 3 types of incongruous words: (a) incongruous words that either shared the same initial auditory fragment as the congruous word (*dolphins*), (b) rhymed with the congruous target (*scholars*), or (c) had initial phonemes differing from those of the highest-cloze probability word (*bureaus*). As long as the auditory input from the target word was consistent with the sentence context (i.e., for the *dol-* portion of *dollars* and *dolphins*), the ERPs for the two conditions were similar. However, as soon as the auditory signal for the congruous and incongruous sentence completions diverged, so did their ERPs. For the incongruous conditions (b) and (c), where the initial phonemes differed from those of the expected completion, the ERPs began to diverge much earlier than for the *dolphins* condition, condition (a). From these results, Van Petten et al. concluded that semantic processing of a word begins even before it is uniquely identified and that there is a continuous mapping from linguistic input onto semantic representations.

These ERP results suggested that verbal processing may begin prior to receiving all the relevant input. Subsequent studies have more directly explored the various levels at which anticipatory processing could occur. For instance, prediction need not be at the level of specific word forms, but could instead or also be at the level of meaning. So even if individuals were not anticipating a specific lexical form, they could be anticipating semantic features of the word most likely to appear in a given context. Federmeier & Kutas (1999) demonstrated just this in an ERP study in which expected sentence completion targets were compared to those for within and between category violations in high and low constraint sentences. For example, a high constraint context such as "*He caught the pass and scored another touchdown. There was nothing he enjoyed more than a good game of...*" was followed by one of three possible continuations: the expected item ("*football*"), an unexpected item from within the same category ("*baseball*"), or an unexpected item ("*monopoly*"), from a different category. The researchers showed that although both types of unexpected items showed a larger N400 than to the expected item ("*football*"), the N400 to the within category violation ("*baseball*") was smaller than that to the between category violation ("*monopoly*"). This pattern of results, where within category violations were easier to process semantically, was observed for high constraint sentences such as the example sentence provided here, but not for the low constraint sentences. Although within and between category violations were judged implausible for both high and low constraint sentences, the within category violation N400 was reliably reduced only when the target noun was highly constrained. The researchers suggested that this pattern of results could only be explained by the greater overlap in perceptual and semantic features of the expected exemplar with the within category violation exemplar compared to the between category violation exemplar. They proposed that in high constraint sentences, contextual information had already acted via semantic memory to preactivate some of the features of the expected exemplar.

Studies by Wicha, Moreno and Kutas (2003, 2004) and by van Berkum et al. (2005), have also demonstrated syntactic anticipation by capitalizing on grammatical gender manipulations in Dutch and Spanish, respectively. These ERP experiments used pre-nominal gender marking that either agreed or disagreed with an expected noun or depiction of a noun in a particular sentence context. In the Wicha et al. studies, native Spanish speakers received constraining sentences that contained a gender-marked article followed by either a noun or an embedded line drawing. The noun or line drawing target could be either an expected continuation or a semantically incongruent continuation of the same gender class as the expected continuation. In half of the sentences, the gender of the pre-nominal article was manipulated to be incongruent with the gender of the following noun or picture. Similarly, van Berkum et al. conducted an auditory ERP study using gender marking on pre-nominal adjectives in Dutch (for words only), but without gender mismatches between pre-nominal adjectives and nouns. In both studies, an ERP difference (albeit somewhat different in timing and distributional detail across studies) at the pre-nominal word between the prediction consistent and inconsistent conditions indicated that individuals had already formed an expectation for representations specifying words' semantic and syntactic properties (lemmas).

ERPs have also been instrumental in finding evidence for preactivation at the level of specific phonological word forms. DeLong et al. (2005) took advantage of a phonological regularity in English whereby the singular indefinite article is phonologically realized as *an* before words beginning with vowel sounds (e.g., *an airplane*, *an eagle*) and as *a* before words beginning with consonant sounds (*a kite*, *a carrot*). Participants read sentences such as "*The day was breezy so the boy went outside to fly...*", where *kite* is the expected noun and by extension *a* is the expected article. Participants also saw sentences such as "*Because it frequently rains in London, Nigel always carries ...*", where *umbrella* is the expected noun and *an* the expected article. The experimental design assumes that if readers are predicting a specific upcoming noun, then these expectations should be violated when they get a contextually less likely (but still plausible) article (and noun) such as *an airplane* in the case of the first example or *a newspaper* in the case of the second. Given comprehenders' background knowledge about entities like boys, breezy days, outdoor activities, and flying objects, it is not difficult to see why *kite* and *airplane* might differ in how well they fit with the schemas or event knowledge that the sentential context "brings to mind" via semantic memory processes. It is exactly this line of reasoning that led to the original hypothesis of the N400 indexing the ease or difficulty of contextual integration processes in the first place. However, whereas the nouns *kite* and *airplane* differ in their semantics, the indefinite articles immediately preceding each do not, possessing identical semantics ("some one thing or other"). Since the indefinite articles' semantics are identical and the two forms differ only in phonological form, frequency of usage and length, there is no reason for one to be differentially difficult to integrate into the mental representation of any particular sentence context, unless people are forming predictions for specific word forms.

We tested this possibility with sentences of varying constraint leading to expectations for particular consonant-initial or vowel-initial nouns with offline expectancy (cloze probability) ratings ranging from highly probable to highly unlikely, based on the percentage of individuals who continued the truncated sentences with that particular word in an offline norming questionnaire. Using broad ranges of cloze probabilities (article cloze probabilities ranged from 0-96%, nouns ranged from 0-100%) allowed us to conduct correlational analyses to determine whether there was a systematic relationship between ERPs at the article and their offline cloze probabilities.

In line with previous research (Kutas & Hillyard, 1984), unexpected nouns were associated with a greater posterior negativity between 200 and 500 ms relative to expected nouns, the amplitude of which was inversely correlated with noun cloze probability. These data thus demonstrate that the different degrees of constraint in these materials are reflected in offline expectancies and in modulations of N400 amplitude in the usual way, but do not speak to the issue of prediction per se. To address that question we turned to the indefinite articles. Just as for the nouns, high cloze articles were associated with less negativity between 200-500 ms post-article onset than lower cloze articles. A comparison of ERP waveforms after a median split on their offline cloze probabilities revealed a very similar pattern for articles as for nouns, although much smaller for articles (Figure 5a). Moreover, the amplitude of this negativity was highly correlated with the article's offline cloze probability, although again slightly lower than for nouns (Figure 5b). Also similar to the nouns, the maximum article correlations were not randomly distributed, but rather clustered over the posterior sites where N400 effects are typically seen (Figure 5c). So at least over certain scalp areas, a large percentage of the variance (up to 52%) in N400 amplitude for the indefinite articles was accounted for by the average probability that individuals would continue the sentence context with that article.

In short, these results offered evidence of lexical prediction, indicating that people do use sentence context to form graded predications for specific upcoming words. These findings also refute the idea that, as some have suggested, prediction is limited to highly constraining contexts, with only a single lexical item activated when its representation exceeds some threshold given a very constraining context. Even in moderately constraining sentence contexts at least one and perhaps multiple items seem to be pre-activated but to varying degrees.

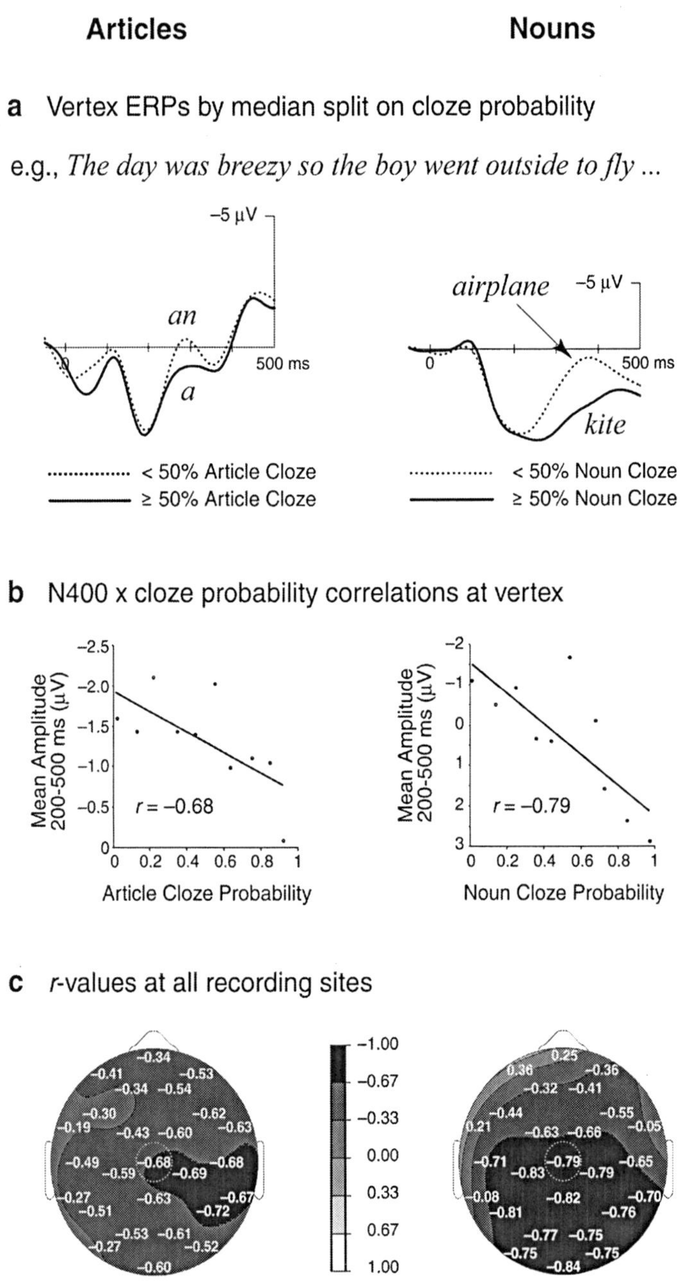

Figure 5. ERP waveforms and correlations between N400 amplitude and cloze probability for articles (left) and nouns (right) showing that specific words are predicted during language comprehension. (a) ERPs at the vertex recording site according to a median split on cloze probabilities. Both articles and nouns with cloze probability less than 50% elicit a greater negativity between 200-500 ms post-stimulus

onset (N400) than those with cloze probability greater than or equal to 50%. (b) There are strong inverse relations between the items' cloze probabilities and mean N400 amplitudes at MiCe for both the articles and the nouns. The solid lines in the scatter diagrams indicate the best fitting regression line. (c) The r-values calculated as in (b) for each electrode site. Analyses indicated that both articles and nouns show a focus of maximal correlations over centro-parietal sites[v].

The studies described here relating to predictive language processing indicate that in the course of sentence comprehension, semantic memory for a particular item is likely not just triggered at the time point when the phonological word form or linguistic item is received. Rather, information of all sorts, both linguistic and extra-linguistic, is actively accessed and integrated to continually update representations of contexts which dynamically constrain linguistic expectations at a variety of different levels (e.g., semantic/conceptual, syntactic, phonological) and aid in meaning construction. While preactivation of linguistic information could be inherently difficult to observe – because we must capture evidence of processing for an event that has not yet occurred – ERPs offer one method of tracking online updating and provide a means of distinguishing between qualitative and quantitative differences. In combination with clever experimental designs, then, the ERP methodology will continue to play an important role in delineating the time course of language processing.

6. CONTEXTUAL ACTIVATION OF INFORMATION IN SEMANTIC MEMORY

In DeLong et al. (2005) we suggested that probabilistic pre-activations are supported by semantic memory, which includes experiential knowledge about people, places, things and events accessed by linguistic input (see also, Kutas & Federmeier, 2000). Although our knowledge of the precise cognitive and neural mechanism involved in activating information in semantic memory remains relatively under-specified, we believe that words and various structures in sentences act as cues that activate different types of information in semantic memory and are thus involved in constructing word and sentence meanings. Some researchers have attempted to use the ERP technique to test specific hypotheses about the types of information that words may activate. Ferretti, Kutas, and McRae (2007), for example, used

ERPs to investigate the hypothesis that information in verbs, such as verb aspect, activates knowledge about events in semantic memory, including which individuals usually take part in the event, the typical locations where those events occur, and the instruments involved. In turn, the availability of this information at different time points across the course of a sentence is presumed to influence how sentence representations are built in real time. The grammatical category of aspect captures some ways in which languages use morphology to refer to the temporal structure of events, in this case as ongoing versus completed. Imperfective aspect, which in English is marked with a verbal form of *be* + a main verb ending with *-ing* (e.g., *was skating*), makes specific reference to the internal structure of events by focusing on their ongoing development. The imperfective makes no reference to an event's completion, highlighting the internal phases of dynamic events instead. Perfect aspect, in contrast, is used to refer to some time period that follows an event and emphasizes the resultant phase or states. In English, this aspectual category is marked by *to have* + a past participle (e.g., *have skated*). Perfect aspect functions to indicate the continuing relevance of a past situation for the present or for some other reference time. One can consider the causal (and temporal) structure of events to include the initiating conditions (beginning), the actual event (middle), and the resultant states (end). Related to each are the various entities, objects, and locations that typically characterize these events. Importantly, the entities and objects relating to particular events will be more or less salient during their different causal components. For instance, location and instrument information are often salient during ongoing events, but not after they are completed. The authors proposed that if this is indeed the case, then there should be differences in the processing of location information when events are linguistically signaled as ongoing compared to when they are signaled as having been completed, and that among other measures, this should be reflected in the accompanying electrical brain activity.

Ferretti et al. collected ERP evidence consistent with this view. Using sentences such as "*The girl was skating/had skated in the rink/ring*" that varied in both aspect (imperfective or perfect) and typicality (high or low) of the location of the verb-related activity, they observed that the N400s were smallest to nouns representing typical locations of particular activities (e.g., *rink*) in imperfective sentences and largest to atypical locations (e.g., *ring*) in imperfective sentences (Figure 6). By contrast, N400s to location nouns completing perfect aspect sentences were less sensitive to location information. These results suggest that the imperfective form of the verb leads to specific expectations about where the events denoted by the verb will occur, whereas location expectancies are less well formed (and/or more difficult to integrate into the sentence representation once the location is known) for sentences in the perfect aspectual form, presumably because locations are generally less expected. In addition to the N400 findings at the location nouns, ERPs throughout the sentence varied as a function of verb aspect. This effect manifested as a sustained frontal negativity spanning the prepositional phrases that was larger following perfect than imperfective aspect verbs. These over-sentence averages indicate that processing differences began with the verbs, if not before.

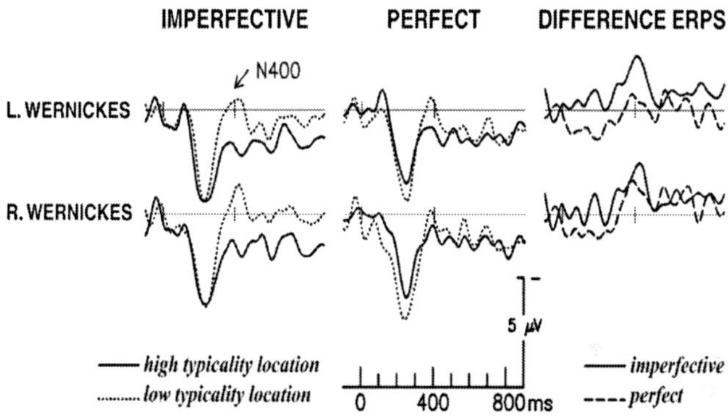

Figure 6. Grand averages for the four experimental conditions at Wernickes (LDPa, RDPa) electrode sites. Column 1 shows the averages for high and low typicality locations for imperfective aspect, and Column 2 shows the averages for high and low typicality locations for perfect aspect. Column 3 shows the difference waves (high – low typicality) for each of the two aspects[vi].

Verb aspect is just one instance of the type of linguistic information that is likely to activate comprehenders' background knowledge of the world and influence sentence processing in real time. ERP recordings show us that this is the case by offering a neural view into how linguistic stimuli cue information in semantic memory to help in constructing word and sentence meaning. The cognitive electrophysiology literature abounds with examples of this sort, where ERPs have been used to examine factors believed to influence language comprehension processes or to test alternative accounts of various psycholinguistic phenomena, in normal and abnormal individuals of all ages.

7. CONCLUSIONS AND FUTURE DIRECTIONS

In this chapter we have presented five varied groups of experimental examples demonstrating how ERPs can provide and have provided insights into different types of language processing. Each subset of studies benefited in a unique way from either the type of information that the electrophysiological measures afforded or from an inherent feature of the methodology itself. In some cases, the sensitivity of the ERP revealed differences that were not readily, if at all, manifest in corresponding behavioral measures. In others, the factor that made the ERP technique the most appropriate solution was that no external responses were required. In yet other studies, the continuous nature of the ERP measurements allowed critical monitoring at different time points of more temporally extended cognitive events. In all cases, the ERP's millisecond-level resolution and the amassed knowledge of the functional correlates of different ERP components were vital in designing the experiments and analyzing and interpreting the data collected. Although we have discussed many of these components throughout the chapter, focusing on the N400, but also mentioning the P1, N1, P3b, P300, P600 and MMN, there are others, both sensory/perceptual and more cognitive, that did not make the cut due to limited space and scope. In ways similar to the studies included here, these unmentioned components have served as useful tools in delineating the cognitive architectures associated with particular perceptual, behavioral, and linguistic phenomena.

Although this chapter has featured studies that capitalize on the strengths of (scalp-recorded) ERPs, the methodology is certainly not the only game in town when it comes to studying language processing. However, with exception to their most obvious deficiencies – a lack of spatial resolution and more superficial depth of recording than neuroimaging techniques such as PET or fMRI – ERPs rank respectably high on a number of characteristics when directly compared to other methodologies. Even with respect to spatial resolution and neural source localization, ERPs have improved in recent years with the use of more densely arrayed electrode caps and more sophisticated inverse modeling software tools. As is often noted, ERPs have an unbeatable temporal resolution and temporal span. In addition, the technique is relatively noninvasive, with the primary inconvenience in some of the older systems being the requisite mild scalp abrasion and administration of electrolyte gel. ERPs are also inexpensive when contrasted with either hemodynamic methods or MEG (although clearly a behavioral study, when appropriate and sufficient, would offer a more economical solution). A final practical advantage of ERPs is that they are relatively convenient to use across a wide variety of population groups, from infants to elderly, and for different patient populations in clinical, laboratory, and in some cases, even residential settings. And unlike MEG or fMRI, ERPs do not require head restraint, although none of these measures tolerates much head movement without additional computations. Even after enumerating these benefits of ERPs, it is worth keeping in mind that recent advances in combining methodologies make these either/or distinctions less relevant than they might have been even five years ago. As cognitive neuroscientists, we would all like to have our methodological cake and eat it, too – temporal *plus* spatial resolution, not one or the other. It is unlikely that ERP measures for studying language processing will be rendered obsolete anytime soon; rather, it is more probable that in the future there will be an even greater emphasis on converging methods, with ERPs (and various electroencephalographic measures more generally) continuing to play an irreplaceable role.

Certainly with respect to language processing, we have demonstrated that even on their own, electrophysiological recordings have come a long way from those early days of monitoring differences in language-related suppression of alpha activity between the cerebral hemispheres. For the most part, the experiments described in this chapter are meant to be representative examples of clever and sophisticated ways in which ERPs can be utilized to reveal how the brain extracts meaning from visually and auditorily presented linguistic stimuli. At least a few of these studies will likely, over time, establish themselves as landmark experiments, perhaps by merit of their designs, but more likely through the novelty of their findings. Although their subject matter is diverse, each serves to fit a small piece of the huge puzzle of figuring out not only how language is neurally instantiated in the brain, but how it works, for instance, in combination with the brain's attentional system, during various states of consciousness, and under the pressures of natural language time constraints. And similar to the aforementioned inter-methodology cross-talk that we assume will play an ever larger role in future neurolinguistic research, equally important is the idea that language researchers working within the ERP methodology stay apprised of other electrophysiological findings outside their specific areas of study. In this way, we can begin, in tandem with our individual endeavors, to gain a more "big picture" understanding of how the brain negotiates the linguistic world.

8. ACKNOWLEDGEMENTS

Some of the work described herein and K.A. Delong were supported by grants NICHD22614 and AG08313 to M.K. This report was written in part while M. Kutas was a Lady Davis Fellow at Hebrew University, Jerusalem.

REFERENCES

Bastuji, H., Perrin F., & Garcia-Larrea, L. (2002). Semantic analysis of auditory input during sleep: Studies with event related potentials. *International Journal of Psychophysiology Special Issue:* Event-Related Potential Measures of Information Processing during Sleep, *46*, 243-255.

Brualla, J., Romero, M. F., Serrano, M., & Valdizán, J. R. (1998). Auditory event-related potentials to semantic priming during sleep. *Electroencephalography & Clinical Neurophysiology: Evoked Potentials, 108*, 283-290.

DeLong, K. A., Urbach, T. P., & Kutas. M. (2005). Probabilistic word pre-activation during language comprehension inferred from electrical brain activity. *Nature Neuroscience, 8*, 1117-1121.

Federmeier, K. D., & M. Kutas. (1999). A rose by any other name: Long-term memory structure and sentence processing. *Journal of Memory and Language, 41*, 469-495.

Ferretti, T. R., Kutas, M., & McRae, K. (2007). Verb Aspect and the Activation of Event Knowledge. Journal of Experimental Psychology: Learning, Memory, and Cognition, *33*, 182-196.

Ibáñez, A., López V., & Cornejo, C. (2006). ERPs and contextual semantic discrimination: Degrees of congruence in wakefulness and sleep. *Brain and Language, 98*, 264-275.

Kamide, Y., Altmann, G. T. M., & Haywood, S. L. (2003). The time-course of prediction in incremental sentence processing: Evidence from anticipatory eye movements. *Journal of Memory and Language, 49*, 133-156.

Kotchoubey, B. (2005). Apallic syndrome is not apallic: Is vegetative state vegetative? *Neuropsychological Rehabilitation, 15,* 333-356.

Kutas, M., & Federmeier, K. D. (2000). Electrophysiology reveals semantic memory use in language comprehension. *Trends in Cognitive Science, 4,* 463-470.

Kutas, M., & Hillyard, S. A. (1980). Reading senseless sentences: Brain potentials reflect semantic incongruity. *Science, 207*, 203-205.

Kutas, M., & Hillyard, S. A. (1984). Brain potentials during reading reflect word expectancy and semantic association. *Nature, 307,* 161-163.

Kutas, M., K. D. Federmeier, J. Staab, and R. Kluender. (In press). Language. In J. T. Cacioppo, L. Tassinary, & G. Berntson (Eds.), Handbook of Psychophysiology, 3rd edition. Cambridge: Cambridge University Press.

McCarthy, G., & Nobre, A. C. (1993). Modulation of semantic processing by spatial selective attention. *Electroencephalography & Clinical Neurophysiology: Evoked Potentials, 88,* 210-219.

McLaughlin, J., Osterhout, L., & Kim, A. (2004). Neural correlates of second-language word learning: Minimal instruction produces rapid change. *Nature Neuroscience, 7,* 703-704.

Naccache, L., Puybasset, L., Gaillard, R., Serve, E., & Willer, J. (2005). Auditory mismatch negativity is a good predictor of awakening in comatose patients: A fast and reliable procedure. *Clinical Neurophysiology, 116,* 988-990.

Paavilainen, P., Simola, J., Jaramillo, M., Näätänen, R., & Winkler, I. (2001). Preattentive extraction of abstract feature conjunctions from auditory stimulation as reflected by the mismatch negativity (MMN). *Psychophysiology, 38,* 359-365.

Perrin, F., Bastuji, H., & García-Larrea, L. (2002). Detection of verbal discordances during sleep. *Neuroreport: For Rapid Communication of Neuroscience Research, 13,* 1345-1349.

Perrin, F., García-Larrea, L., Mauguière, F., & Bastuji, H. (1999). A differential brain response to the subject's own name persists during sleep. *Clinical Neurophysiology, 110,* 2153-2164.

Pulvermüller, F., Shtyrov, Y., Kujala, T., & Näätänen R. (2004). Word-specific cortical activity as revealed by the mismatch negativity. *Psychophysiology, 41,* 106-112.

Raymond, J. E., Shapiro, K. L., & Arnell, K. M. (1992). Temporary suppression of visual processing in an RSVP task: An attentional blink? *Journal of Experimental Psychology: Human Perception and Performance, 18,* 849-860.

Saarinen, J., Paavilainen, P., Schöger, E., & Tervaniemi, M. (1992). Representation of abstract attributes of auditory stimuli in the human brain. *Neuroreport: An International Journal for the Rapid Communication of Research in Neuroscience, 3,* 1149-1151.

Sanders, L. D., & Neville, H. J. (2003). An ERP study of continuous speech processing. I. Segmentation, semantics, and syntax in native speakers. *Cognitive Brain Research, 15,* 228-240.

Sanders, L. D., Newport, E. L. & Neville, H. J. (2002). Segmenting nonsense: An event-related potential index of perceived onsets in continuous speech. *Nature Neuroscience, 5,* 700-703.

Schoenle, P. W., & Witzke, W. (2004). How vegetative is the vegetative state? Preserved semantic processing in VS patients–evidence from N400 event-related potentials. *NeuroRehabilitation 19(4),* 329-34.

Stanovich, K. E., & West, R. F. (1979). Mechanisms of sentence context effects in reading: Automatic activation and conscious attention. *Memory & Cognition, 7,* 77-85.

Stickgold, R., Scott, L., Rittenhouse, C., & Hobson, J. A. (1999). Sleep-induced changes in associative memory. *Journal of Cognitive Neuroscience, 11,* 182-193.

Van Berkum, J. J. A., Brown, C. M., Zwitserlood, P., Kooijman, V., & Hagoort, P. (2005). Anticipating upcoming words in discourse: evidence from ERPs and reading times. *Journal of Experimental Psychology: Learning, Memory, and Cognition, 31,* 443-467.

Van Petten, C., Coulson, S., Rubin, S., Plante, E., & Parks, M. (1999). Time course of word identification and semantic integration in spoken language. *Journal of Experimental Psychology: Learning, Memory, and Cognition, 25,* 394-417.

Vogel, E. K., Luck, S. J., & Shapiro, K. L. (1998). Electrophysiological evidence for a postperceptual locus of suppression during the attentional blink. *Journal of Experimental Psychology: Human Perception and Performance, 24,* 1656-1674.

Wicha, N. Y. Y., Moreno, E. M., & Kutas, M. (2003). Expecting gender: An event related brain potential study on the role of grammatical gender in comprehending a line drawing within a written sentence in Spanish. *Cortex, 39,* 483-508.

Wicha, N. Y. Y., Moreno, E. M. & Kutas, M. (2004). Anticipating words and their gender: An event-related brain potential study of semantic integration, gender expectancy, and gender agreement in Spanish sentence reading. *Journal of Cognitive Neuroscience, 16,* 1272-1288.

---

[i] From Electrophysiological evidence for a postperceptual locus of suppression during the attentional blink, by Vogel, E. K., Luck, S. J., & Shapiro, K. L., 1998, *Journal of Experimental Psychology: Human Perception and Performance*, *24*, 1656-1674. Copyright 1998 by APA. Reprinted with permission.

[ii] From Electrophysiological evidence for a postperceptual locus of suppression during the attentional blink, by Vogel, E. K., Luck, S. J., & Shapiro, K. L., 1998, *Journal of Experimental Psychology: Human Perception and Performance*, *24*, 1656-1674. Copyright 1998 by APA. Reprinted with permission.

[iii] Adapted with permission from Macmillan Publishers Ltd: McLaughlin, J., Osterhout, L., & Kim, A. (2004). Neural correlates of second-language word learning: minimal instruction produces rapid change. *Nature Neuroscience*, *7*, 703-704.

[iv] Figures 4a and 4b adapted with permission from Macmillan Publishers Ltd: McLaughlin, J., Osterhout, L., & Kim, A. (2004). Neural correlates of second-language word learning: minimal instruction produces rapid change. *Nature Neuroscience*, *7*, 703-704.

[v] Figure first published in Probabilistic word pre-activation during language comprehension inferred from electrical brain activity, by DeLong, K. A., Urbach, T. P., Kutas, M., 2005, *Nature Neuroscience, 8*, 1117-1121.

[vi] From Verb aspect and the activation of event knowledge, by Ferretti, T. R., Kutas, M., & McRae, K. (2007). *Journal of Experimental Psychology: Learning, Memory, and Cognition*, *33*, 182-196. Copyright 2007 by APA. Adapted with permission.

7

PROCESSING THE GRAMMATICAL FUNCTION OF WORDS IN SENTENCE READING

Electrophysiological Evidence

Mark Leikin

Neurocognitive Research Laboratory, Faculty of Education, University of Haifa, Haifa 31905 Israel

Abstract: The paper reviews several recent electrophysiological studies by Leikin and Breznitz that investigated the processing of the grammatical function of words by dyslexic and normal Hebrew-speaking adult readers. The findings of the studies showed that among normal and dyslexic readers, processing various elements within sentences may be affected by the grammatical roles of target words. It was found that normal Hebrew-speaking readers tended to utilize a predicate-oriented morphologically based strategy to identify the grammatical function of words. But the morphologically based strategy reaches its full scope only in the presence of the verb, which plays a central role in Hebrew sentences. Apparently, readers use several different procedures to identify a word's grammatical functions. Selection of a particular strategy seems to be influenced by various factors, including the syntactic and lexical-morphological characteristics of the stimuli and the reader's reading skills.

Results of ERP studies of processing the grammatical function of words suggest that N100/P200, P300, and P600 ERP components are sensitive to processes of identification and analysis of target words in accordance with their grammatical functions. Thus, we suggest that changes in these ERP components are associated with processes contributing to the first stage of syntactic parsing.

It has also been shown that significant differences, reflected by the ERP measures, exist in sentence processing between normal and dyslexic readers. Dyslexic readers demonstrated not only higher amplitudes and longer latencies of N100/P200, P300, and P600 ERP components but also tended to use a word-order strategy for identifying the grammatical functions or words.

Key words: Event Related Potentials (ERP), brain activity, syntactic processing, grammatical functions, dyslexia, Hebrew

1. INTRODUCTION

According to many psycholinguists (e.g., Ferstl & Flores d'Arcais, 1999; Frazier, 1987; Perfetti, 1999), sentence comprehension is a complex task that involves several cognitive processes and drawn on various information sources, both linguistic and non-linguistic. Moreover, interpretation seems to develop without waiting for the ends of words, phrases, or sentences. In particular, the act of sentence understanding requires, among other things, the processing of words within sentences in a way that assigns immediate syntactic categorization to words, enabling attribution of their grammatical functions or roles (i.e., subject, predicate, and object). The results of this processing are used in turn to construct a single preliminary phrase structure (Mitchel, 1987). The grammatical functions and syntactic structure of a sentence as a whole carry meanings of their own, and these meanings must be extracted by the reader in the process of comprehending a sentence (Kako, 1999; Leikin & Breznitz, 1999). Thus, identification of the grammatical roles of words appears to be one of the central steps in sentence processing.

2. IDENTIFICATION OF THE GRAMMATICAL FUNCTION OF WORDS

Strong evidence exists that syntactic parsing is a two-stage process (Mitchel, 1994). Common to most models of parsing (e.g., Altmann, Garnham, & Dennis, 1992; Frazier & Rayner, 1982; Tanenhaus & Carlson, 1989) is the view that syntactic categorization is performed in the first stage of parsing. The controversy is between the garden path theory (e.g., Frazier, 1987), which states that the parser uses syntactic information exclusively, and the interactive model (e.g., MacDonald, Pearlmutter, & Seidenberg, 1994), according to which non-syntactic content can also influence the first pass.

Theoretically, each of the grammatical functions of the words contributes differently to sentence comprehension (e.g., Gordon & Chan, 1995). Two main grammatical functions, subject and predicate, appear to play a central role in sentence processing. Identification of these core points of syntactic structure appears to be a very important, even critical task for understanding the sentence.

Current literature suggests that identification of the grammatical function of words may be possible by reference to different sources of information, such as word order, inflectional morphology, and the lexical-morphological properties of the individual words (Ferstl & Flores d'Arcais, 1999; Hahne, Mueller, & Clahsen, 2006; Perfetti, 1999). But the various sources of information seem to contribute differently to this process in different languages. It has been suggested (Kempe & MacWhinney, 1999) that the higher the availability of a cue, the larger the processing benefits associated with the presence of this cue and the smaller the impact of other converging information. In English, for example, the syntactic order of sentence components is usually fixed, so word order has great importance for sentence processing (Bates, Devescovi, & D'Amico, 1999). The situation is different when the syntactic structures are not necessarily in fixed order, as for example in Hebrew and Russian (Berman, 1985; Wade, 1994).

3. THE HEBREW LANGUAGE

In general, Hebrew is closer to languages with pragmatic word order than to those with grammatical word order (Berman, 1985). The most characteristically Semitic feature of Hebrew is its derivational morphology (Deutsch, Frost, Pollatsek, & Rayner, 2005; Ephratt, 1985). Most content words can be broken down into two basic components: root and pattern. The root, the semantic core of the word, is an ordered sequence of consonants (usually three); the pattern is a sequence of vowels or vowels and consonants (e.g., *GiBoR*, "hero"). Semantic information conveyed by the pattern is considerably less transparent than the information provided by the root. Verb patterns differ from those of other content words. Verbs are formed according to seven patterns (*binyanim*, "conjugations"); nouns and adjectives can occur in any of several dozen different patterns (*mishkalim*, "declensions"). The verb patterns denote such predicate-argument relations as transitivity, voice, causativeness, etc. The noun patterns specify lexical classes (e.g., action nouns, agents, and instruments). Except cases in which a verb appears in the infinitive, it is inflected by tense, gender, number, and (in all but present tense) person. Thus the verb provides some information about the subject, and in some cases can express subject information. Usually the verb also determines the selection of prepositions, which frequently appear in the role of object markers. The verb, therefore, provides a great deal of information that is essential for sentence comprehension.

Thus, recognition of lexical-morphological characteristics of the words (word-form information) seems to provide important syntactic information in Hebrew (Leikin, 2002; Shimron, & Sivan, 1994). "Lemma information" (Levelt, 1989), detailed lexical-syntactic information about the word, may be used by the parser to categorize the words syntactically (Mitchel, 1987). That is, the parser can use information about argument structures that different verbs can take part in and about the thematic roles of syntactic arguments (e.g., the necessity for a subject and direct object). Using the lexical entry for a word together with other sources of information (e.g., incremental presuppositions during word-by-word reading), the parser can attribute syntactic functions to words in sentences (Leikin, 2002). Several studies investigating the role of morphological units in the Hebrew mental lexicon have suggested that verbs and nouns are organized differently (Deutsch, Frost, & Forster, 1998; Frost, Forster, & Deutsch, 1997; Frost & Grainger, 2000). Deutsch et al. (1998) concluded that word patterns in the nominal system do not govern the process of the lexical system, whereas verbal-pattern morphemes have a role in lexical organization within the verbal system. Therefore, the differences between verbs and nouns are not only important for sentence structure interpretation but are also prominent from the morphological point of view and more available in the terms of processing. In addition, the effectiveness of morphological processing was found to play an important role in reading and writing in Hebrew (Ben Dror, Bentin, & Frost, 1995; Cohen, Schiff, & Gillis-Carlebach, 1996; Levin, Ravid, & Rapaport, 1999).

The issue of identification of the grammatical function of words has been poorly studied, and most evidence has been derived from behavioral measures that provide information about cognitive processes only at the conclusion of the processing sequence. Strategies used to identify the grammatical function of words and the neurophysiological mechanisms of these processes have been relatively well-studied only for Hebrew as L1 (Leikin, 2002; Leikin & Breznitz, 1999) and partially for English as L1 and L2 (Leikin, under review). These studies showed that Event-Related Potentials (ERP) appeared to be a promising technique for examining this issue.

4. ERP AND THE CONTRIBUTION OF THE GRAMMATICAL FUNCTION OF WORDS TO SENTENCE PROCESSING

Active neurons in the brain produce electrical activity that can be measured by electrodes placed on the scalp. Psycholinguists are concerned with isolating the electrical activity associated with a specific task (ERPs) from the background activity, with the aim of identifying the electrical components associated with a given linguistic stimulus (for reviews, see Kutas & Schmitt, 2003). Current research has demonstrated that ERP measurement has useful applications in reading research (Bentin, 1989; Perfetti & Liu, 2005). Several ERP components have been identified that appear to distinguish certain types of brain activity associated with different cognitive processes. The components found most relevant in the context of reading are N100-P200, P300, and N400. These components provide information about the timing (latencies) and intensity (amplitudes) of stimulus evaluation (N100-P200), response selection (P300), and lexical integration (N400). N100-P200 are considered to be related to perceptual processing (Brandeis & Lehmann, 1994; Breznitz, 2005) and have also been shown to discriminate between grammatical classes: nouns and verbs, open and closed class words (e.g., Friederici, 1999; Pulvermuller, Preissl, Lutzenberger, & Birbaumer, 1996). P300 appears to be associated with stimulus classification and updating in short-term memory (Donchin, 1981), and can also be elicited by morphosyntactic violations (Coulson, King, & Kutas, 1998; Pulvermuller, 1999). N400 is regarded as a manifestation of lexical integration and the integration process necessary to form a meaningful representation of the sentence (Federmeier, Segal, Lombrozo & Kutas, 2000; Kutas & Van Petten, 1994).

Recently, two types of findings have been reported concerning syntactic ERP effects. The first is a late positivity – P600 (e.g., Friederici, Harne, & Douglas, 2002). This finding suggests that more controlled syntactic parsing processes can be acquired in several grammatical domains. The second refers to the processes underlying ELAN or LAN – left-anterior negativity (e.g., Kotz & Friederici, 2003), and seem to be relatively difficult to acquire if the L2 has been learned late in life (Mueller, 2005). P600 seems to reflect a higher level of control than (E)LAN (Hahne & Friederici, 1999).

Recent ERP studies by Breznitz and Leikin (2000, 2001; Leikin, 2002; Leikin & Breznitz, 1999, 2001) used the ERP technique to examine the contribution of the grammatical function of words to sentence processing and the processes of identification of these grammatical functions among regular Hebrew-speaking adult readers. Brain activity was examined during the processing of various parts of a sentence. The obtained effect concerned the amplitudes and latencies of the N100/P200, P300, and P600 components. This effect was manifested in the form of clear differences between three central parts of the sentence (subject, predicate, and object), with the largest differences observed for the predicate. The findings suggested further that changes in ERP amplitudes and latencies did not relate to ordinal word position and word-class differences between target words but were associated with the grammatical functions of the words. The effect was understood as an indication of the processes involved in the identification of the grammatical function of words (Leikin, 2002). Hebrew-speaking readers tended to utilize the predicate-oriented morphologically-based strategy for processing the grammatical functions of words. This strategy was reflected by the descending order of grammatical function of words, according to the level of their activation: predicate > subject > direct object ≥ modifier. This strategy was thought to be language-related and complicated to a degree even for native Hebrew speakers (Leikin & Breznitz, 2001). This strategy seems to develop at relatively later stages of language/reading acquisition (Leikin, unpublished study; Sokolov, 1984). Moreover, Hebrew-speaking readers use several other procedures to process the grammatical function of words, including word-order strategy (Breznitz & Leikin, 2001; Leikin, 2002). Selection of a particular strategy seems to be influenced by different factors, including the lexical-morphological characteristics of the stimuli.

Regarding syntactic-order strategy, Leikin and Breznitz (1999) suggested that in Hebrew word order does not significantly influence the process of identification of grammatical functions, or at least plays a less important role than other sources of information. Based on results of word-by-word reading in the experiment and significant lexical-morphological differences between verbs and nouns in Hebrew, the study suggested that Hebrew-speaking readers tend to use a morphologically based strategy for identification of main grammatical functions. This suggestion was tested more carefully in another study (Leikin, 2002) in which the point of special interest was the potential influence of lexical factor and word position on identification of the grammatical function of words.

The same methodological paradigm was used in Leikin (2002) as in Leikin & Breznitz (1999), but the stimulus material was changed so that sentences included common invariable words with interchangeable *syntactic functions* and *positions* within the sentences.

The results showed a significant main effect for the three sentence elements only in latencies of P200, P300, and P600, and these latencies were significantly longer for subjects than for other sentence elements. In other words, the strategy for identifying the grammatical function of words was different. In contrast to previous study, the patterns of brain activation were neither predicate-oriented nor fully word-order based (i.e., subject > predicate = object).

Modification of differences in activation patterns were attributed to the character of the stimulus sentences in the experiment. Previous results (Leikin & Breznitz, 1999) were obtained by means of stimulus sentences that included verbs with the function of predicate and different prepositions. In the later study (Leikin, 2002), in each group of three sentences the same word (noun) appeared in all three grammatical roles and in three different positions in the sentence. As a result, one third of the sentences were verbless. Moreover, the lexical-morphological characteristics of the words, which played different grammatical roles, were equalized to some degree. Finally, the only preposition that appeared in the sentences was *et,* the object marker in Hebrew syntax. It was suggested therefore that the activation pattern obtained was due to the reduction of lexical-morphological differences between three central sentence elements. The reduction seemed especially critical for verbless sentences, where the absence of the verb could cause a relative decrease in brain activation in response to the predicate, and an equalization in intensity and timing measures for the predicate and object. The new findings confirmed the assumption (Leikin & Breznitz, 1999) that Hebrew readers used a verb-oriented morphologically based strategy for identifying the grammatical function of words.

Regarding the ERP components, these studies (Leikin, 2002; Leikin & Breznitz, 1999) suggested that changes in N100/P200, P300, and P600 amplitudes and latencies are associated with processes contributing to the first stage of syntactic parsing. These ERP components therefore appear to be sensitive to processes of identification and analysis of the target words according to their grammatical roles.

5. SENSITIVITY OF ERP COMPONENTS TO THE PROCESSES OF THE FIRST STAGE OF SYNTACTIC PARSING

N100-P200 is a compound that comprises a negative wave occurring 100 msec after stimulus onset and a positive wave occurring 200 msec post-stimulus. It is held to be related to perception (Regan, 1989; Brandeis & Lehmann, 1994) and correlates positively with measures of reading ability (Harter, 1991). N100 was formerly deemed to be associated with search processes and the identification of core points in sentences requiring information and focusing of attention (e.g., Brandeis & Lehmann, 1994). But a component that resembles the N100, a small anterior negativity (at about 125-180 msec), has also been found in response to syntactic violations (Friederici, Pfeifer, & Hahne, 1993; Neville, Nicol, Barss, Forster, & Garrett, 1991). It has been proposed (Friederici & Mecklinger, 1996; Gunter, Stowe, & Mulder, 1997) that both N100 and N200 ERP components are syntactic-related and associated with automatic syntactic analysis (primarily processes of structuring the language input). The findings of Leikin and Breznitz (1999) also suggest that N100 is sensitive to language processing, particularly to identification of word-form information (i.e., the lexical-morphological features of the words).

P200 is known to be responsive to verb/noun distinctions (Pulvermuller et al., 1996; Preissl, PulvermÜller, Lutzenberger, & Birbaumer, 1995). It is possible that such distinctions may be based on the lexical-semantic or lexical-morphological properties of the words. Because lexical-semantic distinctions relate mostly to N400 (e.g., Federmeier, et al. 2000; Kutas, Lindamood, & Hillyard, 1984), P200 and N100 seem to be sensitive to the lexical-morphological characteristics of the words, as shown in Leikin (2002).

P300 is a positive wave that occurs approximately 300 msec post-stimulus. It occurs in response to rare and relevant events, and appears to be associated with stimulus classification and updating in short-term memory (Brandeis & Lehmann, 1994; Donchin, 1981; Halgren, 1990). Regarding the issue under study, it has been hypothesized (Leikin, 2002; Leikin & Breznitz, 1999) that P300 reflects operations involving the classification of target words, in particular based on their lexical-morphological properties.

P600 has been found previously only in response to syntactic violations, and therefore has been regarded as a metric of syntactic anomaly (e.g., Osterhout, Holcomb, & Swinney, 1994; Osterhout & Holcomb, 1995). Specifically, it was thought to be related to syntactic complexity and probability, and to the processes of syntactic re-analysis (Gunter et al., 1997; Friederici & Mecklinger, 1996; Hagoort, Brown, & Groothusen, 1993), or indicating the difficulty of syntactic integration (Kaan, Harris, Gibson, & Holcomb, 2000). The results obtained by Leikin (2002) suggest, however, that P600 may be sensitive not only to processes of the second stage of syntactic parsing but also to procedures involved in the first pass.

Thus, the findings of Leikin (2002) and Leikin & Breznitz (1999) show that N100/P200, P300, and P600 seem to reflect an operation involved in the processing of words according to their grammatical roles in the sentence. These ERP components appear to be sensitive to the processing of lexical-morphological (word-form) and word-syntactic types of information. It was therefore proposed that if dyslexic readers are characterized by syntactic and morphological "weakness" (see, for example, Ben Dror et al., 1995; Casalis & Louis-Alexandre, 2000; Deutsh & Bentin, 1996; Gottardo, Stanovich, & Siegel, 1996; Joanisse, Manis, Keating, & Seidenberg, 2000; Leikin & Assayag, 2004; Leikin & Aven-Zur, 2006), this would be reflected in different activation patterns from those of normal readers.

6. ERP AND DYSLEXIA

Until recently there have been few studies of dyslexia using ERP methods. But available evidence from electrophysiological studies indicates that specific processing stages are affected by developmental dyslexia. Differences in information processing are reflected in variations in the spatial patterns of neural activity in the brain and in an altered time course (Brandeis, Vitacco, & Steinhausen, 1994; Breznitz, 1999; Riccio & Hynd, 1996). For example, several word recognition studies found differences in early and later ERP waves between dyslexic children and their normally reading controls, although the available data are not conclusive (Brandeis et al., 1994; Riccio & Hynd, 1996). Stelmack, Saxe, Noldy-Cullum, Campbell, and Armitage (1988) found that in contrast to normal readers, reading-disabled boys exhibited greater P200 amplitudes during a visual word recognition task. Taylor and Keenan (1990) obtained the opposite results during a lexical decision task: in dyslexic children P200s were observed to be of lower amplitude than in normally reading children. Evidence of longer N200 latencies among dyslexic children was also obtained. These investigators (Taylor & Keenan, 1990) observed reduced P300 amplitudes and longer P300 latencies in dyslexic children, as opposed to Stelmack and colleagues (1988) who found no evidence of P300 differences between dyslexic and control groups.

Recently, ERP measurement has been used in studying the contribution of the grammatical function of words to sentence processing by dyslexic Hebrew-speaking adult readers (Breznitz & Leikin, 2000, 2001; Leikin, 2002; Leikin, under review). The most important finding of these studies was the significant difference in ERP measures between dyslexic and normal readers in the process of identifying the grammatical function of words.

Breznitz and Leikin (2000) used the same method to investigate the process of identifying the grammatical function of words in dyslexic readers that they had used with normal readers (Leikin & Breznitz, 1999). Similarly to normal readers, essential differences were observed in the contribution of the grammatical function of words to sentence processing by dyslexic group. But dyslexic readers exhibited consistently higher amplitudes and longer latencies in both the N100 and P300 ERP components than did the controls. Higher amplitudes are thought (Taylor & Keenan, 1990) to represent greater effort in the brain during processing of information. Longer latencies are interpreted as reflecting a slower processing speed (Breznitz, 2003). The results seem to indicate that processing of words according to their grammatical functions is slower among dyslexic readers and demands greater effort. Note, however, that the increase in intensity and timing was dissimilar for different sentence elements and different ERP components. Differences between sentence elements were attributed to (Breznitz & Leikin, 2000; Leikin & Breznitz, 1999) the effect of the grammatical function of words. But the inconsistent mode of activation of different ERP components is probably a characteristic of dyslexic readers (Leikin, 2002).

Simultaneously, despite the noted variability in the patterns of brain activity, the results revealed a tendency of dyslexic readers to use a simpler method of identifying the grammatical function of words, namely word order. This is not the most efficient strategy for linguistic processing in Hebrew (Leikin & Breznitz, 1999), and it is typically used during the early stages of language development among Hebrew-speaking children (Berman, 1985; Sokolov, 1984). In the case of adult dyslectic readers, however, even this strategy demanded greater effort by the brain and involved a slower speed of information processing, as reflected by N100 and P300 amplitudes and latencies.

Breznitz and Leikin (2000) showed that in both normal and dyslexic readers, variations in ERP waves were due to the specific grammatical function of words. The observed patterns of brain activity seem to reflect a process of syntactic parsing (first pass), specifically a process of identification of the grammatical roles of words, and the application of this information to further syntactic processing of the sentence. In both groups, identification of grammatical functions was by means of the lexical-morphological properties of the words (word-form information), although dyslexic readers apparently also took into account word order. Thus, the syntactic processing "weakness" in dyslexia may be interpreted, at list partly, as a morphologically based difficulty in identifying the grammatical function of words by means of their lexical-morphological properties (Leikin & Even Zur, 2006).

These suggestions were further examined by Leikin (2002) controlling the lexical properties of the words (which played different grammatical roles) and their position in the sentence (see above). Dyslexic readers exhibited consistently higher amplitudes and longer latencies of P200, P300, and P600 than did normal readers in all sentence elements. The increase of ERP amplitudes and latencies among dyslexic readers was only partly consistent with the data obtained by Taylor and Keenan (1990) and by Stelmack et al. (1988) in lexical decision and visual word recognition tasks. But these results confirmed previous data by Breznitz and Leikin (2000) concerning the increase of N100 and P300 amplitudes and latencies during processing of the grammatical function of words by dyslexic readers. This effect, which appeared consistently in a few ERP components in the two experiments, suggests that dyslexic readers processes some sentence elements differently from normal readers (Leikin, 2002; Leikin, under review).

The activation patterns (processing strategies) that adult dyslexic readers used revealed differences between them and normal readers. The findings indicated a change of activation patterns from those observed in the previous research (Breznitz & Leikin, 2000). Breznitz and Leikin (2000) showed that different grammatical functions had a different effect on sentence processing, reflected in a different level of brain activation. Two distinct patterns of brain activation, with a few small variations. The first, a predicate-oriented pattern, was more evident in normal readers; the second, a word-order pattern (e.g., subject > predicate > direct object = preposition = modifier), was used mostly by dyslexic readers. By contrast, the patterns of brain activation obtained in Leikin (2002) and Leikin and Mizrahi (unpublished manuscript) were neither predicate-oriented nor fully word-order patterns and were manifested only in latency measures (as it was evident in the group of normal readers as well). In the group of normal readers this related to significantly longer P200, P300, and P600 latencies for subjects (i.e., subject > predicate = object, that is, similar to the word-order pattern). The same pattern was also revealed by P200 latency in the dyslexic group. P300 and P600 latency changes reflected another pattern (i.e., object > predicate = subject). The patterns of brain activation with reference to the grammatical function of words were partly different in dyslexic and normal readers. These data confirm the assumption (Breznitz & Leikin, 2000) that similarly to normal readers, dyslexic readers identify the grammatical function of words at least partly by means of the lexical-morphological properties of the words, while they are simultaneously affected by word order as well.

The results demonstrated significant differences in sentence processing (identification of the grammatical function of words) between dyslexic and normal readers, as reflected in ERP measures. Results appear to confirm the hypothesis (Breznitz & Leikin, 2000) of a syntactic/morphological processing "weakness" in dyslexia. Note, however, that this weakness is manifested in difficulties identifying and processing word-form information (the lexical-morphological properties of the words).

7. CONCLUSION

The findings of ERP studies showed that processing different elements within sentences may be affected by the grammatical roles of target words in both normal and dyslexic readers. Normal Hebrew-speaking readers tended to utilize the predicate-oriented morphologically based strategy to identify the grammatical function of words. But the morphologically based strategy gains full expression only in the presence of the verb, which in Hebrew sentences plays the central role. Apparently, readers use several different procedures to identify the grammatical role of a word, and the selection of a given strategy seems to be affected by various factors, including the syntactic and lexical-morphological characteristics of the stimuli and the reader's skill.

The results of ERP studies suggest that N100/P200, P300, and P600 ERP components are sensitive to processes of identification and analysis of the target words according to their grammatical roles. It is possible that changes in these ERP components are associated with processes contributing to the first stage of syntactic parsing.

Significant differences were found in sentence processing by normal and dyslexic readers, reflected in ERP measures. Dyslexic readers demonstrated not only higher amplitudes and longer latencies of the N100/P200, P300, and P600 ERP components, but also tended to use word-order strategy for identifying the grammatical functions of words, contrary to normal readers. This strategy appears to be less efficient for linguistic processing in Hebrew and represents a more primitive mode of identifying the syntactic function of words. These findings confirm the hypothesis of a syntactic processing weakness in dyslexia.

REFERENCES

Adams, M. J. (1990). *Beginning to read: Thinking and learning about print.* Cambridge, MA: MIT Press.

Altmann, G. T. M., Garnham, A., & Dennis, Y. (1992). Avoiding the garden path: Eye movements in context. *Journal of Memory and Language*, *31*, 685-712.

Badian, N. A., Duffy, F. H., Als, H., & McAnulty, G. B. (1991). Linguistic profiles of dyslexic and good readers. *Annals of Dyslexia*, *41*, 221-245.

Bates, E., Devescovi, A., & D'Amico, S. (1999). Processing complex sentences: A cross-linguistic study. *Language and Cognitive Processes*, *14*, 69-123.

Ben Dror, I., Bentin, S., & Frost, R. (1995). Semantic, phonological, and morphological skills in reading disabled and normal children: Evidence from perception and production of spoken Hebrew. *Reading Research Quarterly, 30*, 876-893.

Ben-Dror, I., Bentin, S., & Frost, R. (1995). Semantic, phonologic, and morphologic skills in reading disabled and normal children: Evidence from perception and production of spoken Hebrew. *Reading Research Quarterly*, *30*, 876-893.

Bentin, S. (1989). Orthography and phonology in lexical decision: Evidence from repetition effects at different lags. *Journal of Experimental Psychology, Learning, Memory, and Cognition*, *15*, 61-72.

Bentin, S., Deutsch, A., & Liberman, I. Y. (1990). Syntactic competence and reading ability in children. *Journal of Experimental Child Psychology*, *48*, 147-172.

Berman, R. (1985). The acquisition of Hebrew. In D. Slobin (Ed.), *The Crosslinguistic Study of Language Acquisition* (Vol. 1, pp. 255-371). Hillsdale, NJ: Erlbaum.

Bernal, J., Harmony, T., Rodrigues, M., Reyes, A., Yanez, G., Fernandez, T., Galan, L., Silva, J., Fernandez, B., Rodrigues, H., Guerrero, V., & Marosi, E. (2000). Auditory event-related potentials in poor readers. *International Journal of Psychophysiology, 36(1)*, 11-23.

Birnboim, S. (1995). Acquired surface dyslexia: The evidence from Hebrew. *Applied Psycholinguistics, 16*, 83-102.

Brandeis, D., & Lehmann, G. (1994). ERP mapping: A tool for assessing language disorders. In H. J. Heenze & T. F. Monte (Eds.), *Cognitive Electrophysiology* (pp. 242-250). Boston, MA: Binkhauser.

Brandeis, D., Vitacco, D., & Steinhausen, H. C. (1994). Mapping brain electric micro-states in dyslexic children during reading. *Acta Paedopsychiatrica International Journal of Child and Adolescent Psychiatry, 56*, 239-247.

Breznitz, Z. (2003). Speed of phonological and orthographic processing as factors in dyslexia: Electrophysiological evidence. *Genetic, Social, and General Psychology Monographs, 129(2)*, 183-206.

Breznitz, Z. (2005). Brain Activity During Performance of Naming Tasks: Comparison Between Dyslexic and Regular Readers, *Scientific Studies of Reading, 9(1)*, 17-42.

Breznitz, Z., & Leikin, M. (2000). Syntactic Processing of Hebrew Sentences in Normal and Dyslexic Readers: Electrophysiological Evidence. *The Journal of Genetic Psychology, 161(3)*, 359-380.

Breznitz, Z., & Leikin, M. (2001). Effects of Accelerated Reading Rate on Processing Words' Syntactic Functions by Normal and Dyslexic Readers: Event Related Potentials Evidence. *The Journal of Genetic Psychology, 162(3)*, 276-296.

Casalis, S., & Louis-Alexandre, M. (2000). Morphological analysis, phonological analysis and learning to read French: A longitudinal study. *Reading and Writing, 12,* 303-335.

Cohen, A., Schiff, R., & Gillis-Carlebach, M. (1996). Complexity of morphological, syntactic and narrative characteristics: A comparison of children with reading difficulties and children who can read [Hebrew]. *Megamot, 37(3)*, 273-291.

Coulson, S., King, J., & Kutas, M. (1998). Expect the unexpected: Event-related brain response to morphosyntactic violations. *Language and Cognitive Processes, 13(1),* 21-58.

Coulson, S., King, J. W., & Kutas, M. (1998). Expect the unexpected: Event-related brain response to morphosyntactic violations. *Language and Cognitive processes, 13*, 21-58.

Deutsch, A., & Bentin, S. (1996). Attention factors mediating syntactic deficiency in reading-disabled children. *Journal of Experimental Child Psychology, 63*, 386-415.

Deutsch, A., Frost, R., & Forster, K. I. (1998). Verbs and nouns are organized and accessed differently in the mental lexicon: Evidence from Hebrew. *Journal of Experimental Psychology: Learning, Memory, and Cognition, 24(5)*, 1238-1255.

Deutsch, A., Frost, R., Pollatsek, A., & Rayner, K. (2005). Morhological preview benefit effects in reading: Evidence from Hebrew. *Language and Cognitive Processes, 20(1/2)*, 341-371.

Donchin, E. (1981). Surprise! ... Surprise? *Psychophysiology, 18*, 493-513.

Ephratt, M. (1985). *Root-Pattern Array: Main Tool for Hebrew Word Formation* [in Hebrew]. Doctoral thesis. Jerusalem: The Hebrew University.

Federmeier, K. D., Segal, J. B., Lombrozo, T., & Kutas, M. (2000). Brain responses to nouns, verbs, and class-ambiguous words in context. *Brain, 123*, 2552-2566.

Ferstl, E. C., & Flores d'Arcais, G. (1999). The reading of words and sentences. In A. D. Friederici (Ed.) *Language Comprehension: A Biological Perspective* (pp. 175-210). Berlin: Springer.

Frazier, L. (1987). Sentence processing: A tutorial review. In M. Coltheart (Ed.), *Attention and Performance, XII: The Psychology of Reading* (pp. 559-586). Hove, UK: Erlbaum.

Frazier, L., & Rayner, K. (1982). Making and correcting errors during sentence comprehension: Eye movements in the analysis of structurally ambiguous sentences. *Cognitive Psychology, 14*, 178-210.

Friederici, A. D. (1999). The neurobiology of language processing. In A. D. Friederici (Ed.) *Language Comprehension: A Biological Perspective* (pp. 265-304). Berlin: Springer.

Friederici, A. D., & Mecklinger, A. (1996). Syntactic parsing as revealed by brain responses: First-pass and second-pass parsing processes. *Journal of Psycholinguistic Research, 25*, 157-176.

Friederici, A. D., Harne, A., & Douglas, S. (2002). Distinct neuropsychological pattewrns reflecting aspects of syntactic complexity and syntactic repair. *Journal of Psycholinguistic Research, 31(1)*, 45-63.

Friederici, A. D., Pfeifer, E., & Hahne, A. (1993). Event-related brain potentials during natural speech processing: Effects of semantic, morphological and syntactic violations. *Cognitive Brain Research, 1*, 183-192.

Frost, R., & Granier, J. (2000). Cross-linguistic perspectives on morphological processing: An introduction. *Language and Cognitive Processes, 15(4/5)*, 321-328.

Frost, R., Forster, K. I. & Deutsch, A. (1997). What can we learn from the morphology of Hebrew: A masked priming investigation of morphological representation. *Journal of Experimental Psychology: Learning, Memory, and Cognition, 23*, 829-856.

Gordon, P., & Chan, D. (1995). Pronouns, passives, and discourse coherence. Journal of Memory and Language, *34(2)*, 216-231.

Gottardo, A., Stanovich, K. E., & Siegel, L. S. (1996). The relationships between phonological sensitivity, syntactic processing, and verbal working memory in the reading performance of third-grade children. *Journal of Experimental Child Psychology, 63*, 563-582.

Gunter, T. C., Stowe, L. A., & Mulder, G. M. (1997). When syntax meets semantics. *Psychophysiology, 34*, 660-676.

Hagoort, P., Brown, C., & Groothusen, J. (1993). The syntactic positive shift as an ERP-measure of syntactic processing. *Language and Cognitive Processes, 8*, 439-483.

Hahne, A., & Friederici, A. D. (1999). Processing a second language: late learners' comprehension mechanisms as revealed by event-related brain potentials. Bilingualism: *Language and Cognition, 4(2)*, 123-141.

Hahne, A., Mueller, J., & Clahsen, H. (2006). Morpholigical processing in a second language: Behavioral and Event-related brain potential evidence for storage and decomposition. *Journal of Cognitive Neuroscience, 18(1)*, 121-134.

Halgren, E. (1990). Insights from evoked potentials into the neuropsychological mechanisms of reading. In A. B. Scheibel & A. F. Wechsler (Eds.), *Neurobiology of Higher Cognitive Function* (pp. 103-149). New York: Guilford Press.

Harter, M. R. (1991). Event-related potential indices: Learning disabilities and visual processing. In J. E. Obrzut & G. W. Hynd (Eds.), *Neuropsychological Foundations of Learning Disabilities* (pp. 437-473). New York: Academic Press.

Joanisse, M. F., Manis, F. R., Keating, P., & Seidenberg, M. S. (2000). Language deficits in dyslexic children: Speech perception, phonology, and morphology. *Journal of Experimental Child Psychology, 77(1)*, 30-60.

Kaan, E., Harris, A., Gibson, E., & Holcomb, P. J. (2000). The P600as an index of integration difficulty. *Language and Cognitive Processes, 15*, 159-201.

Kako, E. T. (1999). The event semantics of syntactic structure (meanings of words, grammatical roles). *Dissertation Abstracts International: Section B. The Sciences and Engineering, 59*, 6085.

Kempe, V., & MacWhinney, B. (1999). Processing of morphological and semantic cues in Russian and German. *Language and Cognitive Processes, 14*, 129-171.

Kotz, S. A., & Friederici, A. D. (2003). Electrophysiology of normal and pathological language processing. *Journal of Neurolinguistics, 16(1)*, 43-58.

Kutas, M., & Besson, M. (1999). Electrical signs of languages in the brain. In C. Fuchs & S. Robert (Eds.), Language Diversity and Cognitive Representation (pp. 159-178). Philadelphia: John Benjamins.

Kutas, M., Lindamood, T., & Hillyard, S. A. (1984). Word expectancy and event-related brain potentials during sentence processing. In S. Kornbloom & J. Requin (Eds.), *Preparatory States and Processes* (pp. 217-237). Hillsdale, NJ: Erlbaum.

Kutas, M., & Schmitt, B. (2003). Language in microvolts. In M. T. Banich & M. Mack (Eds.), *Mind, brain, and language* (pp. 171-209). Mahwah, NJ: Erlbaum.

Kutas, M., & Van Petten, G. K. (1994). Psycholinguistic electrified: Event-related brain potential investigations. In M. N. Gernsbacher (Ed.), *Handbook of Psycholinguistics* (pp. 83-143). San Diego: Academic Press.

Leikin, M. (2002). Processing Words' Syntactic Functions in Normal and Dyslexic readers. *Journal of Psycholinguistic Research, 31(2)*, 145-163.

Leikin, M. (under review). Syntactic processing in two languages by native and bilingual adult readers: An ERP study.

Leikin, M., & Assayag, O. (2004). Expression of syntactic complexity in Hebrew sentence comprehension: A comparison between dyslexic and normal readers. *Reading and Writing, 17(7-8)*, 801-821.

Leikin, M., & Even-Zur, H. (2006). Difficulties in L2 Hebrew reading among Russian-Speaking second graders. *Journal of Psycholinguistic Research*. 2006, *35(6)*.

Leikin, M., & Breznitz, Z. (1999). Syntactic processing of Hebrew sentences: ERP measures. *Genetic, Social, and General Psychology Monographs, 2*, 173-191.

Leikin, M., & Breznitz, Z. (2001). Effects of Accelerated Reading Rate on Syntactic Processing of Hebrew Sentences: Electrophysiological Evidence. *Genetic, Social, and General Psychology Monographs, 127(2)*, 193-209.

Levelt, W. J. M. (1989). *Speaking: From Intention to Articulation*. Cambridge, MA: MIT Press.

Levin, I., Ravid, D., & Rapaport, S. (1999). Developing morphological awareness and learning to write: A two-way street. In T. Nunes (Ed.), *Integrating research and practice in literacy*. Amsterdam: Kluwer.

MacDonald, J. L., Bock, J. K., & Kelly, M. N. (1993). Word order and world order: Semantic, phonological, and metrical determinants of serial position. *Cognitive Psychology, 25*, 188-230.

MacDonald, J. L., Pearlmutter, N. J., & Seidenberg, M. S. (1994). The lexical nature of syntactic ambiguity resolution. *Psychological Review, 101*, 676-703.

Mitchel, D. C. (1987). Reading and syntactic analysis. In J. Beech & A. Colley (Eds.), *Cognitive Approaches to Reading* (pp. 87-112). Chichester: Wiley.

Mitchel, D. C. (1994). Sentence parsing. In M. N. Gernsbacher (Ed.), *Handbook of Psycholinguistics* (pp. 375-409). San Diego: Academic Press.

Molfese, D. L., Burger-Judisch, L. M., & Gill, L. A. (1996). Electrophysiological correlates of noun-verb processing in adults. *Brain and Language, 54*, 388-413.

Mueller, J. L. (2005). Electrophysiological correlates of second language processing. *Second Language Research, 21, 2*, 152-174.

Muente, T. F., Wieringa, B. M., Weyerts, H., Szentkuti, A., Matzke, M., & Johannes, S. (2001). Differences in brain potentials to open and closed class words: Class and frequency effects. *Neuropsychologia, 39*, 91-102.

Neville, H. J., Nicol, J. L., Barss, A., Forster, K. I., & Garrett, M. F. (1991). Syntactically based sentence processing classes: Evidence from event-related brain potentials. *Journal of Cognitive Neuroscience, 3*, 151-165.

Osterhout, L., & Holcomb, P. J. (1995). Event-related potentials and language comprehension. In M. D. Rugg & M. G. H. Coles (Eds.), *Electrophysiology of Mind: Event-related Brain Potentials and Cognition* (pp. 171-215). Oxford: Oxford University Press.

Osterhout, L., Holcomb, P. J., & Swinney, D. A. (1994). Brain potentials elicited by garden-path sentences: Evidence of the application of verb information during parsing. *Journal of Experimental Psychology: Learning, Memory, and Cognition, 20*, 786-803.

Perfetti, C. A. (1999). Comprehending written language: a blueprint of the reader. In C. M. Brown & P. Hagoort (Eds.), *The Neurocognition of Language* (pp. 167-208). Oxford: Oxford University Press.

Perfetti, C. A., & Liu, Y. (2005). Orthography to phonology and meaning: Comparisons across and within writing systems. *Reading-and-Writing, 18(3),* 193-210.

Preissl, H., Pulvermüller, F., Lutzenberger, W., & Birbaumer, N. (1995). Evoked potentials distinguish between nouns and verbs. *Neuroscience Letters, 197*, 81-83.

Pulvermüller, F. (1999). Words in brains language. *Behavioral Brain Science, 22*, 253-336.

Pulvermüller, F., Preissl, H., Lutzenberger, W., & Birbaumer, N. (1996). Brain rhythms of language: nouns versus verbs. *European Journal of Neuroscience, 8,* 937-41.

Regan, D. (1989). *Human Brain Electrophysiology: Evoked-Potentials and Evoked Magnetic Fields in Science and Medicine.* New York: Elsevier.

Riccio, C. A. & Hynd, G. W. (1996). Neuroanatomical and neurophysiological aspects of dyslexia. *Topics in Language Disorders, 16*, 1-13.

Shankweiler, D., Crain, S., Brady, S., & Macaruso, P. (1992). Identifying the causes of reading disabilities. In P. B. Gough, L. C. Ehri & R. Treiman (Eds.), *Reading Acquisition* (pp. 275-305). Hillsdale, NJ: Erlbaum.

Share, D. L., & Leikin, M. (2004). Developmental dyslexia in the Hebrew language. In I. Smythe, J. Everatt & R. Salter (Eds.), *International Book of Dyslexia* (pp. 113-121), Second Edition. Wileys.

Shimron, J., & Sivan, T. (1994). Reading proficiency and orthography: Evidence from Hebrew and English. *Language Learning, 44,* 5-27.

Siegel, L. S. (1993). The development of reading. In H. Reese (Ed.), *Advances in Child Development and Behavior* (Vol. 24, pp. 63-97). San Diego, CA: Academic Press.

Sokolov, J. L. (1984). Development in the functionality of grammatical cues in Hebrew sentence comprehension. *Papers and Reports on Child Language Development, 23*, 115-124.

Stelmack, R. M., Saxe, B. J., Noldy-Cullum, N., Campbell, K. B., & Armitage, R. (1988). Recognition memory for words and event-related potentials: A comparison for normal and disabled readers. *Journal of Clinical and Experimental Neuropsychology, 10*, 185-200.

Tanenhaus, M. K., & Carlson, G. N. (1989). Lexical structure and language comprehension. In W. D. Marslen-Wilson (Ed.), *Lexical Representation and Processes* (pp. 529-561). Cambridge MA: MIT Press.

Taylor, M. J., & Keenan, N. K. (1990). Event-related potentials to visual and language stimuli in normal and dyslexic children. *Psychophysiology, 27*, 318-327.

Tunmer, W. E., & Hoover, W. (1992). Cognitive linguistic factors in learning to read. In P. B. Gough, L. C. Ehri & R. Treiman (Eds.), *Reading acquisition* (pp. 175-214). Hillsdale, NJ: Erlbaum.

Van Petten, C. (1995). Words and sentences: Event-related brain potential measure. *Psychophysiology, 32*, 511-525.

Wade, T. L. B. (1994). *A comprehensive Russian grammar.* Oxford, UK: Blackwell.

8

TIMING THE METAPHORIC BRAIN

Contribution of ERPs and Source Localization to Understainding Figurative Language

Abraham Goldstein[1,2], Yossi Arzouan[1] and Miriam Faust[1,2]

[1]Gonda Brain Research Center, [2]Department of Psychology, Bar Ilan University, Ramat Gan 52900, Israel

Abstract: In a series of studies we examined the processing of unfamiliar metaphors using event related potentials (ERPs). We compared the patterns of brain electrical activity elicited by processing two-word expressions denoting literal, conventional metaphoric, and novel metaphoric meaning, as well as unrelated word pairs. Novel metaphors were drawn from poetry texts. The subjects performed a semantic judgment task in which they decided whether each word pair conveyed a meaningful expression. N400 amplitude to the second word of the pair varied as a function of expression type: literal expressions produced the smallest N400, unrelated pairs elicited the largest N400, and metaphoric expressions elicited N400 of intermediate amplitude. ERPs elicited by novel metaphors differed from those elicited by conventional metaphors both on N400 amplitude and scalp distribution. The effect of expression type was not reflected equally across the scalp, and each showed a particular time course and scalp distribution. These findings are consistent with recent brain imaging studies and complement them by adding the temporal dynamics dimension. The contribution to current models of figurative language processing will be discussed.

Key words: Event Related Potentials, N400, figurative language, metaphors, fMRI, LORETA

1. INTRODUCTION

Cognitive processes, such as language comprehension, are fast and complex and involve the interplay of multiple brain areas. Consequently, the use of behavioral measures such as accuracy and reaction time alone, which are the end-product of the various mechanisms, cannot give a full representation of the processing dynamics. Inferences about processing stages can be made by experimental manipulation of variables affecting those mechanisms, but they produce only a crude representation of the actual processes. Similarly, brain imaging techniques based on haemodynamic measures, such as fMRI and PET, are more than adequate for determining the brain regions involved in cognitive processes, but their temporal resolution is too low to capture the dynamical aspects. Typical fMRI studies summarize brain activity in the order of seconds, which in cognitive activity terms is too long. Although fMRI techniques keep improving and have occasionally reached sub-second resolution, disentangling the time course of the various processes involved requires temporal resolution in the order of milliseconds. Electrophysiological recordings, such as event-related potentials (ERPs), possess such temporal resolution, and if used correctly can contribute to our understanding of cognitive mechanisms in the brain.

In this chapter we will show how ERPs can enhance our models of one of the most interesting phenomena of human cognition: figurative language. Using ERPs as 'brain stethoscopes', which provide a dynamic depiction of the processing of information by the brain, we attempt to elucidate a key question in language: whether the comprehension of metaphors, particularly unfamiliar ones, is achieved by the same mechanisms used for understanding literal expressions.

People encounter and use metaphoric expressions regularly in their daily lives. Expressions such as "that lawyer is a shark" are not meant to be taken literally but entail an alternative meaning. For example, when we say that 'brain waves are stethoscopes' we do not mean to say that brain waves (the topic or target of the metaphor) are really stethoscopes (the vehicle or base). Instead, our intention is to suggest that some properties of stethoscopes can be attributed to brain waves; just as cardiologists use stethoscopes to study the workings of the heart, neuroscientists can use brain waves to study the workings of the brain. It is of no surprise that several different models have been postulated to explain how the brain deals with such duality. One of the main issues that distinguish between the various models is whether metaphorical expressions are processed using the same mechanisms that are used for understanding literal meanings. A further matter is the degree of involvement of the right hemisphere (RH) in understanding figurative meaning.

According to the standard pragmatic model (Grice, 1975), the literal meaning of a phrase has to be discarded before attempting to arrive at the metaphorical meaning. Literal and figurative meanings are processed in qualitatively different manners, with precedence for the literal one which is always automatically processed. Thus, when we hear the phrase 'brain waves are stethoscopes', we first try to access the literal meaning and only after failing we try to find a metaphorical one. In contrast, other models (e.g., Glucksberg, 2003; Gibbs, 1984) hold a parallel-processing view, in which both metaphoric and literal meanings are processed concurrently and involve the same mechanisms. Furthermore, according to these models, processing non-literal language does not require initial processing of the literal meaning and the metaphoric meaning can be accessed directly.

Empirical studies measuring reading or comprehension time have usually favored the direct-access approach, and have found no differences in the time it takes to understand literal and metaphoric expressions (Harris, 1976; McElree & Nordlie, 1999), especially following sufficient context (Inhoff et al., 1984; Shinjo & Myers, 1987). Other behavioral studies have also shown that both metaphorical and literal meanings are activated immediately (Keysar, 1989; Blasko & Connine, 1993), even when the literal meaning was by itself acceptable (Gildea & Glucksberg, 1983), demonstrating that metaphors are understood as quickly as literal expressions. However, behavioral results have not provided a clear-cut solution to how metaphors are processed.

Comprehension of unfamiliar or novel metaphors, such as those used in poetry and other creative texts, has been, for the most part, overlooked, in spite of findings suggesting that novel metaphors are processed differently than conventional ones (Blank, 1988). Thus, the claim that figurative and literal meaning is accessed concurrently is based largely on studies of conventional metaphors. However, a few models have proposed distinct operations for novel and conventional metaphors. The graded salience hypothesis (Giora, 1997) posits that the factor determining precedence of access is salience. The salient meaning, either figurative or literal, is the one always processed first. The figurative meaning in conventional metaphors is commonly more salient than the literal one, thus in most 'dead' metaphors the figurative meaning is accessed first. Also, context can make either the figurative or the literal meaning more salient. In contrast, when a novel or unfamiliar metaphor is encountered, the salient meaning is the literal one, and the figurative meaning is inferred later by contextual mechanisms.

An additional model (Bowdle & Gentner, 2005) posits different processing of novel and conventional metaphors. According to the structural-mapping theory (Gentner, 1983), metaphors are comprehended by establishing correspondences between partially isomorphic conceptual structures of the target and base. This comparison process is elicited when comprehending novel metaphors. As metaphors get conventionalized they become associated with a metaphoric category and may be processed using categorization as well. Categorization is more rapid and less computationally costly than comparison but requires an existing metaphoric category. When a novel metaphor (phrased as metaphor and not as simile) is encountered, an initial categorization attempt fails in lack of a well-defined category. Novel metaphors are thus processed sequentially, and the comparison process begins after determining that the literal meaning cannot be sensibly applied.

A related unresolved question concerns the amount of resources required to process metaphors. Even if metaphors are processed automatically and using the same mechanisms as literal language they seem to require extra effort or entail processing costs during comprehension (Noveck, Bianco, & Castry, 2001). As noted by Coulson and Van Petten (2002), equivalent processing time does not necessarily mean equivalent effort. Although the majority of models suggest that comprehending metaphorical language places heavier demands on the comprehension process, most of the empirical work has aimed to determine the directness of access ignoring the possibility of differential resource demands. Furthermore, relatively coarse measures such as reading or comprehension times might not be accurate enough to detect subtle differences in processing demands.

2. METAPHORS AND ERPS

Electrophysiological recordings can help improve our understanding of the time course of metaphoric expressions processing by providing measures of brain activity with very high temporal resolution. Different processes are reflected as different ERP components, whereas variations in effort or difficulty are manifested as amplitude or latency differences in a specific component. Only a handful of studies have investigated metaphors using ERPs (Bonnaud, Gil, & Ingrand, 2002; Coulson, & Van Petten, 2002; Iakimova, Passerieux, Laurent, & Hardy-Bayle, 2005; Kazmerski, Blasko, & Dessalegn, 2003; Laurent, Denhieres, Passerieux, Iakimova, & Hardy-Bayle, 2006; Pynte, Besson, Robichon, & Poli, 1996; Tartter, Gomes, Dubrovsky, Molholm, & Stewart, 2002). As most of the ERP research on language processes, these studies have focused on a particular ERP component, the N400, which is a negative deflection peaking approximately 400 ms after stimulus presentation. The amplitude of the N400 has been shown to vary systematically with the processing of semantic information and can be thought of as a general index of the ease or difficulty of retrieving stored conceptual knowledge associated with a word (Kutas & Federmeier, 2000). Retrieval difficulty is dependent on the stored representation itself (word class, frequency, etc.) and on retrieval cues provided by immediate and discourse context (Kutas et al., in press).

When studying metaphoric language using ERPs, subjects are usually presented short sentences with literal meaning (e.g., 'Those animals are lions', 'The camel is a desert animal') and sentences with metaphorical meaning ('Those fighters are lions', 'The camel is a desert taxi'). ERPs are usually time-locked to the final word of the sentence, which carries the meaning type and is presented separately. In general, final words of sentences with metaphorical meaning elicit N400s of greater amplitude than final words of sentences with literal meaning (Coulson & Van Petten, 2002; Kazmerski et al., 2003; Pynte et al., 1996; Tartter et al., 2002;).

When compared to anomalous sentences or scrambled metaphors ('The camel is a desert table'), ending words of metaphors elicit reduced N400 amplitude (tarter, kazmerski). Tartter et al. (2002) reported that at an earlier time window (200 ms) final words of anomalous expressions and metaphors elicit similar waveforms which are different from those elicited by literal expressions. Disregarding cloze probability and frequency differences between anomalous, metaphoric, and literal sentences, this could indicate that metaphors are initially viewed by the brain as semantic anomalies. Nevertheless, by the time the N400 is elicited the metaphorical meaning has been already accessed, as reflected by the reduced N400 of metaphors relative to anomalous sentences.

The fact that metaphoric meaning can be accessed early on in the processing course does not necessarily mean that it is mandatory.

In a sentence verification task Kazmerski et al. (2003) found N400 differences between metaphoric and anomalous expressions only in participants with high IQ scores but not in participants with low IQ scores, even though in a subsequent test all participants were able to comprehend the metaphorical meaning. Thus, apparently only subjects that had enough available resources to handle metaphoric as well as literal meaning gained access to the figurative sense, whereas individuals with lower resources performed the task without accessing the metaphoric meaning.

In general, apart from a quantitative increase in N400 amplitude, ERP waveforms elicited by target words show no indication of qualitatively different processing of metaphoric and literal sentences. This suggests that accessing the meaning of words in metaphoric expressions is performed using the comprehension mechanisms used for literal language comprehension, but it requires more effort. This continuity claim is further supported by Coulson and Van Petten (2002). They presented subjects with sentences that ended with words used literally, metaphorically, or in an intermediate "literal mapping" condition which made it easier for subjects to bridge the domains of base and target. They found a gradual increase in N400 amplitude from literal to literal mapping to metaphors. Final words in sentences requiring a mapping between two concrete and literal concepts (literal mappings) elicited N400 amplitudes halfway between those elicited by literal and metaphorical sentences. This was thought to reflect a processing continuity such that literal and figurative processing occur in the same time course and involve the same mechanisms. However continuity does not mandate processing equivalence and metaphoric access is more effortful (Coulson & Van Petten, 2002).

Accessing the figurative meaning of a metaphor can be facilitated by preceding contextual information, and is reflected in decreased N400 amplitudes to target words of metaphoric expressions following relevant context (Pynte et al., 1996, Exps 3,4). The salience of the metaphoric expression can also affect the ease of meaning extraction as illustrated in a semantic judgment task (Laurent et al., 2006). In that experiment subjects judged the semantic relatedness of a probe word to the meaning of a salient or non-salient idiomatic expression. Probe words having a metaphorical relation with a salient idiom elicited N400 of reduced amplitudes as compared to probes metaphorically related to non-salient idioms or probes literally related to the idiom. These findings agree with the graded salience hypothesis

(Giora, 1997) which claims that salience, and not figurativity per se, is what determines precedence of access. Whenever the metaphoric meaning is made salient, either by context or familiarity, it should be accessed more readily accessed.

Regarding processing stages later than the retrieval of the semantic information of words, findings in the literature are less consistent. The late positive component (LPC) or P600 usually appears following the N400 and has been thought to reflect sentence-level integration (Kaan, Harris, Gibson, & Holcomb, 2000) or re-analysis (Friederici, 1995) and memory retrieval processes (Paller & Kutas, 1992; Rugg, Cox, Doyle, & Wells, 1995). Coulson & Van Petten (2002) reported larger LPCs for endings of metaphoric sentences, compared to literal and literal-mapping endings. This was interpreted as reflecting recovery and integration of additional material from semantic memory. In contrast, Pynte et al. (1996) did not find significant LPC differences between literal expressions and conventional metaphors, or between conventional and unfamiliar metaphors. However, they do report an effect of context relevance. Metaphors that were preceded by irrelevant context elicited larger N400s and smaller LPCs than those following relevant context, regardless of familiarity.

In sum, ERPs seem to favor a parallel access view, and demonstrate early, yet not obligatory, access to metaphorical meaning. The difficulty of access of the metaphoric meaning appears to be modulated by context and saliency. When encountered with a sentence in which the metaphorical meaning is salient, due to context or familiarity, the metaphorical meaning is accessed with relative ease. The ERP findings are consistent with behavioral data which support these models, and they assist on pinpointing the processing stages at which metaphorical meaning is achieved. As will be demonstrated in the following section, the usefulness of the ERP method can be increased by estimating the neural generators of the waveforms using source localization techniques.

3. HEMISPHERIC DIFFERENCES

The involvement of the right hemisphere (RH) in understanding figurative meanings has recently attracted growing attention. Although the RH has been classically thought to be irrelevant to language processing, recent behavioral, neuropsychological and imaging studies have shown evidence of the unique contribution of the RH in integrating information to understand discourse themes and ambiguous expressions such as jokes and metaphors. For example, RH damaged patients have been found to show difficulties in understanding connotative meanings of words and appreciating metaphors (Brownell, Potter, Michelow, & Gardner, 1984; Brownell, Simpson, Bihrle, Potter, & Gardner, 1990). Similarly, studies using divided visual field presentation with normal subjects have found that distant and metaphoric meanings are maintained significantly longer in the RH than in the LH (Anaki, Faust, & Kravetz, 1998; Chiarello, 1991; Schmidt, DeVuse, & Seger, in press) and thus may provide the means to comprehend the non-literal meaning of discourse and sentences. However, the empirical evidence is inconsistent. Other neuropsychological studies have found deficits in metaphor in LH as well as in RH damaged patients (Chobor & Schweiger, 1998; Gagnon, Goulet, Giroux, & Joanette, 2003). Furthermore, additional studies show even a greater specific impact of LH damage in metaphor comprehension (Zaidel, Zaidel, Oxbury, & Oxbury, 1995; Zaidel, Kasher, Soroker, & Batori, 2002).

Recent brain imaging studies have shown activation in RH areas when subjects are given metaphorical expressions (Ahrens et al., in press; Bottini et al., 1994; Mashal, Faust, & Hendler, 2005; Mashal, Faust, Hendler, & Jung-Beeman, in press; Stringaris et al., 2006). However, other fMRI studies have found no evidence for RH activation in metaphoric language processing, and, instead, showed increased activation in LH areas (Eviatar & Just, 2006; Lee & Dapretto, 2006; Rapp, Leube, Erb, Grodd, & Kircher, 2004; Stringaris et al., in press).

These contradictory findings might be due to differences in the stimuli and tasks used in the various studies. First, a distinction should be made between conventional (familiar) metaphors and novel (unfamiliar) ones. According to various models (Giora, 1997; Bowdle & Gentner, 2005), the mechanisms used for comprehending conventional metaphors are different from those used on novel ones. Two fMRI studies that distinguished between conventional and novel metaphors (Mashal et al., in press; Ahrens et al., in press) have indeed reported more RH activity when processing novel metaphors as compared to conventional metaphoric expressions. Studies which used only familiar metaphors (Lee & Dapretto, 2006; Stringaris et al. in press) or did not make a distinction (Rapp et al., 2004; Rapp, Leube, Erb, Grodd, & Kircher, in press) did not find more RH activity when extracting metaphoric relative to literal meaning. Thus, the type of stimuli used may determine the hemispheric activity pattern.

However, a major factor contributing to the inconsistencies might be the low temporal resolution of the measuring devices. Imaging techniques aggregate the brain activity over time-epochs of a few seconds, which in cognitive processing terms is too long. Relatively small changes in RH activity occurring only at determined time frames might go undetected if activity is averaged over a whole epoch or if it is measured only at fixed stages. Consequently, hemispheric asymmetries would have to be large-scaled or long-lasting to be detected by using those methods. Changes in asymmetry patterns over time are thus not easily captured using fMRI. In order to reveal the dynamics of hemispheric activity the temporal resolution of electrophysiological techniques is necessary.

ERP experiments so far have not tested deliberately the RH involvement in metaphor comprehension. Most studies report symmetric scalp distribution of ERP components, and only one study (Tartter et al., 2002) reports a small right topographic effect in one of the experiments. However, recently, Sotillo et al. (2005) used a source localization algorithm on ERPs and found differential RH activity when processing words related to the metaphorical meaning of a preceding sentence. In that study, participants were presented novel metaphoric phrases (e.g., '*Green lung of the city*') followed by a word that could ('*park*') or could not ('*semaphore*') be defined by the phrases and had to indicate the degree of correspondence (high/low). Low-resolution brain electro-magnetic tomography (LORETA) was applied to the N400 component elicited by the target words. LORETA is a discrete linear solution for the EEG inverse problem which calculates the three-dimensional current density distribution of the neural generators in the brain under the assumption that for each voxel the current density should be as close as possible to the average current density of the neighboring voxels ('contiguity') (Pascual-Marqui, 1999; Pascual-Marqui, Michel, & Lehmann, 1994; Pascual-Marqui, Esslen, Kochi, & Lehmann, 2002). The LORETA solutions revealed that related words elicited the highest activation relative to unrelated words at the posterior part of the right middle/superior temporal gyrus (Sotillo et al., 2005).

Source localization methods can be used to add the temporal dimension to hemispheric asymmetries. In a series of recent studies (Arzouan, Goldstein & Faust, 2007), we investigated the asymmetric activity elicited by word-pair expressions denoting literal (e.g., *burning fire*, *problem resolution*), conventional metaphoric (e.g., *lucid mind*, *transparent intention*), novel metaphoric (e.g., *ripe dream*, *conscience storm*) meanings, as well as unrelated (e.g., *indirect blanket, wisdom wash)* word pairs (because of Hebrew grammar, the order of words in the translated examples was actually reversed). The novel metaphoric expressions were drawn from poetry texts. The list was pre-tested for metaphoricity, familiarity, length, frequency, class and concreteness using subjective ratings from a different group of participants. Apart from word-pair metaphoricity and familiarity, words in the four conditions were balanced for the rest of the measures. The two-word expressions were presented in a random order, one word at a time, each for 200 ms with an interval of 200 ms between words. Participants were instructed to "judge whether the presented two-word expression conveys a meaning (be it literal or metaphoric) or does not convey a meaning as a pair," and press a corresponding key. ERPs to the second word of the expression were derived and entered into a neural-source estimation algorithm (LORETA), and current density at each brain area was compared between expression types.

Figure 1 shows the LORETA solutions of the grand average of 28 right-handed native Hebrew speakers for each expression type at the N400 window (325-425 ms after second word presentation). Computations were made using a three-shell spherical head model registered to the Talairach space of the brain's gray matter. The procedure yielded current densities for 2394 voxels, with a spatial resolution of 7 mm and a temporal resolution on the order of 4 milliseconds. Anatomical labeling of voxels is performed according to the MNI305 atlas (Collins, Neelin, Peters, & Evans, 1994). As can be seen in the figure, unrelated word pairs and novel metaphoric expressions elicited activity at the right temporal regions (upward pointing arrows) whereas literal and conventional metaphoric expressions did not. However, the left supramarginal gyrus (SMG) was activated only by literal expressions and conventional metaphors (downward pointing arrows).

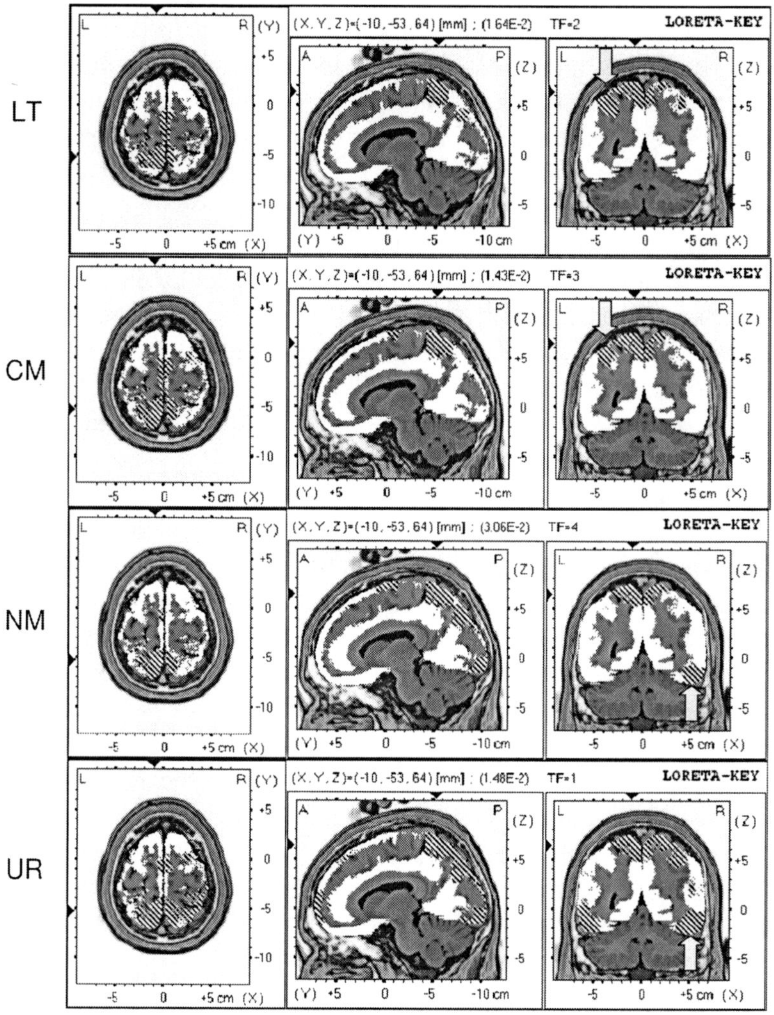

Figure 1. LORETA solution views of the average N400 distribution for each condition. Areas of significant activation are shown with slanted-lines pattern. Upward pointing arrows indicate right temporal areas activated in the novel metaphor and unrelated conditions. Downward pointing arrows indicate left supramarginal regions activated in the literal and conventional metaphor conditions. EEG was recorded using a 65-chanel geodesic net (Electrical Geodesics Inc.) at a 250 Hz sampling rate using a 0.1-100 Hz bandpass filter. Data were further filtered (40 Hz) and referenced to an average reference offline. ERPs were time-locked to the onset of the second word of the pair. Epochs were 1000 ms long with a 100 ms pre-stimulus baseline. Trials with eye movement and other artifacts were removed.

Current density estimates at frontal and temporal regions of interest known to be involved in language task were further analyzed in order to compare the activation of the left and right homologues for the various expression types. In the temporal regions (inferior, middle, and superior gyri) literal and conventional metaphoric expressions showed higher current densities in the LH than the RH, whereas novel metaphors and unrelated pairs showed the opposite pattern. At more anterior regions (inferior, middle, and medial gyri) all expressions showed significantly more activation at the LH homologues. The only exception was the superior frontal gyrus in which novel metaphoric expressions showed a right asymmetry whereas the rest of the expression types elicited more LH activity.

These results are in agreement with those of the imaging studies that have distinguished novel from conventional metaphors. It appears that novel metaphoric expressions activate RH temporal areas more than conventional metaphors or literal expressions. The advantage of ERP data is that it enabled to identify the processing stage at which such hemispheric asymmetries occur. The N400 component is related to general index of the ease or difficulty of retrieving stored conceptual knowledge associated with a word (Kutas & Federmeier, 2000). Understanding novel metaphors requires the retrieval of more semantic information about the words in order to bridge the gap between seemingly unrelated words. And indeed, the RH temporal regions have been found to be involved in integration of semantic information during discourse (Caplan & Dapretto, 2001; St George, Kutas, Martinez, & Sereno, 1999). The neural sources of the scalp-recorded N400 have been estimated to be the left and (though somewhat less) right temporal lobes (Van Petten & Luka, 2006). The contribution of right areas appears to be augmented for the processing of novel metaphors.

An additional approach to examine changes in hemispheric activity over time is to use statistical non-parametric mapping (SnPM; Nichols & Holmes, 2002). In this technique for each condition and on each time point current density was compared to baseline (random and homogenous average level of the 100 ms pre-stimulus activity) on a voxel-by-voxel basis (Sinai & Pratt, 2003), and correcting for multiple comparisons (Holmes, Blair, Watson, & Ford, 1996; Nichols & Holmes, 2002). The number of voxels with t-value above threshold level of p=0.01 were then counted for each hemisphere at each time point to evaluate the contribution of each hemisphere. As can be seen in Figure 2, the fluctuations in the number of supra-threshold voxels were mostly parallel in both hemispheres. Nevertheless, asymmetries occurred during various periods. Novel metaphoric expressions elicited more relative RH activity (as reflected by the number of supra-threshold voxels) at two time windows, 350-450 ms and 550-750 ms approximately, with three prominent peaks at about 425, 600 and 710 ms (see dotted arrows). At those same time windows (and throughout most of the epoch), CM words showed relative greater LH activity (solid arrows). LT and UR expressions elicited more relative LH activity mainly at the first time window. Although this approach estimates the bulk activity of each hemisphere, it does assist on giving a general picture of the dynamics of hemispheric interactions. Apart from revealing the relative LH and RH asymmetries at specific stages, the results indicate that both hemispheres were active during the comprehension process of all expressions as reflected in the absolute current density values and the number of active voxels in each hemisphere.

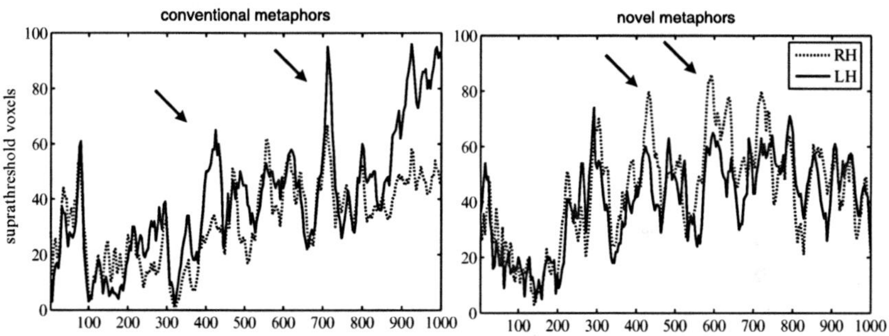

Figure 2. Number of total supra-threshold voxels in the LH (solid lines) and the RH (dotted lines) for conventional and novel metaphors.

An additional advantage of electrophysiological recordings emerges when the time course of activation of a specific area is analyzed. To illustrate this we show here current density estimates for every time-point at the left and right homologues of Brodmann area 22 (superior temporal gyrus, including Wernicke). Figure 3 shows the time course of activation at this area. There is a striking effect of greater novel metaphor activity in the RH between 200 ms to 600 ms post-stimulus relative to the other expression types. However, at the N400 window, novel metaphors elicit significant LH activity as well.

Relatively more LH activity can be seen for literal expressions, conventional metaphors and unrelated pairs at the late parts of the waveform. Metaphors have been shown to activate the RH at temporal gyri (Ahrens et al., in press; Mashal et al., in press; Sotillo et al., 2005; Stringaris, Medford, Giampietro, Brammer, & David, in press), but LH activation have been found as well (Lee & Dapretto, 2006; Rapp et al., 2004). This type of analysis can elucidate the seemingly contradictory results in the brain imaging literature. Precise timing is essential to uncover the patterns of hemispheric activity as well as the differential processing of the various linguistic expressions.

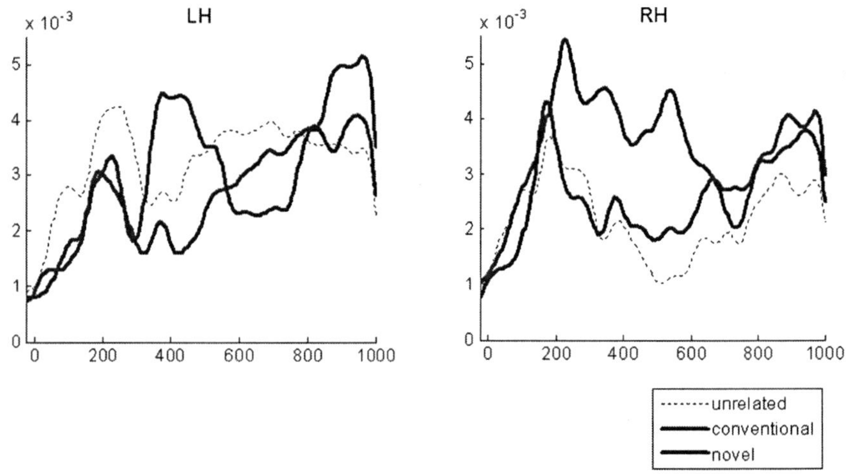

Figure 3. Time course of activity for the various expression types at the superior temporal gyri (Brodmann area 22). Left and right panels show the left and right hemisphere homologues, respectively. Activity is measured in current density units.

The results from spatial-temporal analyses agree with the models of metaphor processing that stress the differential processing of novel and conventional metaphors. The graded salience hypothesis (Giora, 1997) posits that the factor determining precedence of access is salience. The metaphoric meaning of conventional metaphors is usually the salient one and is immediately accessed, whereas a novel metaphoric meaning is less salient and is inferred by contextual mechanisms. The RH has been reported to be sensitive to less salient linguistic material (Burgess & Simpson, 1988; Faust & Chiarello, 1998; Faust & Lavidor, 2003).

Similarly, according to the structural-mapping theory (Gentner, 1983), metaphors are comprehended by establishing correspondences between partially isomorphic conceptual structures of the target and base. This comparison process is elicited when comprehending novel metaphors. As metaphors get conventionalized they become associated with a metaphoric category and may be processed using categorization as well (Bowdle & Gentner, 2005). Categorization is more rapid and less computationally costly than comparison but requires an existing metaphoric category. When a novel metaphor (phrased as metaphor and not as simile) is encountered, an initial categorization attempt fails in lack of a well-defined category. Novel metaphors are thus processed sequentially, and the comparison process begins after determining that the literal meaning cannot be sensibly applied. The greater overall activity and RH asymmetry at the N400 and LPC components elicited by processing novel metaphoric expressions might be a reflection of the structural mapping mechanisms.

4. SUMMARY

Our findings, together with other recent imaging studies, suggest that the literal-figurative hemispheric language dichotomy in its strong form is not an accurate representation of the way the brain derives linguistic meaning (Rapp et al., in press). Both hemispheres are engaged in the comprehension process of both literal and metaphoric expressions, thus simple dichotomies are not an appropriate description. The differential contribution of each hemisphere in literal and figurative language comprehension is relatively subtle and varies during the different processing stages. Previous studies that looked at metaphor processing lacked the temporal precision to uncover this complicated interaction pattern and therefore showed either LH or RH involvement. The addition of the temporal dimension demonstrates that RH mechanisms are necessary, but not sufficient, for understanding metaphoric expressions. Both hemispheres work in concert in a complex dynamical pattern during literal and figurative language comprehension.

Electrophysiological recordings with high temporal resolution together with source localization algorithms such as LORETA are a viable tool for measuring this type of activity patterns. However, interpreting source localization findings should be done with the caveat that they are only estimations of the true neural sources of activity and are acceptable as long as their assumptions are correct.

Nevertheless, convergent results resulting from different methods attest to the validity of each of the techniques used.

In sum, we can describe two strategies of cognitive neuroscience research using a novel metaphor: "Brain scientists are realtors". There are two mantras in the real estate jargon. The first one – "location, location, location" – is generally used in brain imaging studies which place much of the weight on the specific brain areas activated by the particular task at hand. The second real-estate mantra is "timing is everything", and is emphasized in ERP studies that investigate the processing stages revealed while performing the task. In this approach timing and amplitude differences in waveform patterns are the main interest, regardless of their neural generators. We believe that the use of source localization techniques can combine both approaches and generate a more comprehensive depiction of the way our brains work.

REFERENCES

Ahrens, K., Liu, H. L., Lee, C. Y., Gong, S. P., Fang, S. Y., & Hsu, Y. Y. (2007). Functional MRI of conventional and anomalous metaphors in Mandarin Chinese. *Brain and Language*, *100*, 163-171.

Anaki, D., Faust, M., & Kravetz, S. (1998). Cerebral hemispheric asymmetries in processing lexical metaphors. *Neuropsychologia*, *36*, 353-362.

Arzouan, Y., Goldstein, A., & Faust, M. (2007). Dynamics of hemispheric activity during metaphor comprehension: Electrophysiological measures. *NeuroImage*, *36*, 222-231.

Blank, G. D. (1988). Metaphors in the lexicon. *Metaphor and Symbol, 3*, 21-36.

Blasko, D. G., & Connine, C. M. (1993). Effects of familiarity and aptness on metaphor processing. *Journal of Expperimental Psychology. Learning, Memory, and Cognition, 19*, 295-308.

Bonnaud V., Gil, R., & Ingrand, P. (2002). Metaphorical and non-metaphorical links: a behavioral and ERP study in young and elderly adults. *Neurophysiologie Clinique, 32*, 258-268.

Bottini, G., Corcoran, R., Sterzi, R., Paulesu, E., Schenone, P., Scarpa, P., Frackowiak, R. S. J., & Frith, C. D. (1994). The role of the right hemisphere in the interpretation of figurative aspects of language: A positron emission tomography activation study. *Brain*, *117*, 1241-1253.

Bowdle, B., & Gentner, D. (2005). The career of metaphor. *Psychological Review, 112*, 193-216.

Brownell, H. H., Potter, H. H., Michelow, D., & Gardner, H. (1984). Sensitivity to lexical denotation and connotation in brain-demaged patients: A double dissociation. *Brain and Language, 22*, 253-265.

Brownell, H. H., Simpson, T. L., Bihrle, A. M., Potter, H. H., & Gardner, H. (1990). Appreciation of metaphoric alternative word meanings by left and right brain damaged patients. *Neuropsychologia*, *28*, 375-383.

Burgess, C., & Simpson, G. (1988). Cerebral hemispheric mechanisms in the retrieval of ambiguous word meanings. *Brain and Language*, *3*, 86-103.

Caplan, R., & Dapretto, M. (2001). Making sense during conversation: an fMRI study. *NeuroReport*, *12*, 3625-3632.

Chiarello, C. (1991). Interpretation of word meanings in the cerebral hemispheres: One is not enough. In P. J. Schwanenflugel (Eds.), *The psychology of word meanings* (pp. 251-275). Hillsdale, NJ: Erlbaum.

Chobor, K. L., & Schweiger, A. (1998). Processing of lexical ambiguity in patients with traumatic brain injury. *Journal of Neurolinguistics, 11*, 119-136.

Collins, D. L., Neelin, P., Peters, T. M., & Evans, A. C. (1994). Automatic 3D intersubject registration of MR volumetric data in standardized Talairach space. *Journal of Computer Assisted Tomog*raphy, *18*, 192-205.

Coulson, S., & Van Petten, C. (2002). Conceptual integration and metaphor: An event-related potential study. *Memory & Cognition, 30*, 958-968.

Eviatar, Z., & Just, M. A. (2006). Brain correlates of discourse processing: An fMRI investigation of irony and conventional metaphor comprehension. *Neuropsychologia, 44*, 2348-2359.

Faust, M., & Chiarello, C. (1998). Sentence context and lexical ambiguity resolution by the two hemispheres. *Neuropsychologia, 3*, 827-836.

Faust, M., & Lavidor, M. (2003). Semantically convergent and semantically divergent priming in the cerebral hemispheres: Lexical decision and semantic judgment. *Cognitive Brain Research, 17,* 585-597.

Friederici, A. D. (1995). The time course of syntactic activation during language processing: A model based on neuropsychological and neurophysiological data. *Brain and Language, 50*, 259-281.

Gagnon, L., Goulet, P., Giroux, F., & Joanette, Y. (2003). Processing of metaphoric and non-metaphoric alternative meaning of words after right- and left-hemispheric lesion. *Brain and Language*, *87*, 217-226.

Gentner, D. (1983). Structure-mapping: A theoretical framework for analogy. *Cognitive Science*, *7*, 155-170.

Gibbs, R. W. (1984). Literal meaning and psychological theory. *Cognitive Science*, *8(3)*, 275-304.

Gildea, P., & Glucksberg, S. (1983). On understanding metaphor: The role of context. *Journal Verbal Learning and Verbal Behavior*, *22(5)*, 577-590.

Giora, R., (1997). Understanding figurative and literal language: The graded salience hypothesis. *Cognitive Linguistics*, *8*, 183-206.

Glucksberg, S. (2003). The psycholinguistics of metaphor. *Trends in Cognitive Sciences, 7(2)*, 92-96.

Grice, H. P. (1975). Logic and conversation. In P. Cole, J. L. Morgan, (Eds.), *Syntax and semantics: Vol. 3. Speech acts* (pp. 41-58). New York, NY: Academic Press.

Harris, R. J. (1976). Comprehension of metaphors: A test of the two-stage processing model. *Bulletin of the Psychonomic Society*, *8(4),* 312-314.

Holmes, A. P., Blair, R. C., Watson, J. D. G., & Ford, I. (1996). Nonparametric analysis of statistic images from functional mapping experiments. *Journal of Cerebral Blood Flow & Metabolism*, *16*, 7-22.

Iakimova, G., Passerieux, C., Laurent, J. P., & Hardy-Bayle, M. C. (2005). ERPs of metaphoric, literal, and incongruous semantic processing in schizophrenia. *Psychophysiology*, *42*, 380-90.

Inhoff, A. W., Lima, S. D., & Carroll, P. J. (1984). Contextual effects on metaphor comprehension in reading. *Memory & Cognition*, *12(6)*, 558-567.

Kaan, E., Harris, A., Gibson, E., & Holcomb, P. J. (2000). The P600 as an index of syntactic integration difficulty. *Journal of Language and Cognitive Processes*, *15*, 159-201.

Kazmerski, V. A., Blasko, D. G., & Dessalegn, B. G. (2003). ERP and behavioral evidence of individual differences in metaphor comprehension. *Memory & Cognition*, *31*, 673-689.

Keysar, B. (1989). On the functional equivalence of literal and metaphorical interpretations in discourse. *Journal of Memory and Language*, *28(4)*, 375-385.

Kutas, M., & Federmeier, K. D. (2000). Electrophysiology reveals semantic memory use in language comprehension. *Trends in Cognitive Science, 4*, 463-470.

Kutas, M., Van Petten, C., & Kluender, R. (in press). Psycholinguistics Electrified II: 1994-2005. In M. J. Traxler & M. A. Gernsbacher (Eds.), *Handbook of Psycholinguistics Second Edition*. New York, NY: Elsevier Press.

Laurent, J. P., Denhières, G., Passerieux, C., Iakimova, G., & Hardy-Baylé, M. C. (2006). On understanding idiomatic language: The salience hypothesis assessed by ERPs. *Brain Research, 10*, 151-160.

Lee, S. S., & Dapretto, M. (2006). Metaphorical vs. literal word meanings: fMRI evidence against a selective role of the right hemisphere. *Neuroimage, 29(2)*, 536-44.

Mashal, N., Faust, M., & Hendler, T. (2005). The role of the right hemisphere in processing nonsalient metaphorical meanings: Application of Principal Components Analysis to fMRI data. *Neuropsychologia, 43*, 2084-2100.

Mashal, N., Faust, M., Hendler, T., & Jung-Beeman, M. (2007). An fMRI investigation of the neural correlates underlying processing of novel metaphoric expressions. *Brain and Language, 100(2)*, 115-126.

McElree, B., & Nordlie, J. (1999). Literal and figurative interpretations are computed in equal time. *Psychonomic Bulletin & Review, 6(3)*, 486-494.

Nichols, T. E., & Holmes A. P. (2002). Nonparametric permutation tests for functional neuroimaging: a primer with examples. *Human Brain Mapping, 15,* 1-25.

Noveck, I. A., Bianco, M., & Castry, A. (2001). The costs and benefits of metaphor. *Metaphor and Symbol, 16(1-2),* 109-121.

Paller, K. A., & Kutas, M. (1992). Brain potentials during memory retrieval provide neurophysiological support for the distinction between conscious recollection and priming. *Journal of Cognitive Neuroscience, 4,* 375-391.

Pascual-Marqui, R. D. (1999). Review of methods for solving the EEG inverse problem. *International Journal of Bioelectromagnetism 1*, 75-86.

Pascual-Marqui, R. D., Esslen, M., Kochi, K., & Lehmann, D. (2002). Functional imaging with low resolution brain electromagnetic tomography (LORETA): review, new comparisons, and new validation. *Jouranl of Clinical Neurophysiology, 30,* 81-94.

Pascual-Marqui, R. D., Michel, C. M., & Lehmann, D. (1994). Low resolution electromagnetic tomography: a new method for localizing electrical activity in the brain. *International Journal of Psychophysiology, 18*, 49-65.

Pynte, J., Besson, M., Robichon, F. H., & Poli, J. (1996). The time-course of metaphor comprehension: An event-related potential study. *Brain and Language, 55*, 293-316.

Rapp, A. M., Leube, D. T., Erb, M., Grodd, W., & Kircher, T. T. J. (2004). Neural correlates of metaphor processing. *Cognitive Brain Research, 20*, 395-402.

Rapp, A. M., Leube, D. T., Erb, M., Grodd, W., & Kircher, T. T. J. (2007). Laterality in metaphor processing: Lack of evidence from functional magnetic resonance imaging for the right hemisphere theory. *Brain and Language, 100(2)*, 142-149.

Rugg, M. D., Cox, C. J. C., Doyle, M. C., & Wells, T. (1995). Event-related potentials and the recollection of low and high frequency words. *Neuropsychologia, 33,* 471-484.

Schmidt, G. L., DeBuse, C. J., & Seger, C. A. (2007). Right hemisphere metaphor processing? Characterizing the lateralization of semantic processes. *Brain and Language, 100(2)*, 127-141.

Shinjo, M., & Myers, J. L. (1987). The role of context in metaphor comprehension. *Journal of Memory and Language, 26(2),* 226-241.

Sinai, A., & Pratt, H. (2003). High-resolution time course of hemispheric dominance revealed by low-resolution electromagnetic tomography. *Clinical Neurophysiology, 114*, 1181-8.

Sotillo, M., Carretie, L., Hinojosa, J. A., Tapia, M., Mercado, F., Lopez-Martin, S., et al. (2005). Neural activity associated with metaphor comprensión: Spatial análisis. *Neuroscience Letters, 373*, 5-9.

St George, M., Kutas, M., Martinez, A., & Sereno, M. I. (1999). Semantic integration in reading: engagement of the right hemisphere during discourse processing. *Brain*, *122*, 1317-1325.

Stringaris, A. K., Medford, N. C., Giampietro, V. C., Brammer, M. J., & David, A. S. (2007). Deriving meaning: Distinct neural mechanisms for metaphoric, literal, and non-meaningful sentences. *Brain and Language, 100(2)*, 150-162.

Stringaris, A. K., Medford, N. C., Giora, R., Giampietro, V. C., Brammer, M. J., & David, A. S. (2006). How metaphors influence semantic relatedness judgments: The role of the right frontal cortex. *NeuroImage*, *33*, 748-793.

Tartter, V. C., Gomes, H., Dubrovsky, B., Molholm, S., & Stewart, R. V. (2002). Novel metaphors appear anomalous at least momentarily: Evidence from N400. *Brain and Language*, *80*, 488-509.

Van Petten, C., & Luka, B. J. (2006). Neural localization of semantic context effects in electromagnetic and hemodynamic studies. *Brain and Language*, *97(3)*, 279-293.

Zaidel, D. W., Zaidel, E., Oxbury, S. M., & Oxbury, J. M. (1995). The interpretation of sentence ambiguity in patients with unilateral focal brain surgery. *Brain and Language*, *51*, 458-468.

Zaidel, E., Kasher, A., Soroker, N., & Batori, G. (2002). Effects of right and left hemisphere damage on performance of the "Right Hemisphere Communication Battery". *Brain and Language*, *80*, 510-535.

9

EEG CORRELATES OF HEMISPHERIC WORD RECOGNITION

Eran Zaidel[1,2], Andrew Hill[1] and Scott Weems[3]
[1]Department of Pschology, University of California, Los Angeles, USA, [2]Brain Research Institute, University of California, Los Angeles, USA, [3]Center for Advanced Study of Language, University of Maryland, USA.

Abstract: In several experiments, we compared behavioral and electrophysiological correlates of hemifield tachistoscopic presentations of single words and nonwords for lexical decision in English and in Hebrew. The English task showed an overall right visual field advantage for latency and accuracy, which was larger for target words than for nonwords, suggesting independent processing in each hemisphere. The right hemisphere was more sensitive to word frequency than the left, and the left hemisphere was more sensitive to orthographic regularity than the right. All lexical variables (Wordness, Frequency, Regularity, and Word Pronounceability) had physiological correlates, and those correlates were often different in the two hemispheres. Occasionally, the behavioral and physiological measures conflicted and some lexical variables had physiological but no behavioral correlates. The physiological variables can reflect early stages of information processing that are not available to conscious decision. Moreover, different cognitive phenomena may have the same EEG correlates. Thus, gamma changes as a function of Lexicality (Wordness), semantic (Word Frequency), orthographic (Word Regularity), and phonological (Nonword Pronounceability) variables.

The Hebrew lexical decision task showed an overall right visual field advantage, but not the same for target word and nonword, suggesting exclusive specialization in the left hemisphere. The EEG at rest was predictive of subsequent hemispheric specialization for lexical decision.

We also studied hemispheric error monitoring in the English task. We found that while the left hemisphere was superior for lexical decision, the right hemisphere better monitored errors and adapted to them by slowing down and becoming more accurate. Further, error correction in a given trial was negatively correlated with left asymmetry in the alpha amplitude over mid and posterior electrodes. Thus, effective error monitoring seems to require interhemispheric cooperation.

We conclude that the EEG, as currently measured, differentiate all the relevant dimensions of the lateralized lexical decision task, but that it taps different stages of processing. The EEG response in the gamma band multiply determines so that different cognitive states have the same EEG signature. Consequently, a more refined, wider range, and more theoretically informed partitioning of the EEG spectra is now due.

Key words: Event Related Potentials, reading, developmental dyslexia

1. INTRODUCTION

The purpose of this paper is to illustrate that the ongoing EEG is sensitive to and informative about the psycholinguistic variables that characterize hemispheric processing of words. We will try to draw some general theoretical conclusions about the relationship between behavior and electrophysiology from several experiments that offer new data on hemispheric word recognition.

1.1 The hemispheres are "atomic"

It is the underlying assumption of this paper that hemispheric functioning is "atomic." That is to say, it is not possible to understand complex cognitive processes without understanding the selective contribution of the two hemispheres alone and together, to the process. In particular, the two hemispheres interact in complex ways during the processing of any linguistic task, ranging from word recognition to discourse processing. One can study the role of the two hemispheres in language both behaviorally and physiologically. In this paper, we will focus on word recognition and its electrophysiological correlates. It is tempting to monitor brain activity during natural word recognition in free vision using, say, fMRI, but this approach is not optimal for analyzing the independent contributions of the two hemispheres to the process. The reason is that fMRI tends to show peaks of activity rather than secondary processes and its temporal resolution (on the order of seconds) is of an order of magnitude coarser than the cognitive window necessary for understanding psycholinguistic processes (on the order of milliseconds). Moreover, lexical processing in central, full-field vision may reflect the idiosyncratic contributions of the two hemispheres to the task, rather than their linguistic competence.

1.2 Free vision versus half visual field (VF) presentation

The preferred approach is to use lateralized presentation of target words and to monitor the associated cortical activity using dense montage EEG. Here, the stimuli are restricted to one hemisphere by flashing the targets to one visual half-field, the responses are restricted to the same hemisphere by using responses of the hand ipsilateral to the stimulated visual field, and the analysis of the EEG considers only electrodes over the hemisphere opposite the stimulated VF. In this way, we maximally restrict the analysis to one hemisphere at a time. While lateralized word recognition may appear unnatural, it is in fact the usual condition under which words are viewed during normal, fast reading (Melamed & Zaidel, 1993). This type of analysis describes the competence of each hemisphere under conditions of maximal independence from the other and is therefore more illuminating about its capacities and possible strategies than a consideration of full-field alone would allow.

1.3 Dynamic hemispheric independence

The two cerebral hemispheres may be considered two separate and independent cognitive systems each with its own cognitive repertoire—including perception, memory, language, and attention—capable of processing information in parallel. There are multiple forms of possible interaction between the two hemispheres during word recognition. The two hemispheres may process information independently of each other, they may share intermediate results, and one hemisphere may even monitor the performance of the other. We have distinguished two limit case models of hemispheric interaction during word recognition. When each hemisphere processes information projected to it independently of the other, using its own lexical representations and strategies, we refer to the situation as "direct access." A common indication of direct access is a statistically significant interaction between some independent stimulus variable and VF of presentation. For example, in visual word recognition (lexical decision) there usually occurs a significant interaction between word frequency and VF, such that low frequency words exhibit a larger deficit relative to high frequency words in the left visual field (LVF) than in the right visual field (RVF). On the other hand, when one hemisphere is exclusively specialized for processing the information and the stimuli are projected to the "wrong" hemisphere, the targeted stimulus information needs to be relayed through the corpus callosum prior to processing in the specialized hemisphere. This is called the "callosal relay model." For example, phonetic discrimination between voiced and unvoiced stop consonants is a callosal relay task exclusively specialized in the left hemisphere (LH) (Zaidel, Clarke, & Suyenobu, 1990).

1.4 The hemispheric dual route model

The dual route model of naming (in lexical decision) posits two different strategies for naming/recognizing the target word: The "lexical route" recognizes words via their visual entries in a visual lexicon. This strategy develops from experience. Frequent words have priority over infrequent ones. The "nonlexical route" assembles the name by grapheme-phoneme correspondent rules, and it is sensitive to word regularity. The hemispheric dual route model posits an addition that the normal left hemisphere can process target words using either a lexical route or a nonlexical route, whereas the right hemisphere can only use a lexical route. However, we have shown that lexical competence in the normal right hemisphere shows sensitivity to both word frequency and word regularity, but that their effects are observable only when attentional resources are limited (Zaidel, 1998). Here, we ask whether the ongoing EEG is sensitive to dual route variables so that we can infer how the actual performance in the hemisphere differs from its competence.

1.5 EEG

The EEG is characterized by superior temporal resolution, and recent methods for source localization have enriched the method with improved spatial resolution as well. The standard methodology involves Fourier analysis of the waveform in each recording electrode, focusing on the amplitude (power) of several regions in the spectra, usually from 4 Hz to 30 Hz, although more recent studies have examined EEG up to 100 Hz (Tanji, Suzuki, Delorme, Shamoto, & Nakasato, 2005). The EEG signal is assumed to reflect electrical activity in the underlying neo-cortex. Each electrode is influenced by several square millimeters of cortical space and reflects mainly synchronized components of neural activity. However, the activity in a given electrode need not reflect the activity of the directly underlying cortex.

Table 1. Common EEG spectral bands and their putative cognitive significances.

Theta	4-8 Hz	Intrinsic rhythms, non-cognitive, attention.
Alpha	7-13 Hz	Global binder, preparatory, meta cognitive, negatively correlated with specific processing.
Beta	12-25 Hz	Low beta (11.7-15 Hz): "motor alpha." Motor preparation, effortful cognitive processing.
Gamma	30-100 Hz	Activation of cell assemblies; binding, consciousness.

The cognitive significance of each band has yet to be fully understood (Table 1). In particular, each band has multiple cognitive meanings depending on the task and its context. Nonetheless, one generally distinguishes between high and low frequency of oscillations in the EEG response, with lower frequencies suggesting cortical deactivation and higher frequencies representing cognitive engagement, including sensory encoding and higher cognitive processes. Interestingly, even lower bands (e.g., theta: 4-8 Hz) are implicated in high level cognition, particularly the allocation of attention and cognitive load (Klimesch, 1999).

2. A BRIEF REVIEW OF THE LITERATURE

Lutzenberger, Pulvermuller, and Birbaumer (1994) was the first to show greater activation in the gamma band (25-30 Hz) for word presentations compared to nonword presentations during lexical decision. This difference occurred in the time window 320-520 ms, approximately the time at which lexical access is believed to occur. Interestingly, nonwords decreased power in the gamma band whereas words did not increase it. Furthermore, this difference was observed for LH electrodes only. By contrast, Weems et al. (2004a) used lateralized tachistoscopic presentations of the target stimuli and found that both hemispheres showed a relative increase in gamma power for word presentations compared to nonword presentations. Those latter differences occurred only under "strong lateralization" conditions in which one hemisphere received the stimulus information directly, responded to it alone and was paired with electrodes in the contralateral hemisphere.

Pulvermuller, Lutzenberger, and Preissl (1999) further showed that lexical decision of different classes of words elicited different spatial patterns of gamma response. Thus, nouns elicited greater gamma response over visual areas whereas verbs elicited greater gamma response over motor areas. Other gamma band findings vary widely, with Tanji et al. (2005) demonstrating high bilateral temporal gamma (up to 100 Hz) changes during naming tasks, but a preferential left temporal gamma activation in a lexical decision task. Kim and Kim (2006) demonstrated significant increases in gamma (30-50 Hz) in prefrontal, frontal, and temporal sites during word perception, with gamma activity in prefrontal and temporal areas significantly correlated with response time. In a recent review article, Bastiaansen and Hagoort (2006) suggested that language comprehension tasks show both beta (12-30 Hz) and Gamma (above 30 Hz) increases, while alpha band desyncronization may be related more to management of secondary attention required for language processing.

Many other EEG "language laterality" findings can be found in the literature. Tomberg (1999) showed increased complexity of the EEG in the left temporal lobe during reading tasks (involving lateral anterior extrasylvian temporal cortex) with no concomitant change in gamma amplitudes (at 40 Hz). In addition, Weems et al. (2004b) found that hemispheric alpha band asymmetry predicts accuracy of lexical decision, such that increased left asymmetry is related to reduced accuracy, whereas decreased asymmetry facilitates subsequent word recognition.

In addition, EEG coherence measures, indicating the degree of electrophysiological coupling of different cortical sites, show some interesting language-related differences across frequency bands. Weiss and Mueller (2003) found band coherence differences in processing language categories, such that broad changes in coherence in the 1-10 Hz range generally occurred in all language processing, suggesting this range is related to the memory and attention processes subserving linguistic perception. In contrast, they found that perception of concrete nouns relative to abstract nouns increased interhemispheric coherence (in the 13-18 Hz range) between left frontal and right posterior sites, while high-imagery verbs produced greater interhemispheric coherence (in the 11-31 Hz range) coherence measures compared to low-imagery verbs. As might be expected, the left hemisphere is preferentially involved in most EEG and language studies. Interestingly, Bizas et al. (1999) found that regional changes in EEG across different reading tasks was restricted to the left hemisphere. On the other hand, Khader and Rosler (2004) found that visual processing produced a stronger theta band desynchronization at left frontal sites for verbs than for nouns, as well as a smaller theta EEG coherence between left frontal and bilateral posterior sites for verbs than nouns, suggesting different patterns of interhemispheric interactions for processing words of different categories.

We are critically interested in the relationship between behavioral and electrophysiological indices of various psycholinguistic parameters, such as lexical status, word frequency, orthographic regularity, and semantic class. Each measure can correspond to a different stage of processing of a particular stimulus type and together the behavioral and electrophysiological measures complement each other and present a more coherent and complete characterization of the processing sequence.

3. LATERALIZED LEXICAL DECISION TASK IN ENGLISH AND IN HEBREW

3.1 Canonical effects

Here are the tasks that we used for studying the relation between behavioral and electrophysiological correlates of lexical decision in the two hemispheres.

3.1.1 English

Over the past 25 odd years, we have developed an experimental paradigm, which we found to be particularly illuminating about the potential contributions of the two cerebral hemispheres to reading. In this paradigm, character strings representing either words or orthographically pronounceable nonwords are flashed briefly (180 ms) to one visual hemifield or the other. Subjects are required to indicate with the index or middle finger of the left or the right hand whether the target string is a word or a nonword. In order to maximize independent processing by each hemisphere, lateralized underlined targets are accompanied by word or nonword distracters in the opposite VF (Iacoboni & Zaidel, 1996). Stimuli range in length from three to six letters. This task consistently exhibits three canonical effects. First, there is a robust right visual field advantage (RVFA) in both latency and accuracy reflecting left hemisphere (LH) specialization for the task. Second, there is a significant and reliable interaction between target wordness and visual field of target presentation such that words exhibit a greater RVFA than nonwords. This is taken to indicate that the task is direct access and that the right hemisphere (RH) is capable of processing the stimuli albeit less efficiently than the left. Third, the RH seems to monitor errors in the task automatically, slowing down and increasing accuracy following errors (Iacoboni, Rayman, & Zaidel, 1997). Moreover, when explicit error feedback, consisting of a smiling, a frowning or a neutral face, is presented to one visual field or the other only feedback to the LVF (RH) results in error correction consisting of slowing down and increasing accuracy (Kaplan & Zaidel, 2001).

3.1.2 Hebrew

We adapted the lateralized lexical decision experiment to Hebrew and administered it to 28 right-handed, normal young adults who were native Hebrew readers. Since the "look-ahead" during reading fixation in Hebrew occurs mostly for LVF items, we may expect Hebrew to engage a greater RH contribution than in English. Instead, results revealed a robust RVFA, larger than that observed in English. Unlike English, there was no interaction between Target Wordness and Target VF, suggesting that the task may be exclusively specialized in the LH. In that case, LVF targets would be relayed through the corpus callosum to the LH prior to decision. These data are consistent with the conclusion that Hebrew is more lateralized to the LH than English, presumably due to the root structure of lexical items in Hebrew, which engages combinatorial computational processes specialized in the LH.

We have also administered the Hebrew lateralized lexical decision task to two groups of learning disabled Israeli young adults (17 participants in each group). Again, the results showed an RVFA but a similar difference between words and nonwords in each visual field (i.e., no significant Target Wordness x Target VF interaction), consistent with callosal relay. In this case, however, the RVFA (57 ms and 35 ms, respectively, in the two groups) was comparable to English (60 ms).

3.2 Relationship of lateralized lexical decision to reading

Why should we study the lateralized lexical decision task? What will it tell us about normal reading, which appears to be much more complex than lexical decision?

3.2.1 English

We administered the English lateralized lexical decision task as well as the Nelson-Denny reading test to 66 normal young adults. We correlated performance in each VF with the Vocabulary and Reading

Comprehension measures of the Nelson-Denny. Lexical decision performance showed strong relationships with both reading measures. Specifically, Vocabulary performance correlated significantly with LVF word accuracy and with LVF nonword latency, both measures of RH performance in English. There were also significant, though somewhat weaker, correlations between Reading Comprehension and RVF nonword latency.

3.2.2 Hebrew

We correlated the Hebrew lateralized lexical decision task with performance on the MATAL Reading Comprehension Test (A. Ben Simon & Y. Cohen, personal communication, March 28, 2007). Lexical decision performance showed significant relationships of the number of omission errors (in response to reading comprehension questions) with latency (reading speed) measures of the Reading Comprehension Test. Specifically, overall RVF accuracy as well as the RVFA ([R-L]/[R+L]) correlated negatively with number of omissions, and the RVFA correlated positively with reading speed. Interestingly, LVF accuracy and RVF latency both correlated positively with a Rapid Naming Test, which was designed to measure lexical retrieval. Furthermore, LVF accuracy, RVF accuracy, and the RVFA were negatively correlated with the Judging Equations Test, which was designed to measure "procedural knowledge." Thus, in Hebrew, unlike English, the LH rather than the right was more strongly correlated with reading behavior, again consistent with exclusive LH specialization for reading Hebrew.

3.3 Error monitoring

The EEG correlates of lateralized lexical decision are informative about the competence of each hemisphere separately. What can the EEG tell us about how the two hemispheres interact? In order to answer that question, we analyze the EEG correlates of tasks that require interhemispheric interaction and involve interhemispheric control. We focus on the hemispheric division of labor during error monitoring of lexical decision. It is possible to analyze both implicit and explicit error detection and correction in the two hemispheres during the lateralized lexical decision task. We may characterize effective implicit error monitoring by: (1) slowing down following an error, and (2) becoming more accurate after an error. We have shown that RH has a special role in error correction of lexical decision, even though the LH is specialized for the task (Iacoboni et al., 1997). Similarly, we may characterize effective explicit error monitoring by slowing down and becoming more accurate following negative feedback indicating that the previous response was incorrect. We found that only the RH showed evidence for explicit error monitoring.

Negative feedback consisting of unhappy faces in the LVF resulted in slowing down and becoming more accurate on the following trial. Face feedback in the RVF had no effect. Feedback consisting of color patches was again effective only in the LVF, albeit at a lower level than faces. Verbal feedback was not effective in either VF (Kaplan & Zaidel, 2001). We found that implicit error monitoring was not effective in children (Barnea, Zaidel, Greene, Rassis, Raz, Johnstone, & Metzler, 2003) or in patients with schizophrenia (Narr, Green, Capetillo-Cunliffe, Toga, & Zaidel, 2003; Hirschman, Lamschtein, BazBarChana, Barnea, & Zaidel, 2003).

4. HEMISPHERIC ELECTROPHYSIOLOGICAL CORRELATES OF LEXICAL VARIABLES: STATE ANALYSIS

4.1 The normal brain

Is EEG sensitive to psycholinguistic variables? Do EEG correlates reflect the same hemispheric differences that accuracy and reaction time do?

4.1.1 Unilateral versus bilateral targets

In this experiment, we presented lateralized English character strings for lexical decision and measured the ongoing EEG and trial-based ERPs during task performance. We administered the test under two different conditions, (1) unilateral targets and (2) targets with word/nonword distractors in the opposite VF (bilateral targets). At the same time, the EEG was sampled from 32 electrodes over the entire head using a NeuroScan system. We analyzed the data by pairing trials with targets in one VF and responses by the ipsilateral hand. We then analyzed the ongoing EEG in the electrodes over the hemisphere contralateral to the target VF and response hand. In this way, we ensured measuring hemispheric performance under conditions of maximal independence. Behaviorally, bilateral presentations resulted in greater hemispheric independence and in more reliable hemispheric differences. Physiologically, however, the opposite pattern was observed: Unilateral presentations resulted in greater EEG differences between the two hemispheres.

Using unilateral presentations, each hemisphere elicited a larger gamma response for words as compared to nonwords. However, using bilateral presentations, the gamma response for words disappeared. This is likely attributable to "smearing" effects of the EEG due to the distractors. Thus, behaviorally, bilateral presentations enhanced hemispheric independence, whereas physiologically, bilateral presentations reduced our ability to measure independence. This shows the need for converging methodologies.

For spectral analysis, we normalized the EEG responses to the stimuli by measuring frequency-specific EEG response during target relative to baseline time windows. Trials were examined over four time windows: a baseline of 256 ms before stimulus onset, followed immediately by three consecutive non-overlapping 256 ms time windows. Three frequency bands were chosen for analysis: 35-43 Hz (gamma), 27-35 Hz (low-gamma), 11.7-27 Hz (beta), and 7.8-11.7 Hz (alpha) (Figure 1). We report the results of three experiments together (Weems, Zaidel, Berman, & Mandelkern, unpublished, a, b, c).

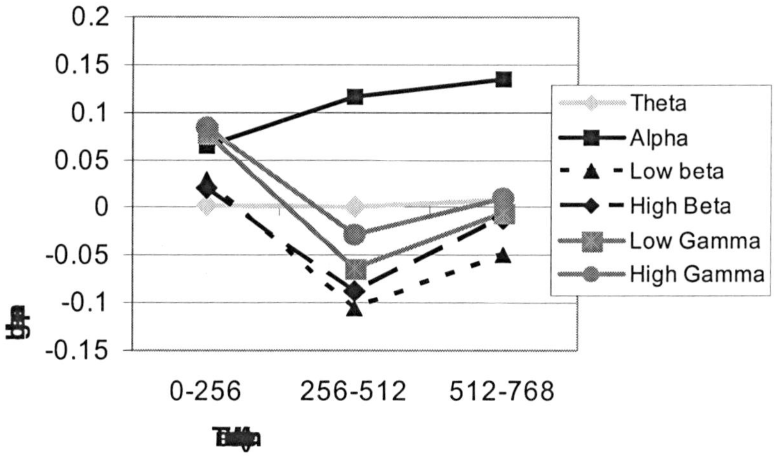

Figure 1. EEG spectral response following target presentation, averaged over both hemispheres (Weems et al., unpublished, a).

Gamma responses in the first time window exceeded that in the second and the third exceeded that of the second. There were larger gamma responses to words than to nonwords. Furthermore, the gamma differences between words and nonwords followed different time courses in the two hemispheres. For the LH, the difference reached significant during the second time window, whereas for the RH, it reached significance in the first and third time windows. Moreover, for the RH, high frequency words elicited a greater gamma response than low frequency words, whereas in the left hemisphere, the low frequency words yielded larger responses than high frequency words (Figure 2). The hemispheric dissociation in physiological response was not mirrored in the behavior. Both hemispheres performed better for high than for low frequency words, although the difference was larger in the RH (Figure 3). Power in the alpha band decreased between the second and the third time windows, and showed larger response over the right than the left hemisphere.

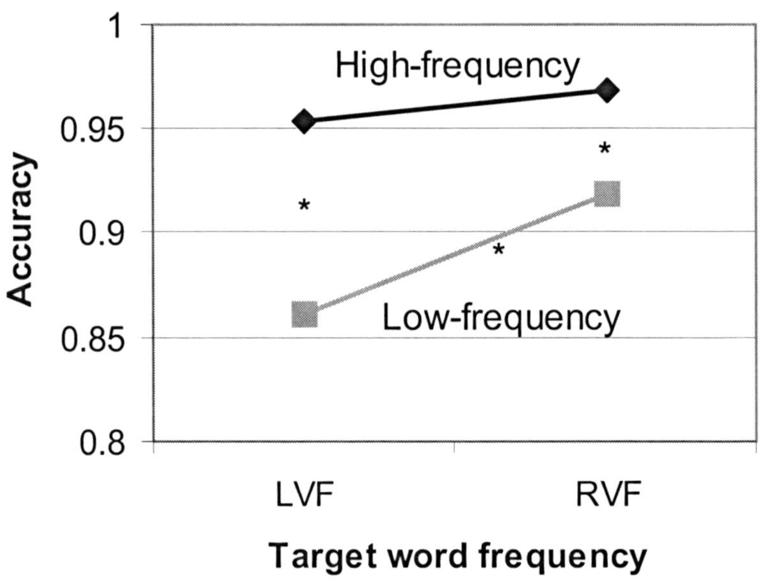

Figure 2a. Accuracy in the two visual fields is a function of word frequency. Low ≤ 20 per million, high frequency ≥ 100 per million written test (Francis & Kucera, 1982) (Weems et al., unpublished, b).

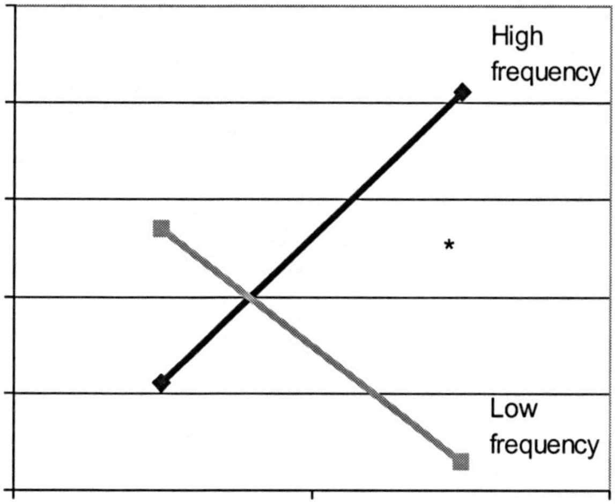

Figure 2b. High gamma band response relative to baseline for high and low-frequency words in the first-time window (0-256 ms), * = p <.01.

Table 2. Summary of significant effects, unilateral EEG (Weems et al., Unpublished manuscript, (b)).

	Behavior	*Gamma*	*Alpha*
Hemispheric specialization (RVFA)	+	-	+
Hemispheric independence (TW x VF)	+	+[1]	-

RVFA = Right visual field advantage
TW = Target wordness
VF = Visual field

[1] word frequency x hemisphere

Orthographic regularity also exhibited a dissociation between behavior and electrophysiology. Weems et al., (unpublished manu-cript, (a)) found no significant effects or interaction of orthographic regularity in either latency or accuracy. However, they found a significant interaction in high gamma response during the second time window between orthographic regularity and target visual field (Figure 3).

In sum, the physiological responses showed interactions between lexical variables and VF of presentation, supporting direct access,

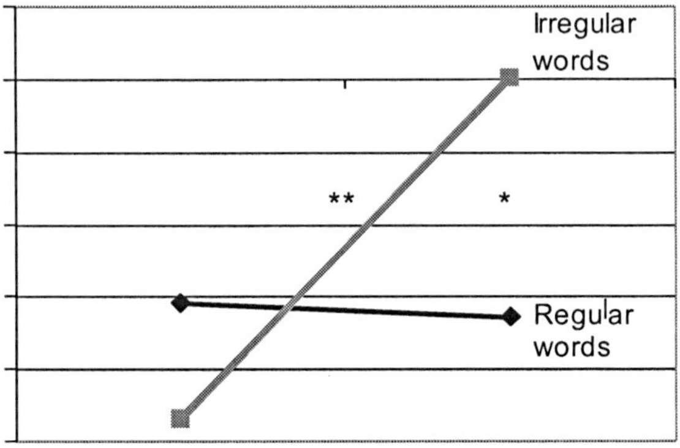

Figure 3. High gamma-band response relative to baseline for regular and irregular words in the 2nd time window (256-512 ms). * = p<.05, ** = p<.005 (Weems et al., unpublished manuscript, (a)).

while the behavioral responses did not (Table 2). In particular, there were both spectral and ERP correlates of hemisphere, of wordness and of word frequency. Of special interest are the dissociations between word frequency and VF, and between orthographic regularity and VF, which were observed in the electrophysiology but not in the behavior (Table 3). In this case, the ongoing gamma was more sensitive than the ERPs and it may have reflected investment of cognitive resources during early processing.

Table 3. Summary of significant effects, unilateral EEG (Weems et al., Unpublished manuscript, (a)).

	Behavior		*EEG*					
			Gamma		Alpha		Beta	Theta
	% error	RT	Power	Coherence	Power	Coherence	Power	Power
Wordness	-	+	+	+	-	+	-	-
VF / hemisphere	+	+	-	+	+	+	-	-
Word frequency	+	+	+	N/A	+	N/A	-	-
Word orthography	-	-	+	N/A	-	N/A	-	-
Nonword pronounce-ability	+	+	-	N/A	+	N/A	+	-

4.2 The split brain

Two patients with complete cerebral commissurotomy from the Bogen-Vogel California series, NG and AA, received the same lateralized lexical decision task with unilateral targets as the normal subjects. Neither patient was able to perform the task above chance in the LVF (RH) using left hand responses. Both patients showed a strong word bias in their behavioral response, and only patient NG showed some tendency for word identification ability, but only for RVF trials. Patient AA revealed a strong word bias and poor sensitivity, with log beta = -0.09 and d' = 2.1. Patient NG also had a strong word bias, with log beta = -0.69 and d' = 0.73.

Patients' ongoing EEG was recorded as in the normal subjects, and again we analyzed the EEG from electrodes over the hemisphere contralateral to the input VF and the responding hand. Thus, only LH electrodes were examined for RVF trials when paired with right hand responses and only RH electrodes for LVF trials when paired with left hand responses. EEG power was averaged over each of the electrodes in the target hemisphere. Separate analyses were conducted for each patient.

In patient AA, gamma response in the first time window exceeded that in both subsequent time windows. Surprisingly, however, amplitude in the gamma range (35-43 Hz) disclosed a significant advantage for nonwords as early as the first time window (0-256 milliseconds) and continuing in the two subsequent windows. The direction of the differential gamma response was opposite to that of previous findings, where words tend to elicit greater high frequency EEG response than nonwords. The greater gamma response for nonwords was observed over the RH but not the left (Figure 4). Thus, in both patients, gamma over the RH showed that, occasionally, the brain knows what the mind does not.

NG also showed greater gamma response in the first time window than in the subsequent two (Figure 4). Again there was a greater gamma response for nonwords than for words. NG's latency data did show faster responses for target words and a significant interaction between Target Wordness and Target VF. This highlights the dissociation between accuracy and latency measures of behavior. Latency may reflect early perceptual processes, whereas accuracy reflects later, conscious, detection as well as response programming. An alternative interpretation of the increase in gamma during the first time window may be that it is largely stimulus independent and indicative of initial processing before the introduction of top-down cognitive interpretation. The decrease in activity in the following two time windows may relate to cognitive processing of the stimulus proper. The subsequent decrease in high frequency response may reflect the fact that activity generated by stimulus-dependent cognitive processing is dwarfed by strong early processing of stimuli.

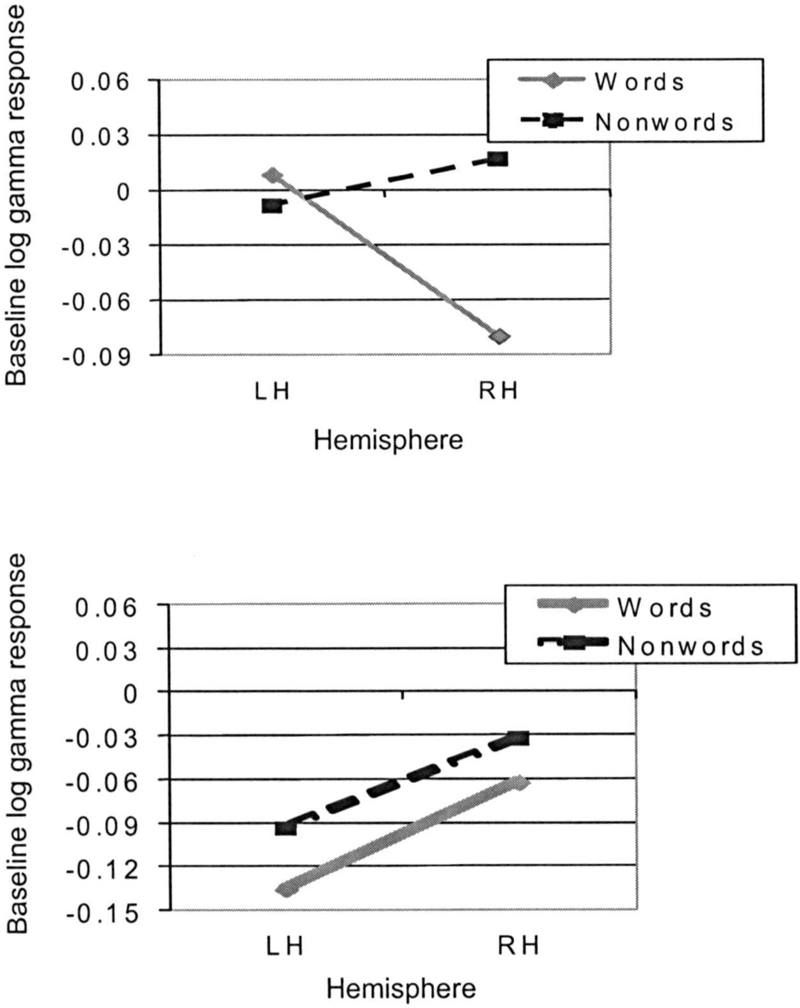

Figures 4a and b. High frequency gamma (35-43 hz.) response relative to baseline for lexical stimuli in the disconnected hemispheres of two split brain patients, AA (left) and NG (right) (Weems et al., unpublished manuscript, (c)).

4.3 The many faces of gamma

Here, electrophysiological response appears to be a more sensitive index of word recognition ability than behavior. It appears that in this case, gamma represents distributional properties of the stimuli rather than awareness of their identities. It follows that, far from representing "consciousness," gamma reflects lexical representation such that items in long-term semantic store require less engagement of processes indexed by gamma (Figure 2). Taken together, the data show that gamma is variously sensitive to lexicality (wordness), semantic variables (word frequency), orthographic variables (regularity), and phonological variables (nonword pronounceability).

5. PHYSIOLOGICAL CORRELATES OF HEMISPHERIC LEXICAL VARIABLES: TRAIT ANALYSIS

In the summers of 2004 and 2005, we tested two groups of learning disabled young adults in Tel Chai College, in Northern Galilee, Israel (Barnea et al., 2005). Each student had a lateralized lexical decision task in Hebrew and had his/her EEG recorded for six minutes at rest. We used a Deymed TruScan system with 19 electrodes placed according to the 10-20 system. The EEG was remontaged relative to whole head reference. We considered the frequency bands: 4-8 Hz (Theta), 8-12 Hz (Alpha), 12-15 Hz (SMR), and 15-18 Hz (low Beta). We also computed the ratios of Theta/Beta and (Alpha left – Alpha right)/(Alpha left + Alpha right) (defined as Alpha asymmetry). Further, we computed regional amplitude by averaging over electrodes: F3, F7 = left front; F4, F8 = right front; Fz = midline frontal; C3, C7 = left motor; C4, C8 = right motor; Cz = midline motor; T3, T5 = left temporal; T4, T6 = right temporal; P3 = left parietal; P4 = right parietal; Pz = midline parietal.

We correlated the amplitude in each of the regions with the LVF (RH score), RVF (LH score), and RVFA of the Hebrew lateralized lexical decision task. The participants were 17 of the learning disabled young adults. Only significant correlation coefficients at $p < .01$ were considered. There were surprising correlations between the EEG at rest and subsequent performance on the lateralized lexical decision. The data are shown in Figure 5. Normalization by whole head made the strongest predictions. The amplitude in the low Beta range in the temporal, motor, and central motor regions on both sides was negatively correlated with hemispheric specialization for language. This suggests that the EEG at rest is diagnostic of individual differences in hemispheric relations (Figure 5).

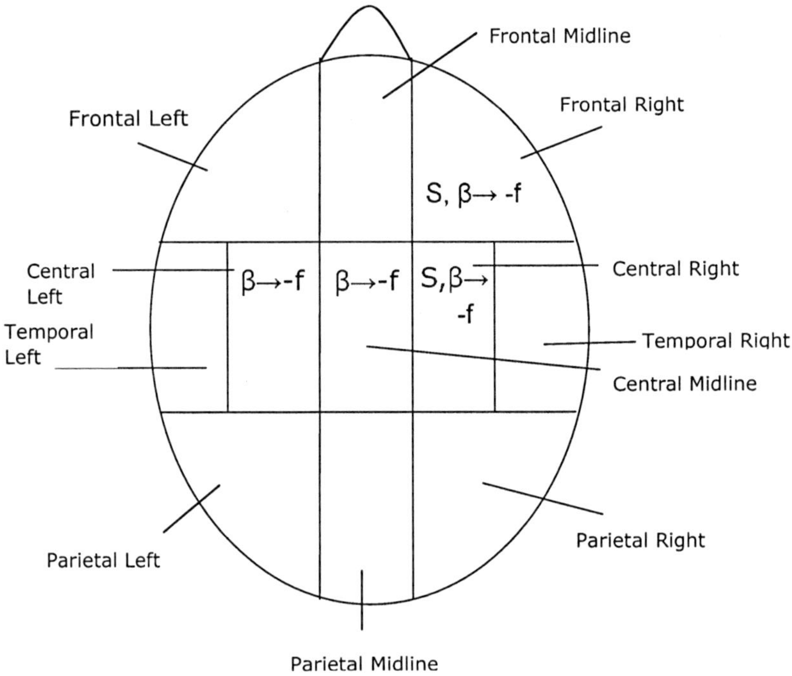

Figure 5. Significant correlations between components of the EEG spectra at rest and hemispheric specialization for lateralized lexical decision (Barnea et al., 2005).

6. PHYSIOLOGICAL CORRELATES OF HEMISPHERIC ERROR MONITORING

We measured Alpha power immediately preceding English lexical decision trials in relationship to accuracy and latency on the lexical decision response for the following trial. We found that greater left asymmetry in alpha amplitude immediately before presentation of a word led to a reduced likelihood for its successful identification (Weems et al., 2004b). Greater left alpha asymmetry was also associated with reduced identification of both words and nonwords lateralized to the RVF. Thus, word recognition appears to be facilitated by a decreased asymmetry in cognitive engagement in the two hemispheres, particularly when the stimuli are lateralized to the

LH (RVF). This result held for both frontal, temporal, and parietal electrodes, and it may well provide a mechanism for implicit error monitoring of the LH by the RH during lateralized lexical decision. Importantly, there was no relationship between implicit error monitoring and performance in either VF alone. Rather, the correlations were significant with the underlying asymmetry in alpha amplitude, suggesting an interaction between the two hemispheres.

Indeed, split brain patients do not self-correct even when they make many errors and are explicitly encouraged to correct them (Kaplan & Zaidel, unpublished). Thus, the EEG also reflects hemispheric dynamics in control operations.

7. CONCLUSION

Lateralized presentations provide a unique window into the linguistic competence of the two cerebral hemispheres. Behavioral dependent variables alone can reveal remarkable lexical competence in the right cerebral hemisphere. Physiological variables provide complementary information about different stages of processing, some of which are not available to conscious decisions. Thus, some physiological variables show evidence of cortical processing sufficient to make a decision much earlier than the corresponding decision occurs, occasionally even when the decision cannot be made altogether. The EEG seems to provide sensitive measures of hemispheric lexical processing. It provides temporal information that goes beyond ERPs. It is sensitive to a variety of psycholinguistic variables ranging from lexicality, semantic, and orthographic dimensions to phonological ones. It is also sensitive to metacognitive, or control, processes, such as error correction. The EEG has important methodological implications. However, the EEG in the service of analyzing hemispheric relations also has important methodological implications. Electrodes over one hemisphere are sensitive to far-field effects from the other side, and given our current state of ignorance, disparate cognitive states often exhibit the same EEG profile.

Nonetheless, our analyses suggest that it is critical to compare brain activation during lateralized presentations with brain activations during more natural, central, presentations in order to develop comprehensive models of interhemispheric interaction in reading that account for development, learning, deficit, and recovery. The former describes cortical activation during maximal hemispheric competence, while the latter describes cortical activation during actual interhemispheric performance. A complete description of reading in the brain must include an account of the control processes that select and incorporate hemispheric components into the decision required by a particular task.

REFERENCES

Barnea, A., Mooshagian, E., & Zaidel, E. (2003). The development of hemispheric specialization and interhemispheric interaction in Hebrew. *Annual Meeting of the Cognitive Neuroscience Society, 10*, 30.

Barnea, A., Zaidel, E., Greene, D., Rassis, A., Raz, A., Johnstone, J., & Metzler, Y. (2005). Effect of neurofeedback on lateralized attention networks in learning-disabled young adults. *Brain & Cognition, 59(3)*, 314-321.

Bastiaansen, M., & Hagoort, P. (2006). Oscillatory neuronal dynamics during language comprehension. *Progress in Brain Research, 159,* 179-96.

Bizas, E., Simos, P. G., Stam, C. J., Arvanitis, S., Terzakis, D., & Micheloyannis, S. (1999). EEG correlates of cerebral engagement in reading tasks. *Brain Topography, 12(2)*, 99-105.

Fiebach, C. J., Friederici, A. D., Muller, K., & von Cramon, D. Y. (2002). fMRI evidence for dual routes to the mental lexicon in visual word recognition. *Journal of Cognitive Neuroscience, 14(1),* 11-23.

Francis, W. N., & Kucera, H. (1982). *Frequency analysis of English usage, lexicon and grammar.* Boston, MA: Houghton Mifflin Co.

Hirschmann, S., Lamschtein, C., BazBarChana, M, Barnea, A., & Zaidel, E. (2003). *Hemispheric specialization and interhemispheric interaction in schizophrenia.* Annual Meeting for the Israeli Society for Neuroscience.

Iacoboni, M., Rayman, J., & Zaidel, E. (1997). Does the previous trial affect lateralized lexical decision? *Neuropsychologia, 35*, 81-88.

Iacoboni, M., & Zaidel, E. (1996). Hemispheric independence in word recognition: Evidence from unilateral and bilateral presentations. *Brain and Language, 53*, 121-140.

Kaplan, J. T., Iacoboni, M., & Zaidel, E. *The neural mechanisms of feedback processing in lexical decision: an fMRI study*. Unpublished manuscript.

Kaplan, J. T., & Zaidel, E. (2001). Error monitoring in the hemispheres: The effect of feedback on lateralized lexical decision. *Cognition, 82*, 157-178.

Kaplan, J. T., & Zaidel, E. *Impaired error correction in the split brain.* Unpublished manuscript.

Khader, P., & Rosler, F. (2004). EEG power and coherence analysis of visually presented nouns and verbs reveals left frontal processing differences. *Neuroscience Letters, 354(2)*, 111-114.

Kim, K. H., & Kim, J. H. (2006). Analysis of induced gamma-band activity in EEG during visual perception of Korean, English, Chinese words. *Neuroscience Letters, 403(3)*, 216-221.

Klimesch, W. (1999). EEG alpha and theta oscillations reflect cognitive and memory performance: a review and analysis. *Brain Research, Brain Research Reviews, 29(2-3),* 169-195.

Lutzenberger, W., Pulvermuller, F., & Birbaumer, N. (1994). Words and nonwords elicit distinct patterns of 30-Hz EEG responses in humans. *Neuroscience Letters, 176(1),*115-8.

Melamed, F., & Zaidel, E. (1993). Language and task effects on lateralized word recognition. *Brain & Language, 45,* 70-85.

Narr, K. L., Green, M. F., Capetillo-Cunliffe, L., Toga, A. W., & Zaidel, E. (2003). Lateralized lexical decision in schizophrenia: Hemispheric specialization and interhemispheric lexicality priming. *Journal of Abnormal Psychology, 112*, 623-632.

Pulvermuller, F., Lutzenberger, W., & Preissl, H. (1999). Nouns and verbs in the intact brain: evidence from event-related potentials and high-frequency cortical responses. *Cerebral Cortex, 9(5),* 497-506.

Tanji, K., Suzuki, K., Delorme, A., Shamoto, H., & Nakasato, N. (2005). High-frequency gamma-band activity in the basal temporal cortex during picture-naming and lexical-decision tasks. *Journal of Neuroscience, 25(13),* 3287-3293.

Tomberg, C. (1999). Focal enhancement of chaotic strange attractor dimension in the left semantic (Wernicke) human cortex during reading without concomitant change in vigilance level. *Neuroscience Letters, 263(2-3),* 177-180.

Weems, S., & Zaidel, E. (2004a). The relationship between reading ability and lateralized lexical decision. *Brain & Cognition, 55(3),* 507-515.

Weems, S., Zaidel, E., Berman, S., & Mandelkern, M. (2004b). Asymmetry in alpha power predicts errors in hemispheric lexical decision. *Clinical Neurophysiology, 115(7),* 1575-1582.

Weems, S., Zaidel, E., Berman, S., & Mandelkern, M. *Behavioral and electrophysiological response for repeated lateralized lexical stimuli.* Unpublished manuscript (a).

Weems, S., Zaidel, E., Berman, S., & Mandelkern, M. *Electrophysiological response to laterally presented lexical stimuli.* Unpublished manuscript (b).

Weems, S., Zaidel, E., Berman, S., & Mandelkern, M. *Gamma response to lexical stimuli in the split-brain: electrophysiological response in absence of behavioral competency.* Unpublished manuscript (c).

Weiss, S., & Mueller, H. M. (2003). The contribution of EEG coherence to the investigation of language. *Brain and Language, 85(2),* 325-43.

Zaidel, E. (1998). Language in the right hemisphere following callosal disconnection. In B. Stemmer & H. Whitaker (Eds.), *Handbook of Neurolinguistics* (pp. 369-383). New York: Academic Press.

Zaidel, E., Clarke, J. M., & Suyenobu, B. (1990). Hemispheric independence: A paradigm case for cognitive neuroscience. In A. B. Scheibel & A. F. Wechsler (Eds.), *Neurobiology of Higher Cognitive Function* (pp. 297-335). New York: Guilford Press.

10

BRAIN MAPPING OF LANGUAGE USING HIGH FREQUENCY GAMMA OSCILLATIONS IN THE ELECTROCORTICOGRAPHY

Alon Sinai

Department of Neurology, The Johns Hopkins University School of Medicine, Baltimore, MD 21287, USA

Abstract: Electrocorticographic (ECoG) recordings, necessary for clinical intervention in epileptic patients, provide a unique opportunity to study the electrophysiological correlates of functional brain activation in more detail than noninvasive recordings. The proximity of ECoG electrodes to EEG sources enhances their spatial resolution, as well as their sensitivity and signal-to-noise ratio, particularly for high frequency EEG activity. ECoG recordings have therefore been used to study the event-related dynamics of brain oscillations in a variety of frequency ranges, and in a variety of functional-neuroanatomic systems, including cortical networks responsible for language. Synchronized gamma oscillations particularly in the high gamma range (>60Hz) was suggested to play a role in binding between cortical regions, essential part of efficient semantic network. The functional response properties of high gamma activity (HGA) are distinct from similar phenomena in lower frequencies. The HGA findings are consistent with its proposed binding role in models of neural computation.

Preliminary studies suggest that interactions between gamma oscillations in macroscopic local field potentials (LFP) generated by different large-scale populations of neurons engaged by the same functional task occur in gamma frequencies at latencies consistent with the timing of task performance. The neuronal mechanisms underlying high gamma activity and its distinctive response properties in humans are still largely unknown, but their research through invasive means is expected to support and expand their potential clinical and research applications, including functional brain mapping, brain-computer interfaces, and neurophysiological studies of human cognition.

In our lab studies we aim to asses HGA and compare it to event related potentials (ERP's) at different stages of linguistic processing from early sensory to late lexical and semantic stages of processing. The results of these studies indicate that HGA which is related to the semantic network activation distinguished spatially and temporally from the early sensory registration. HGA specific to semantic processing occurs mainly in late stages of processing and its cortical distribution is restricted in comparison to ERP's response of the same process.

Key words: electrocorticography, gamma, ERD?ERS, functional mapping, auditory cortex, language

1. INTRODUCTION

Oscillatory activity in the recorded EEG was known for many years as related to states of sleep and awakening. In general synchronization among brain regions in lower frequencies mainly in the alpha band (8-12 Hz) can not be detected in an awake alert state and there is desynchronization of alpha activity in response to stimuli. Synchronization is gradually built up in deep relaxation state and is growing (i.e., slower frequencies) in sleep stages as sleep gets deeper. This synchronous activity is wide spread over large portion of the brain and therefore hard to draw conclusion on functionality of specific region with respect to it. Recent studies suggested oscillatory activity In higher frequency in recordings of single and multiple units, local field potentials (LFP), and large neuronal populations, as well as computer simulations of neural circuits and networks (Gray, 1994; Klimesch, 1999; Lopes da Silva, 1991; Pfurtscheller & Lopes da Silva, 1999; Steriade, Gloor, Llinas, Lopes Da Silva, & Mesulam, 1990). This activity is spatially and temporally restricted. The oscillatory activity most promising as an index of regional cortical processing is that which occurs in the gamma band, operationally defined as >30 Hz. Odor-specific spatial patterns of gamma oscillations (38-80 Hz) were observed in rabbit olfactory cortex (Freeman, 1978), a wider scientific debate developed from experiments linking gamma oscillations with neuronal synchronization and the "temporal correlation hypothesis" (Eckhorn, Bauer, Jordan, Brosch, Kruse, & Reitboeck, 1988; Gray, Konig, Engel, & Singer, 1989; Gray, 1999). Oscillations in the gamma range were suggested to be a mechanism that form a temporal code that dynamically "binds" spatially segregated neurons into assemblies representing higher-order stimulus properties (Singer & Gray, 1995; Von der Malsburg, 1995), leading to a cohort perception. These hypotheses were linked with EEG gamma oscillations by experiments demostrating synchronization of single unit firing bursts with LFP gamma oscillations (Murthy & Fetz, 1992; Sanes & Donoghue, 1993). Modern neuroimaging techniques found activation pattern of multiple brain regions associated with language processing (Binder et al., 1997). Incorporating these findings with the abovementioned theories of binding activity through oscillations may add an important aspect in supporting or disproving models of linguistic processing in the brain.

Gamma band oscillations have been studied extensively in humans with scalp EEG, and more recently with magnetoencephalography (MEG). Event-related synchronization (ERS - a.k.a. *induced gamma activity*) have been observed during auditory (Kaiser, Lutzenberger, Ackerman, & Birbaumer, 2002; Pantev, 1995), visual (Tallon-Baudry, Bertrand, Wienbruch, Ross, & Pantev, 1997), and motor tasks (Pfurtscheller, Flotzinger, & Neuper, 1994a), but the localization of induced gamma activity recorded from the scalp has often been difficult to determine.

The clinical practice of implanting subdural electrodes for the surgical management of intractable epilepsy has provided a unique opportunity to study gamma activity in greater detail than possible with noninvasive recordings. Subdural electrocorticography (ECoG) has improved spatial resolution because of higher spatial sampling (inter-electrode distances of ~1 cm) and the absence of spatial blurring from scalp, skull, and dura mater (Cooper, Winter, Crow, & Walter, 1965; Gevins, et al., 1994). Since the skull acts as a low-pass filter (Pfurtscheller & Cooper, 1975), and artifacts from cranial muscle activity occur in the gamma band (Loring & Sheer, 1984; Akay & Daubenspeck, 1999), the signal-to-noise ratio for gamma band activity in ECoG is much better than that in scalp EEG. This property of subdural ECoG enabled the discovery of event-related activity in a higher gamma frequency range beginning at ~70-80 Hz (Crone, Miglioretti, Goron, Sieracki, et al., 1998b) and including a broad range of higher frequencies that may extend up to ~150 Hz (Crone, Hao, et al., 2001b; Ray, Jouny, Crone, Boatman, Thakor, & Franaszczuk, 2003). This broadband "high gamma" activity (HGA) has been observed during a variety of functional activation tasks, including self-paced and visually cued limb movements (Crone, Miglioretti, Goron, Sieracki, et al., 1998b; Ohara et al., 2000; Pfurtscheller, Graimann, Huggins, Levine, & Schuh, 2003; Leuthardt, Schalk, Wolpaw, ojemann, & Moran, 2004), auditory discrimination (Crone, Hao, et al., 2001b), and word production tasks (Crone, Boatman, Gordon, & Hao, 2001a), ECoG studies have also shown that, compared to event-related activity in other frequency bands, event-related HGA typically occurs in spatial and temporal patterns that are more consistent with functional anatomy and the results of electrocortical stimulation mapping (ESM) (Crone, Miglioretti, Gordon, et al., 1998a, Crone, Miglioretti, Gordon, Sieracki, et al., 1998b; Crone, Hao, et al., 2001b; Crone & Hao, 2002a; Pfurtscheller et al., 2003). In ECoG recordings of auditory association cortex in dominant superior temporal gyrus, HGA was greater and more widespread during speech discrimination than during tone discrimination, whereas auditory evoked responses were not substantially different, suggesting that HGA provided a better index of the cortical processing demands of the tasks (Crone, Hao, et al., 2001b). In addition, although ECoG power in high gamma frequencies was consistently augmented during cortical activation, the power in lower gamma frequencies around the traditional 40 Hz band was sometimes increased and at other times decreased, varying not only across patients, but also across recording sites within patients.

Because of its spatial, temporal, and functional response characteristics, HGA appears to be a promising index of task-related cortical activation with potential applications in functional mapping.

The clinical circumstances that require the implantation of subdural electrodes may be motivated by the need to obtain functional map of the patient's individual anatomy prior to the planned surgical resection. Until recently this has been achieved primarily through ESM, during which a weak electrical current is passed between pairs of the subdural electrodes that have been implanted on the cortical surface. Although this procedure is still considered to be the gold standard for predicting postoperative functional impairments (Ojemann, Ojemann, Lettich, & Berger, 1989; Roux et al., 2003), it has some important drawbacks. The most concerning one is the tendency of the stimulating current to evoke after discharges, which can evolve into clinical seizures (Blume, Jones, & Pathak, 2004; Lesser et al., 1984) that do not accurately reflect the patient's seizure focus (Blume et al., 2004). At times these frequent complications prevent the completion of the ESM mapping. Functional maps based on passive recordings of event-related ECoG gamma activity could potentially avoid this obstacle. In addition, ECoG functional maps could be obtained for all implanted electrode sites at once. In contrast, ESM must be done sequentially on pairs of electrodes, regularly requiring several hours of testing.

To evaluate the potential application of ECoG HGA to functional brain mapping, our lab has compared the maps derived from event-related ECoG spectral changes, particularly those in the gamma band, with maps obtained by ESM through the same subdural electrodes (Crone, Miglioretti, Gordon, et al., 1998a; Sinai, Bowers, et al., 2005b), and we are in the process of making similar comparisons with functional maps obtained with fMRI. Using subdural ECoG to study alpha ERD in greater spatial detail, alpha ERD was observed in regional patterns that are broadly consistent with functional activation in visual (Crone et al., 1994), auditory (Crone, Boatman, et al., 2001a), somatosensory (Ohara et al., 2004), and somatomotor (Crone et al., 1998b) cortices. However, the spatial and temporal patterns of alpha ERD have generally been less specific to the functional anatomy and timing of the tasks than those of high gamma activity (Crone, Miglioretti, Gordon, et al., 1998a; Crone, Miglioretti, Gordon, Sieracki, et al., 1998b; Crone, Boatman, et al., 2001a; Crone & Hao, 2002; Crone et al., 2006).

Differences in the response properties of brain oscillations in different frequency bands may provide insights into differences in their underlying neurophysiological mechanisms. ECoG studies are thus expected to provide basic information about electrophysiological correlates of cortical processing that will facilitate the study of complex cognitive operations such as language by other electrophysiological techniques, e.g., scalp EEG and MEG. Even the most basic language tasks (e.g., naming) can be decomposed into sub-operations that occur within hundreds of milliseconds in spatially distributed, functionally specialized, cortical modules. The dissection of these sub-operations, however, will require not only excellent temporal and spatial resolution, but also reliable indices of task-specific cortical processing. Furthermore, studies of how cognitive sub-operations are integrated in real time will require indices of the dynamic interaction between their cortical modules. Analyses of event-related coherence and other multichannel analyses of oscillatory activity have been used for this purpose in EEG recordings (Andrew & Pfurtscheller, 1996; Ginter et al., 2005) and are being applied to ECoG recordings as well (Korzeniewska, Kus, Franaszczuk, Crainiceanu, & Crone, 2005). ECoG recordings may therefore allow us to test hypotheses regarding the functional significance and potential clinical utility of ECoG gamma activity and other spectral indices of cortical processing in and among functionally activated brain regions. fMRI and PET studies can suggest the participating regions in processing but lack the temporal resolution essential to follow brain activity as it unfold over time. Electrophysiological methods on the other hand have sufficient temporal resolution but suffer from sub-optimal spatial resolution. ECoG of behaving human although restricted mainly to a small population of patient that undergo sub-dural electrode implementation as part of their clinical evaluation for epilepsy, preserve excellent temporal resolution and have improved spatial resolution. Semantic processing was extensively studied using scalp ERP method but much less so, using invasive electrocorticography. Most studies suggest that in late processing stages (>400 msec) associated to semantic representation, the activation pattern of semantic tasks is across modalities (Anderson & Holcomb, 1995; Crone, Hao, et al., 2001b). The same semantic knowledge can be accessed by different modalities, this suggest the existence of a common pathway and thus allows investigation of the brain substrate that is related to the retrieval of a word meaning. ERP studies described a negativity peaking around 400 msec (N400) that is related to semantic processing (Kutas & Hillyard, 1980). N400 is manipulated by semantic relation as well as by many other related factors (priming, word frequency etc.) and has similar scalp distribution across modalities. Current dipole modeling of the source of N400m using MEG (magnetic equivalent of N400) found sources in the vicinity of the superior temporal sulcus (STS) (Simos, Basile, Papanicolaou, 1997). ECoG intracranial recordings suggest multi-generators active in the time frame of N400, widespread over the cortex. The most prominent activity was found in the anterior temporal lobe (Halgren et al., 1994; McCarthy, Nobre, Bentin, & Spencer, 1995; Nobre and McCarthy, 1995 for review see Van Petten & Luka, 2006).

Neuroimaging studies typically demonstrate bilateral activation with often Leftward asymmetry for both written (Frederici, Opitz, & von Cramon, 2000; Frost et al., 1999; Gabrieli, Poldrack, & Desmond, 1998; Petersen, Fox, Posner, Mintun, & Raichle, 1988) and spoken (Binder et al., 1997; Zatorre, Evans, Meyer, & Gjedder, 1992) word recognition. In tasks that require semantic processing the activity most related to semantic and mnemonic processing is taking place in the left prefrontal and temporal regions (Buckner, Koutstaal, Schacter, & Rosen, 2000; Chee, O'Craven, Bergida, Rosen, & Savoy, 1999; Perani et al., 1999; Petersen et al., 1988), and may represent the neural basis of supramodal processing. Conversely, ERPs and MEG provide complementary evidence suggesting that access to the central semantic store is reflected in the N400 component (Kutas & Fediermeier, 2000). This evidence along with the great degree of overlap in the scalp distribution of N400 to spoken and written words suggests the existence of common semantic network that its input originated from the sensory-specific regions (Gomes, Ritter, Tartter, Vaughan, & Rosen, 1997; Hagoort & Brown, 2000). The scalp distribution of the N400 however does not support left hemisphere preferences and in most reports show some right parietal distribution. The relationship between the scalp distribution and a multi-source distribution is nonetheless vague.

We hypothesized that the region that are the core of the amodal semantic network will show as part of their information sharing binding processes high gamma activity in the approximate time frame of the N400. In addition we expect high gamma activity in sensory specific regions earlier to that point and possibly later integration processes that may be reflected in high gamma activity as well and are expected to be in common amodal semantic regions.

2. METHODOLOGICAL CONSIDERATIONS

2.1 Subjects and clinical procedures

The most common reason for invasive EEG recording is for the surgical management of patients with intractable epileptic seizures which have not responded to antiepileptic drugs. Noninvasive scalp EEG monitoring has usually failed to pinpoint the seizure focus, or the focus has been discovered in or near "eloquent cortex" i.e., a cortical region that is presumably responsible for language, vision, or motor function. Implantation of intracranial EEG electrodes is thus indicated for further localization of the seizure focus and/or functional mapping with electrocortical stimulation mapping (ESM).

The major weakness of invasive EEG recordings is that they must be done in patients that have abnormal brain physiology. It is necessary to take a number of precautions to lessen the impact of this concern. In Patients with a brain lesion the experimental tasks are limited to cortical regions that would not likely be affected by the patient's lesion. EEG epochs contaminated by epileptiform activity and/or pathological slowing may also be excluded from analysis. Patient is allowed a recovery time if he has recently had a seizure. Experiments may also have to be suspended if the patient has been given medication to moderate their seizure frequency. These restrictions may result in that a patient may be excluded altogether from the study.

One potential gain of studying the clinical population is that our subjects typically undergo an extensive battery of testing as a part of their preoperative clinical evaluation. This battery typically includes broad neuropsychological testing, an intracarotid amobarbital test, a high-resolution 3-D MRI scan, and a PET scan. Preoperative 3-D MRI scans provide information about lesions that might impact the patient's cognitive performance, and after implantation of intracranial electrodes, they can be co-registered with the patient's 3-D CT scan to demonstrate the location of the implanted electrodes with respect to cortical gyral anatomy (Crone et al., 1998b). Likewise, postoperative 3-D MRI scans can confirm the margins of surgical resection and their relationship with the results of functional mapping with ESM and with ECoG indices of functional activation. In addition to the aforementioned studies, Some of patients are undergoing fMRI studies for preoperative functional mapping. Thus, although the subjects available for testing with invasive EEG cannot be considered truly representative of the normal population, a great deal of information is available regarding their cognitive abilities, cortical physiology, and functional neuroanatomy, and this information can be extremely useful in correlations with the patterns of ERD/ERS and other ECoG indices of functional evaluation. In particular, this patient population provides an unprecedented opportunity to evaluate the results of ECoG functional mapping in relation to the results both ESM and fMRI, and with the accumulation of enough subjects, it should be possible to determine the relative strengths and weaknesses of these techniques for predicting postoperative functional impairments.

2.2 ECoG electrodes, recordings, and signal analyses

The subdural electrodes we used consist of platinum-iridium discs (0.4 mm diameter) embedded in a soft silastic sheet with a circular exposed surface of 2.3 mm diameter and an interelectrode distance of 1-cm (Adtech Medical Instrument Corporation, Racine, WI). These electrodes may be configured as one-dimensional strips of 4-8 electrodes, or as two-dimensional arrays (grids) of electrodes with 2 x 8, 4 x 6, or 8 x 8 dimensions. The surgeon may cut these into smaller grids in order to find an optimal fit of electrodes over cortical regions of interest. Grids with smaller interelectrode distances are available, but to cover the same cortical region, a much greater number of electrodes, and EEG amplifiers, is required. One dimensional subdural strips are 1-cm wide, and several may be passed through single burr holes in the skull. Using several burr holes on one or both sides of the head, subdural strips may be used to sparsely cover a large brain region when there is uncertainty about the lobar localization or lateralization of a patient's seizure focus. When the focus can be narrowed down to a specific cortical region, two-dimensional grids may be implanted. Although they require a more invasive craniotomy, grids are more useful than strips for pinpointing a patient's seizure focus and for comprehensive functional mapping with ESM to define the margins of resection.

To take advantage of the wider bandwidth of invasive EEG recordings, it is important to use a recording system with adequate specifications for the signals of interest. Because we have observed wideband event-related high gamma activity at frequencies consistently reaching up to ~180 Hz, our digital ECoG recordings have typically employed a sampling rate of 1000 Hz. Because high gamma activity has a very low voltage, we use 16-bit A/D converters. Until recently there were no commercially available systems for clinical EEG monitoring that had these specifications, and our experimental ECoG recordings were made with a custom-built 128-channel system that was used in parallel with the clinical video-EEG monitoring system in our Epilepsy Monitoring Unit. However, our current clinical video-EEG system (Stellate, Montreal, Canada) has adequate specifications for both clinical and research ECoG recordings with up to 128 channels.

When performing event-related spectral analysis on intracranial EEG data it is usually appropriate to reformat ECoG data to a reference-independent montage, e.g., the average reference, if only to avoid voltage distributions biased by the location of the reference electrode. This problem can also addressed by using a reference electrode far from the active electrodes in the recording. However, an extracranial reference, e.g., scalp electrodes or linked ears, is problematic because cortical gamma activity overlaps the frequency spectrum of myogenic potentials from scalp muscles. For this reason we typically use one of the intracranial electrodes as a reference, preferably one that is relatively quiet and free of epileptiform activity, and one that is located as far away as possible from the recording area of interest.

To analyze ECoG signals for event-related changes in their power spectrum, i.e., ERD/ERS, a number of approaches are available for decomposition of the signals into the frequency domain and subsequent statistical analysis of frequency dependent event-related changes in signal energy. With advances in computing power and quantitative analytic tools, the band-pass filtering approach used in the pioneering quantitative studies of ERD/ERS (Pfurtscheller & Aranibar, 1977) has been replaced by more comprehensive time-frequency assessments of event-related changes in signal energy (Pfurtscheller and Lopes da Silva, 1999). Here too there are many different approaches to choose from, including ones based on wavelets and Fourier analysis (Pfurtscheller et al., 2003). The one we have adopted recently is one based upon the matching pursuit algorithm for signal decomposition (Ray, Jouny, Crone, Boatman, Thakor, & Franaszczuk, 2003; Zygierewicz , Durka, Klekowicz, Franaszczuk, & Crone, 2005).

3. HIGH GAMMA ERS AND LANGUAGE PROCESSING

Most studies of gamma ERS have focused on functional activation of sensori-motor cortex, there have been however also efforts to use this and other event-related spectral indices of cortical activation to map the brain regions responsible for speech perception and production and other linguistic functions. High gamma ERS in particular has been studied using a variety of tasks designed to activate these regions of the brain in hopes of providing a functional mapping technique capable of complementing or even replacing ESM.

To evaluate ERD/ERS in different frequency bands during activation of auditory association cortex in the language dominant superior temporal gyrus, subdural ECoG was recorded during tone and speech discrimination tasks, and the resulting spatiotemporal patterns of auditory ERPs, alpha ERD, low gamma ERS (35-45 Hz), and high gamma ERS (80-100 Hz) were compared across the two tasks (Crone et al., 2001a). High gamma ERS occurred in a relatively focused spatial distribution concentrated over the dominant superior temporal gyrus, similar to the N100 of the auditory evoked response associated with onset of the stimuli. Likewise the onset of high gamma ERS generally coincided with the N100, but it typically lasted longer. More importantly, however, high gamma ERS occurred with a greater magnitude in association with speech stimuli than with tone stimuli, whereas the amplitude of the N100 did not. This suggested that high gamma ERS reflected the greater cortical processing demands of speech discrimination and/or the greater activation of cortex in the dominant superior temporal gyrus specialized for speech discrimination. In contrast to high gamma ERS, alpha ERD was usually observed in a broader spatial distribution, sometimes extending into suprasylvian frontal and parietal regions temporal regions far removed from the classic boundaries of Wernicke's area. In addition, the temporal course of alpha ERD was slower than that of high gamma ERS, reaching its lowest point later than the peak of high gamma ERS, and recovering more slowly than high gamma ERS. There was also less of a difference between alpha ERD during discrimination of speech and tones.

A particularly surprising finding of the study of ECoG gamma ERS during auditory perception was that 35-45 Hz ERS was present in only two of the four subjects, and in one subject there was ERD instead of ERS in this frequency band. Interestingly, like low gamma ERS, low gamma ERD had a greater magnitude during speech stimuli than during tone stimuli. The explanation for these seemingly inconsistent findings was suggested by the results of exploratory power spectral analyses comparing the ECoG power spectra during 0.5-second baseline and post-stimulus (activated) epochs. Not surprisingly, these analyses demonstrated that relative to the baseline, the power spectrum of the activated epoch had a significant suppression of power in lower frequencies, including alpha and beta bands, and a power augmentation in higher gamma bands. Although there was consistently power augmentation in high gamma frequencies, there was significant variance in the frequency at which there was a crossover between ERD and ERS. This crossover point varied across subjects and even within subjects, there was significant variability across recording sites. Thus, in two subjects the low gamma band (35-45 Hz) fell above the crossover, yielding ERS, and in one subject it fell below it, resulting in ERD. In yet another, the crossover occurred at about 40 Hz, apparently yielding no net change. This observed variability in the direction of power change in the 40 Hz band could explain why 40 Hz ERS has not been consistently observed in subjects studied with scalp EEG.

In many of our recent studies using power spectral analysis we find that high gamma ERS extended well above 100 Hz. The maximum power is typically centered around 80-120 Hz band, but statistically significant power augmentation are also consistently observed up to 150-200 Hz, and in some cases even higher. This extended frequency response has been confirmed in recordings of non-phase-locked gamma

LFP oscillations in monkey auditory cortex during tone bursts (Brosch, Budinger, & Scheich, 2002) and in subdural ECoG recordings of neurosurgical patients listening to deviant auditory stimuli (Edwards, Soltani, Deouell, Berger, & Knight, 2005). In the latter study, high gamma oscillations were reported in the frequency range of 60-250 Hz, centered at ~100 Hz. This extended high gamma frequency response has also been demonstrated during training of a brain-computer interface (Leuthardt et al., 2004).

ECoG study of speech perception demonstrated the potential utility of high gamma ERS for mapping cortical regions necessary for linguistic functions. However, the tasks used were ones that are not routinely tested in the clinical setting and are not typically tested with ESM in patients undergoing epilepsy surgery. The potential of ECoG high gamma activity application for mapping the cortical regions responsible for commonly tested language abilities was tested by recording subdural ECoG during three simple word production tasks that are routinely tested in bedside neurological examinations, as well as during ESM of language cortex. Confrontation naming of pictured objects, repetition of spoken words, and reading of written words are all simple tasks in which the patient makes a spoken verbal response to a stimulus in either the visual or auditory modality. These tasks are differentially affected by aphasia due to acquired lesions, and both picture naming and word reading tasks have been extensively studied by cognitive neuropsychologists. These studies have generated well developed, sometimes competing, models of the cognitive operations necessary for task performance, and the cortical regions responsible for these operations have been studied through lesion analysis and/or functional neuroimaging. Models of these language tasks also include predictions about the temporal dynamics of different stages of processing, including whether these stages occur in sequence, in parallel, or in a cascading relationship with one another.

High gamma activity during word production tasks was illustrated in a patient with normal hearing and speech, who was also fluent in sign language (Crone et al., 2001b). This made it possible for the patient to respond to the word production tasks with either spoken or signed responses. Because the picture naming and word reading tasks used visual stimuli while the word repetition task used auditory stimuli, it was possible to contrast the spatiotemporal patterns of high gamma ERS associated with different modalities of input (visual vs. auditory stimuli) and output (spoken vs. signed responses). The observed spatial distribution of high gamma ERS during these tasks was consistent with general principles of human functional neuroanatomy. For example, the earliest gamma responses occurred over auditory association cortex in superior temporal gyrus during auditory word repetition and over temporal-occipital cortex during visual object naming and word reading. Late gamma responses occurred over tongue area of sensorimotor cortex when responses were spoken, and over hand areas when responses were signed, and the latency of these late gamma responses covaried with the patient's different response latencies for the different tasks. In addition, there was generally good correspondence between high gamma ERS and maps of the same or similar language tasks derived from ESM. Gamma responses were also seen at times that were intermediate between those associated with word stimuli and responses, and based upon their locations in perisylvian regions typically associated with language function, it was postulated that these responses reflected intermediate stages of linguistic processing, e.g., lexical semantics. In contrast to these high gamma ERS responses, alpha ERD was observed to occur in a broader spatial distribution and with a temporal course that less closely matched that of task performance (Crone & Hao, 2002). In particular the onset of alpha ERD was usually delayed with respect to high gamma ERS and lasted much longer. High gamma ERS therefore appeared to be better suited for making contrasts between the neural substrates of different language tasks (Crone et al., 2006).

A recent study of high gamma ERS during lexical semantic processing provides another illustration of its utility for researching the neural substrates of human language (Sinai, Franaszczuk, & Crone, 2005a). Lexical semantic judgments are expected to depend on modality-specific, as well as modality-independent, lexical semantic processing. Patients with subdural grids were asked to judge whether sequentially presented pairs of words were semantically related or not, and to respond with a forced choice button press. Word pairs were presented in either visual or auditory modalities during separate blocks, and event-related time-frequency plots for different conditions (visual/auditory; semantically related/non-related) were compared within subjects. The results for one subject are illustrated in Fig. 1. In all 12 subjects high gamma ERS was observed in at least one recording site in a modality-specific pattern, i.e., only during auditory stimuli or only during visual stimuli. This modality-specific pattern was typically observed at early latencies. Modality-independent energy changes i.e., during stimuli of either modality, sensitive to the semantic relation between stimuli were observed in 9 out of the 12 patients. These responses were typically earlier to the auditory than to the visual stimuli and were modulated by the semantic relatedness of the word stimuli in each pair. This modulation typically consisted of a greater magnitude following presentation of semantically unrelated word pairs than following semantically related pairs. The region this pattern was observed most frequently was the left inferior frontal gyrus (Fig. 1 and 2), but was also observed in left superior temporal gyrus, supramarginal gyrus, and basal temporal cortex. In some cases the high gamma response to semantically related pairs outlasted the response to unrelated pairs in spite of having a lower magnitude. Our findings of high gamma power augmentation in response to words presented in both the auditory and the visual modality support and extend the suggested model of common amodal semantic network (Booth et al., 2002; Marques, 2006; Vandenberghe, Price, Wise, Josephs, & Frackowiak, 1996); (but see also (Federmeier & Kutas, 2001). This activation pattern also suggests that distinct regions that are engaged in semantic processing oscillate in high gamma frequencies possibly as way of binding activity in the relevant neuronal assembly as previously suggested (Engel, Konig, Kreiter, Schillen, & Singer, 1992; Fitzgibbon, Pope, Mackenzie, Clark, & Willoughby, 2004; Freeman & Barrie, 2000). By manipulating the semantic relation between stimuli we demonstrated greater HGA to semantically non-related pairs compared to semantically related pairs. This effect may suggest larger cell assembly involved in the response to non-related word pairs in analogous way to the enlargement of the N400 ERP component to similar manipulation (Holcomb, 1988; Sinai & Pratt, 2002). A potential interpretation of these findings is that although semantically unrelated pairs require a more extensive search of lexical semantic networks, semantically related pairs are associated with more prolonged activation of these networks, perhaps due to feedback from semantically related representations in other cortical regions. Language related activation from its early sensory components to semantic representation and perception was studied extensively using the entire inventory of research techniques. The general framework supported by most literature is of distributed network that has multiple interactions (Mesulam, 1990). This notion embraces early modality specific components subsequently accessing an amodal semantic

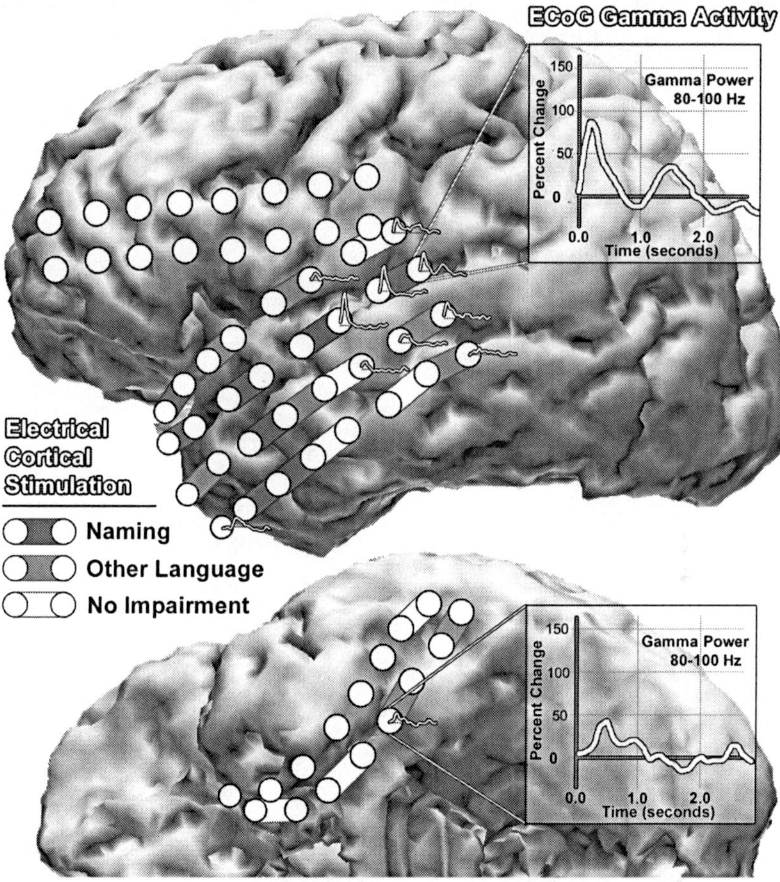

Figure 1. Comparison of event-related ECoG high gamma activity (HGA) with electrocortical stimulation mapping (ESM) in an individual subject. White circles denote electrode sites where ECoG was recorded. Yellow plots show the magnitude of HGA as a percentage change (y-axis) with respect to baseline. The onset of the pictured object to be named occurred 400 milliseconds after disappearance of a fixation point at 0 seconds (x-axis). Colored bars join electrode pairs where ESM was performed, color-coded for the occurrence and types of functional effects. Note that ESM was not performed at some sites where ECoG was recorded (pain was encountered at some temporal-occipital sites. ESM at three sites over middle temporal gyrus was done in reference a distant silent site to rule out language function at these sites.

system. In this study we supplied additional support and extension of this view by demonstrating high gamma oscillations that correspond specifically to semantic relation between words in a pair. These effects appear in most of the patients and takes place more often in regions not associated with specific modality. The temporal pattern of the semantic specific activity show two major time frame in which this effect take place, 400-600 msec and around 1200 msec after the onset of second stimulus in the pair. The spatial distribution of these amodal semantic relation sensitive regions was mainly in inferior frontal and anterior temporal regions with variation of the exact location between subjects. The activation in these sites tend to be larger to auditory stimuli compared to visual stimuli.

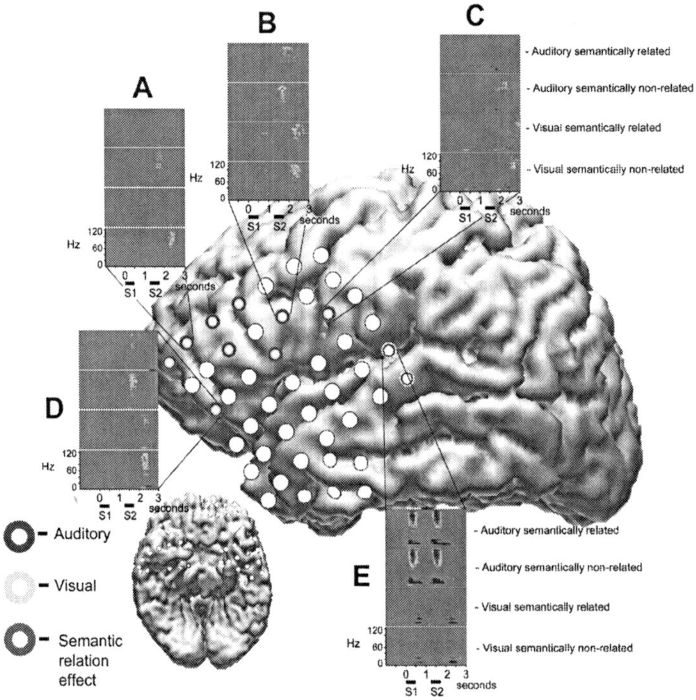

Figure 2. Left and bottom view of a subject brain image (co-registration of pre-operative 3D-MRI and post-implantation CT scan). Electrodes are shown as white disks. Red circles denote sites with differential high gamma activity (HGA, >70 Hz) between semantically related pairs and non-related pairs. Blue and yellow circles denote HGA to auditory or visual stimuli respectively. Representative time-frequency plots A-E are presented. Sites A-D show an effect of semantic relatedness. Non-related word pairs are associated with greater HGA compared with semantically related stimuli, most apparent at late latencies. The latencies of HGA responses to visual stimuli are typically longer than those to auditory stimuli. Site E shows HGA responses and event-related desynchronization at lower (alpha/beta) frequencies almost exclusively during presentation of auditory (spoken) stimuli, with no difference based upon semantic relatedness. Note that the only site with responses confined to visual stimuli was located over occipital-temporal cortex.

To investigate the clinical utility of high gamma ERS for mapping language cortex, we recently compared its spatial patterns during picture naming with ESM maps of naming in the same clinical subjects undergoing epilepsy surgery (Sinai, Bowers, et al., 2005b). ESM remains the gold standard for predicting postoperative functional impairment in these patients. However, ESM is often associated with afterdischarges and stimulated seizures, which sometimes preclude complete functional mapping of cortical regions to be resected. In addition, ESM must be done sequentially at pairs of electrodes, whereas subdural ECoG mapping can be done simultaneously at all electrode sites.

Subdural ECoG signals were recorded in 13 subjects while they verbally named sequentially presented line drawings of objects, and the resulting signals were analyzed for high gamma ERS (80-100 Hz) at each recording site using traditional band-pass-filtering. Routine clinical ESM mapping at each cortical site utilized a subset of the same naming stimuli used for ECoG. If ESM disrupted mouth-related motor function, i.e., if it affected the mouth, lips, or tongue, naming could not be tested with ESM at the same cortical site. The maps of language derived from ESM and high gamma ERS are illustrated for one subject in Fig. 3. Because naming during ECoG involved these

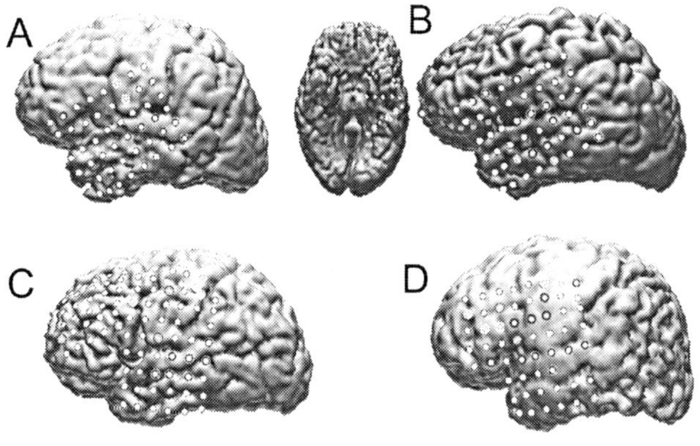

Figure 3. Examples of 4 patients with electrode grids over left hemisphere. High gamma responses are indexed with the same convention as in Figure 2. Most sites that show an effect of semantic relatedness were in inferior prefrontal regions and, in a few patients, in lateral temporal regions.

muscles of articulation, the sensitivity and specificity of ECoG high gamma ERS were estimated relative to both ESM-induced impairments of naming and disruption of mouth-related motor function by ESM. The average number of electrode sites with statistically significant high gamma ERS was 12 per patient. When sensitivity/specificity estimates were made separately in each patient for the 12 electrode sites with greatest high gamma ERS, the specificity of high gamma ERS with respect to ESM (the "gold standard") was 78% for naming and 81% for mouth-related motor function, whereas the equivalent sensitivities were 38% and 46%, respectively. When ESM maps of naming and mouth-related motor function were combined, the specificity and sensitivity of high gamma ERS with respect to ESM were 84% and 43%, respectively.

Although our study suggested that the sensitivity of high gamma ERS is too low to offer a replacement to the established ESM procedure, there were methodological limitations to our comparison of these two mapping techniques that might have biased our estimates of sensitivity/specificity (Sinai, Bowers, et al., 2005b). Furthermore, problems with the ESM procedure itself may limit its utility as a gold standard against which other mapping methods, including fMRI (Roux et al., 2003), are compared. Previous studies of ESM in motor cortex (Nii, Uematsu, Lesser, & Gordon, 1996) and language cortex (Krauss et al., 1996; Luders et al., 1991) have suggested that it may sometimes overestimate functionally critical cortex and underestimate cortex that is safe for resection. It is possible that ESM in a functionally silent region can impair function through a distant effect on eloquent cortex. This effect could take place by trans-synaptic interference with normal network activity in essential cortex and/or by diaschisis from deactivation of functionally interconnected cortex. Indeed, studies of afterdischarges during ESM have shown that they often spread to electrodes outside the immediate site of stimulation current (Blume et al., 2004; Lesser et al., 1984; Motamedi et al., 2002). In addition to the effects of afterdischarges in distant cortical regions, there is a more general potential for ESM to exert distant effects outside the stimulating current field. Matsumoto et al. (2004) recently found that single pulses at intensities typical for ESM produce cortical-cortical evoked potentials (CCEPs) at sites several centimeters away from the stimulating electrodes.

The apparently low sensitivity of high gamma ERS with respect to ESM in our study could have also resulted from a limitation in the sensitivity of subdural ECoG recordings for high gamma activity. This is an important consideration given the low amplitude of high gamma activity both at baseline and during cortical activation. Because the amplitudes of field potential oscillations logarithmically decline with increasing frequency, it is assumed that as the frequency of these oscillations increases, the neuronal aggregates generating them are smaller and/or more dispersed (Menon et al., 1996; Singer, 1993). Thus, it is possible that the spatial sampling of subdural electrode grids (1-cm center-to-center) is inadequate for capturing all event-related gamma activity, and that some of this activity is "falling between the cracks."

Another potential limitation of high gamma ERS for both clinical and research applications, is that interpretation of its magnitude is problematic. There can be no *a priori* knowledge of what magnitude of ERS is indicative of cortical processing or more fundamentally, of how much cortical processing is necessary and sufficient for function. Like fMRI and other activation-based techniques, ECoG activation mapping requires the setting of a threshold that must be derived either empirically or arbitrarily. Beyond these theoretical considerations, however, the basic methods for calculating event-related changes in signal energy are also problematic with respect to gamma ERS. Because ERS is calculated as a ratio or percentage of signal energy in baseline and activated epochs, the magnitude of ERS depends on the energy of activity in the baseline, which is typically very low for gamma frequencies (Pfurtscheller, Graimann, Huggins, Levine, & Schuh, 2003).

Most experimental data from animals on gamma oscillations have emphasized their role in the dynamic formation of neuronal assemblies allowing parallel distributed processing within and across functional anatomic domains. From these data it has been hypothesized that functional interactions between different cortical regions will be accompanied by gamma activity and that this gamma activity will demonstrate a coherent or causal relationship between interacting regions. This general hypothesis has been tested by many investigators using a variety of methods. Most of this work has focused on low gamma frequencies, especially 40 Hz. However, given the ECoG data on high gamma ERS at individual cortical sites, it is reasonable to question whether high gamma activity is also involved in interactions between these cortical sites.

Language processing during speech production likely requires the cooperation of distributed cortical resources in perisylvian regions of the dominant temporal, frontal, and parietal lobes. The short-time direct directed transfer function (SdDTF) was used to estimate event-related causal interactions between multiple ECoG signals during auditory word repetition and other speech production tasks (Korzeniewska, 2005). These studies have suggested that causal interactions between cortical regions do occur at high gamma frequencies and that different word production tasks are associated with different patterns of interactions. These interactions can be distinguished by the latencies and frequencies at which they occur, the cortical regions involved, and the directionality of causal influences between regions. Future studies utilizing multi-channel ECoG analyses are expected to provide additional information about dynamic interactions across distributed cortical networks during language and other cognitive operations, as well as the role of gamma oscillations in these interactions.

4. CONCLUSIONS

ECoG recordings from intracranial electrodes in humans are possible only under unusual clinical circumstances. Research studies utilizing these recordings generally do not pose additional risks to clinical subjects and may provide valuable insights into human brain physiology. In the study of linguistic processing this is exceptional opportunity to investigate the brain "in action" from close proximity. The superior spatial resolution and signal-to-noise ratio of invasive recordings allow more detailed investigations of electrophysiological phenomena previously observed with noninvasive EEG recordings. In addition, invasive EEG studies have allowed the discovery of event-related responses in gamma frequencies that were previously undisclosed by scalp EEG.

Results of the studies of high gamma ERS to date suggest its role as an index of cortical activation with functional response properties that distinguish it from those of event-related potentials and other event-related spectral changes, e.g., ERD/ERS in alpha, beta, theta, and even low gamma (30-50 Hz) bands. Compared to ERD/ERS in alpha and beta bands, high gamma ERS appears to occur in spatial and temporal patterns that are more discrete and more consistent with the putative location and timing of task-related cortical activation. The response properties of ERS in high gamma frequencies (greater than ~60 Hz) also appear to be distinct from those of ERS in low gamma frequencies, but the dividing line between these two phenomena is not yet clear.

Because high gamma ERS has now been observed in several different functional neuroanatomical domains with relatively consistent functional response properties, it is tempting to generalize to other, yet unexplored domains and to postulate that it is a general purpose index of cortical activation. However, it still remains to be determined whether the functional properties of this particular index will vary with the cytoarchitectonics, functional connectivity, and types of processing in different cortical regions. The neuronal elements and neurophysiological mechanisms specifically responsible for high gamma ERS are yet to be elucidated and will likely require additional studies in animals. However, based upon previous studies of gamma activity in animals, it seems reasonable to speculate that high gamma activity in humans is generated by the cooperative activity of distributed neuronal assemblies engaged in cortical information processing. The broadband nature of high gamma ERS could potentially reflect the aggregate activity of many such neuronal assemblies operating in parallel at more or less distinct frequencies. Our preliminary studies of event-related causal interactions among ECoG signals also suggest that activity, and perhaps information, is transmitted across neural networks in a variety of frequencies in the high gamma range.

ECoG high gamma ERS has a potential clinical applications to patients undergoing surgery for epilepsy. In addition its research applications may extend our ability to understand brain functionality, particularly in the language domain. Nevertheless, there is still a need for improved techniques of both recording and analysis of the data. It is also necessary to compare the functional mapping results with other imaging techniques (e.g., fMRI) and to better understand the physiological significance of this oscillations. With further improvements in ECoG recording and analysis, high gamma ERS could make it a useful index of cortical activation in brain-computer interfaces utilizing implanted subdural electrodes (Leuthardt et al., 2004).

High gamma ERS applications in both clinical and research settings would be vastly expanded if it could be recorded non-invasively. Recent studies using MEG suggest that this may be possible (Kaiser & Lutzenberger, 2004; Bauer, Oostenveld, Peeters, & Fries,

2006). If so, the questions generated by invasive ECoG studies of high gamma ERS, e.g., its generalizability as an index of cortical processing in normal humans across different functional neuroanatomic domains, may be more fully addressed.

5. ACKNOWLEDGEMENTS

The work reviewed herein was done at Johns Hopkins University under the supervision of Nathan E. Crone and was supported by NINDS R01 NS040596 with Dr, Crone as the principal investigator. The authors wish to thank Piotr Franaszczuk, for his fundamental assistance in developing the analysis methods.

ABBREVIATIONS

EEG = electroencephalography; ECoG = electrocorticography; ESM = electrocortical stimulation mapping; fMRI = functional magnetic resonance imaging; MEG = magneto-encephalography; ERD/ERS = event-related desynchronization/event-related synchronization.

REFERENCES

Akay, M., & Daubenspeck, J. A. (1999). Investigating the contamination of electro-encephalograms by facial muscle electromyographic activity using matching pursuit. *Brain and Language*, *66*, 184-200.

Anderson, J. E., & Holcomb, P. J. (1995). Auditory and visual semantic priming using different stimulus onset asynchronies: an event-related brain potential study. *Psychophysiology*, *32*, 177-90.

Andrew, C., & Pfurtscheller, G. (1996). Event-related coherence as a tool for studying dynamic interaction of brain regions. *Electroencephalography and Clinical Neurophysiology*, *98*, 144-148.

Bauer, M., Oostenveld, R., Peeters, M., & Fries, P. (2006). Tactile spatial attention enhances gamma-band activity in somatosensory cortex and reduces low-frequency activity in parieto-occipital areas. *The Journal of Neuroscience, 26*, 490-501.

Binder, J. R., Frost, J. A., Hammeke, T. A., Cox, R. W., Rao, S. M., & Prieto, T. (1997). Human Brain Language Areas Identified by Functional Magnetic Resonance Imaging. *The Journal of Neuroscience, 17*, 353-362.

Blume, W. T., Jones, D. C., & Pathak, P. (2004). Properties of after-discharges from cortical electrical stimulation in focal epilepsies. *Clinical Neurophysiology*, *115*, 982-989.

Booth, J. R., Burman, D. D., Meyer, J. R., Gitelman, D. R., Parrish, T. B., & Mesulam, M. M. (2002). Modality independence of word comprehension. *Human Brain Mapping*, *16*, 251-61.

Bragin, A., Engel, J., Jr., Wilson, C. L., Fried, I., & Buzsaki, G. (1999). High-frequency oscillations in human brain. *Hippocampus*, *9*, 137-142.

Brosch, M., Budinger, E., & Scheich, H. (2002). Stimulus-related gamma oscillations in primate auditory cortex. *Journal of Neurophysiology, 87*, 2715-2725.

Buckner, R. L., Koutstaal, W., Schacter, D. L., & Rosen, B. R. (2000). Functional MRI evidence for a role of frontal and inferior temporal cortex in amodal components of priming. *Brain, 123*, 620-640.

Chee, M. W., O'Craven, K. M., Bergida, R., Rosen, B. R., & Savoy, R. L. (1999). Auditory and visual word processing studied with fMRI. *Human Brain Mapping, 7*, 15-28.

Cooper, R., Winter, A. L., Crow, H. J., & Walter, W. G. (1965). Comparison of subcortical, cortical and scalp activity using chronically indwelling electrodes in man. *Electroencephalography and Clinical Neurophysiology, 18*, 217-228.

Crone, N. E., Boatman, D., Gordon, B., & Hao, L. (2001a). Induced electrocorticographic gamma activity during auditory perception. *Clinical Neurophysiology, 112,* 565-582.

Crone, N. E., & Hao, L. (2002). Functional dynamics of spoken and signed word production: A case study using electrocorticographic spectral analysis. *Aphasiology, 16*, 903-926.

Crone, N. E., Hao, L., Hart, J., Jr., Boatman, D., Lesser, R. P., Irizarry, R., & Gordon, B. (2001b). Electrocorticographic gamma activity during word production in spoken and sign language. *Neurology, 57*, 2045-2053.

Crone, N. E., Hart, J., Jr., Boatman, D., Lesser, R. P., & Gordon, B. (1994). Regional cortical activation during language and related tasks identified by direct cortical electrical recording. *Brain and Language, 47*, 466-468.

Crone, N. E., Miglioretti, D. L., Gordon, B., & Lesser, R. P. (1998a). Functional mapping of human sensorimotor cortex with electrocorticographic spectral analysis. II. Event-related synchronization in the gamma band. *Brain, 121*, 2301-2315.

Crone, N. E., Miglioretti, D. L., Gordon, B., Sieracki, J. M., Wilson, M. T., Uematsu, S., & Lesser, R. P. (1998b). Functional mapping of human sensorimotor cortex with electrocorticographic spectral analysis. I. Alpha and beta event-related desynchronization. *Brain, 121*, 2271-2299.

Crone, N. E., Sinai, A., & Korzeniewska, A. (2006). Chapter 19 High-frequency gamma oscillations and human brain mapping with electrocorticography. *Progress in Brain Research, 159*, 275-95.

Eckhorn, R., Bauer, R., Jordan, W., Brosch, M., Kruse, W., Munk, M., et al. (1988). Coherent oscillations: A mechanism of feature linking in the visual cortex? Multiple electrode and correlation analyses in the cat. *Biological Cybernetics, 60*, 121-130.

Edwards, E., Soltani, M., Deouell, L.Y., Berger, M. S., & Knight, R. T. (2005). High gamma activity in response to deviant auditory stimuli recorded directly from human cortex. *Journal of Neurophysiology, 94*, 4269-4280.

Engel, A. K., Konig, P., Kreiter, A. K., Schillen, T. B., & Singer, W. (1992). Temporal coding in the visual cortex: new vistas on integration in the nervous system. [Review]. *Trends in Neurosciences, 15*, 218-226.

Federmeier, K. D., & Kutas, M. (2001). Meaning and modality: influences of context, semantic memory organization, and perceptual predictability on picture processing. *Journal of Experimental Psychology. Learning, Memory and Cognition, 27*, 202-24.

Fitzgibbon, S. P., Pope, K. J., Mackenzie, L., Clark, C. R., & Willoughby, J. O. (2004). Cognitive tasks augment gamma EEG power. *Clinical Neurophysiology, 115*, 1802-9.

Freeman, W. J. (1978). Spatial properties of an EEG event in the olfactory bulb and cortex. *Electroencephalography and Clinical Neurophysiology, 44*, 586-605.

Freeman, W. J., & Barrie, J. M. (2000). Analysis of spatial patterns of phase in neocortical gamma EEGs in rabbit. *Journal of Neurophysiology, 84*, 1266-78.

Friederici, A. D., Opitz, B., & von Cramon, D. Y. (2000). Segregating semantic and syntactic aspects of processing in the human brain: an fMRI investigation of different word types. *Cerebral Cortex, 10*, 698-705.

Frost, J. A., Binder, J. R., Springer, J. A., Hammeke, T. A., Bellgowan, P. S., Rao, S. M., et al. (1999). Language processing is strongly left lateralized in both sexes. Evidence from functional MRI. *Brain, 122(Pt. 2)*, 199-208.

Gabrieli, J. D., Poldrack, R. A., & Desmond, J. E. (1998). The role of left prefrontal cortex in language and memory. *Proceedings of the National Academy of Sciences of the United States of America, 95*, 906-13.

Gevins, A., Cutillo, B., Desmond, J., Ward, M., Bressler, S., Barbero, N., et al. (1994). Subdural grid recordings of distributed neocortical networks involved with somatosensory discrimination. *Electroencephalography and Clinical Neurophysiology, 92*, 282-290.

Ginter, J., Jr., Blinowska, K. J., Kaminski, M., Durka, P. J., Pfurtscheller, G., & Neuper, C. (2005). Propagation of EEG activity in the beta and gamma band during movement imagery in humans. *Methods of Information in Medicine, 44*, 106-113.

Gomes, H. W., Ritter, V. C., Tartter, H. G., Vaughan Jr., & Rosen, J. J. (1997). Lexical processing of visually and auditorily presented nouns and verbs: evidence from reaction time and N400 priming data. *Cognitive Brain Research, 6*, 121-134.

Gray, C. M. (1994). Synchronous oscillations in neuronal systems: mechanisms and functions. *Journal of Computational Neurosciences, 1*, 11-38.

Gray, C. M. (1999). The temporal correlation hypothesis of visual feature integration: still alive and well. *Neuron, 24*, 31-47, 111-125.

Gray, C. M., König, P., Engel, A. K., & Singer, W. (1989). Oscillatory responses in cat visual cortex exhibit inter-columnar synchronization which reflects global stimulus properties. *Nature, 338*, 334-337.

Hagoort, P., & Brown, C. M. (2000). ERP effects of listening to speech: semantic ERP effects. *Neuropsychologia, 38*, 1518-30.

Halgren, E., Baudena, P., Heit, G., Clarke, J. M., Marinkovic, K., & Clarke, M. (1994). Spatio-temporal stages in face and word processing. I. Depth-recorded potentials in the human occipital, temporal and parietal lobes [corrected]. *Journal of Physiology Paris, 88*, 1-50.

Holcomb, P. J. (1988). Automatic and attentional processing: an event-related brain potential analysis of semantic priming. *Brain and Language, 35*, 66-85.

Kaiser, J., & Lutzenberger, W. (2004). Frontal gamma-band activity in magneto-encephalogram during auditory oddball processing. *Neuroreport, 15*, 2185-2188.

Kaiser, J., Lutzenberger, W., Ackermann, H., & Birbaumer, N. (2002). Dynamics of gamma-band activity induced by auditory pattern changes in humans. *Cerebral Cortex, 12*, 212-221.

Klimesch, W. (1999). EEG alpha and theta oscillations reflect cognitive and memory performance: a review and analysis. *Brain Research Review, 29*, 169-195.

Korzeniewska, A., Kus, R., Franaszczuk, P., Crainiceanu, C., & Crone, N. E. (2005). Dynamic high-gamma interactions during language-related task performance. *Epilepsia, 46*, 312-324.

Krause, C. M., Lang, A. H., Laine, M., Kuusisto, M., & Porn, B. (1996). Event-related EEG desynchronization and synchronization during an auditory memory task. *Electro-encephalography and Clinical Neurophysiology, 98*, 319-326.

Krauss, G. L., Fisher, R., Plate, C., Hart, J., Uematsu, S., Gordon, B., et al. (1996). Cognitive effects of resecting basal temporal language areas. *Epilepsia, 37*, 476-483.

Kutas, M., & Federmeier, K. D. (2000). Electrophysiology reveals semantic memory use in language comprehension. *Trends in Cognitive Sciences, 4*, 463-470.

Kutas, M., & Hillyard, S. A. (1980). Reading senseless sentences: brain potentials reflect semantic incongruity. *Science, 207*, 203-205.

Lebrun, N., Clochon, P., Etevenon, P., Baron, J. C., & Eustache, F. (1998). Effect of environmental sound familiarity on dynamic neural activation/inhibition patterns: an ERD mapping study. *Neuroimage, 8*, 79-92.

Lesser, R. P., Lüders, H., Klem, G., Dinner, D. S., Morris, H. H., & Hahn, J. (1984). Cortical afterdischarge and functional response thresholds: results of extraoperative testing. *Epilepsia, 25*, 615-621.

Leuthardt, E. C., Schalk, G., Wolpaw, J. R., Ojemann, J. G., & Moran, D. W. (2004). A brain-computer interface using electrocorticographic signals in humans. *Journal of Neural Engineering, 1*, 63-71.

Lopes da Silva, F. (1991). Neural mechanisms underlying brain waves: from neural membranes to networks. *Electroencephalography and Clinical Neurophysiology, 79,* 81-93.

Loring, D. W., & Sheer, D. E. (1984). Laterality of 40 Hz EEG and EMG during cognitive performance. *Psychophysiology, 21*, 34-38.

Luders, H., Lesser, R. P., Hahn, J., Dinner, D. S., Morris, H. H., Wyllie, E., et al. (1991). Basal temporal language area. *Brain, 114*, 743-754.

Marques, J. F. (2006). Specialization and semantic organization: evidence for multiple semantics linked to sensory modalities. *Memory & Cognition, 34*, 60-7.

Matsumoto, R., Nair, D. R., LaPresto, E., Najm, I., Bingaman, W., Shibasaki, H., et al. (2004). Functional connectivity in the human language system: a cortico-cortical evoked potential study. *Brain, 127*, 2316-2330.

McCarthy, G., Nobre, A. C., Bentin, S., & Spencer, D. D. (1995). Language-related field potentials in the anterior-medial temporal lobe: I. Intracranial distribution and neural generators. *Journal of Neuroscience, 15*, 1080-9.

Menon, V., Freeman, W. J., Cutillo, B. A., Desmond, J. E., Ward, M. F., Bressler, S. L., et al. (1996). Spatio-temporal correlations in human gamma band electrocorticograms. *Electroencephalography and Clinical Neurophysiology, 98*, 89-102.

Mesulam, M. M. (1990). Large-scale neurocognitive networks and distributed processing for attention, language, and memory. *Annals of Neurology, 28*, 597-613.

Motamedi, G. K., Lesser, R. P., Miglioretti, D. L., Mizuno-Matsumoto, Y., Gordon, B., Webber, W. R., et al. (2002). Optimizing parameters for terminating cortical afterdischarges with pulse stimulation. *Epilepsia, 43*, 836-846.

Murthy, V. N., & Fetz, E. E. (1992). Coherent 25- to 35-Hz oscillations in the sensorimotor cortex of awake behaving monkeys. *Proceedings of the National Academy of Sciences of the United States of America, 89*, 5670-5674.

Nii, Y., Uematsu, S., Lesser, R. P., & Gordon, B. (1996). Does the central sulcus divide motor and sensory functions? Cortical mapping of human hand areas as revealed by electrical stimulation through subdural grid electrodes. *Neurology, 46,* 360-367.

Nobre, A., & G. McCarthy (1995). Language-related field potentials in the anterior-medial temporal lobe: II. Effects of word type and semantic priming. *Journal of Neuroscience, 15*, 1090-1098.

Ohara, S., Crone, N. E., Weiss, N., & Lenz, F. A. (2004). Attention to pain modulates electrocorticographic event-related desynchronization during cutaneous laser stimulation in humans. *Clinical Neurophysioogy, 115*, 1641-1652.

Ohara, S., Ikeda, A., Kunieda, T., Yazawa, S., Baba, K., Nagamine, T., et al. (2000). Movement-related change of electrocorticographic activity in human supplementary motor area proper. *Brain, 123*, 1203-1215.

Ojemann, G., Ojemann, J., Lettich, E., & Berger, M. (1989). Cortical language localization in left, dominant hemisphere. An electrical stimulation mapping investigation in 117 patients. *Journal of Neurosurgery, 71*, 316-326.

Pantev, C. (1995). Evoked and induced gamma-band activity of the human cortex. *Brain Topography, 7*, 321-330.

Perani, D., Schnur, T., Tettamanti, M., Gorno-Tempini, M., Cappa, S. F., & Fazio, F. (1999). Word and picture matching: a PET study of semantic category effects. *Neuropsychologia, 37*, 293-306.

Petersen, S. E., Fox, P. T., Posner, M. I., Mintun, M., & Raichle, M. E. (1988). Positron emission tomographic studies of the cortical anatomy of single-word processing, *Nature, 331*, 585-589

Pfurtscheller, G., & Aranibar, A. (1977). Event-related cortical desynchronization detected by power measurements of scalp EEG. *Electroencephalography and Clinical Neurophysiology, 42*, 817-826.

Pfurtscheller, G., & Berghold, A. (1989). Patterns of cortical activation during planning of voluntary movement. *Electroencephalography and Clinical Neurophysiology, 72,* 250-258.

Pfurtscheller, G., & Cooper, R. (1975). Frequency dependence of the transmission of the EEG from cortex to scalp. *Electroencephalography and Clinical Neurophysiology, 38,* 93-96.

Pfurtscheller, G., Graimann, B., Huggins, J. E., Levine, S. P., & Schuh, L. A. (2003). Spatiotemporal patterns of beta desynchronization and gamma synchronization in corticographic data during self-paced movement. *Clinical Neurophysiology, 114*, 1226-1236.

Pfurtscheller, G., & Lopes da Silva, F. H. (1999). Event-related EEG/MEG synchronization and desynchronization: basic principles. *Clinical Neurophysiology, 110*, 1842-1857.

Pfurtscheller, G., Flotzinger, D., & Neuper, C. (1994a). Differentiation between finger, toe and tongue movement in man based on 40 Hz EEG. *Electroencephalography and Clinical Neurophysiology, 90*, 456-460.

Pfurtscheller, G., Neuper, C., & Mohl, W. (1994b). Event-related desynchronization (ERD) during visual processing. *International Journal of Psychophysiology, 16*, 147-153.

Ray, S., Jouny, C. C., Crone, N. E., Boatman, D., Thakor, N. V., & Franaszczuk, P. J. (2003). Human ECoG analysis during speech perception using matching pursuit: a comparison between stochastic and dyadic dictionaries. *IEEE Transactions Biomedical Engineering, 50*, 1371-1373.

Roux, F. E., Boulanouar, K., Lotterie, J. A., Mejdoubi, M., LeSage, J. P., & Berry, I. (2003). Language functional magnetic resonance imaging in preoperative assessment of language areas: correlation with direct cortical stimulation. *Neurosurgery, 52*, 1335-1345; discussion, 1345-1337.

Sanes, J. N., & Donoghue, J. P. (1993). Oscillations in local field potentials of the primate motor cortex during voluntary movement. *Proceedings of the National Academy of Sciences of the United States of America, 90*, 4470-4474.

Simos, P. G., Basile, L. F., & Papanicolaou, A. C. (1997). Source localization of the N400 response in a sentence-reading paradigm using evoked magnetic fields and magnetic resonance imaging. *Brain Research, 762*, 29-39.

Sinai, A., Bowers, C. W., Crainiceanu, C. M., Boatman, D., Gordon, B., Lesser, R. P., et al. (2005b). Electrocorticographic high gamma activity versus electrical cortical stimulation mapping of naming. *Brain, 128*, 1556-1570.

Sinai, A., Franaszczuk, P., & Crone, N. E. (2005a). Electrocorticographic spectral responses during auditory vs. visual lexical semantic processing. *Epilepsia, 46*, 71-72.

Sinai, A., & Pratt, H. (2002). Electrophysiological evidence for priming in response to words and pseudowords in first and second language. *Brain and Language, 80*, 240-52.

Singer, W. (1993). Synchronization of cortical activity and its putative role in information processing and learning. *Annual Review of Physiology, 55*, 349-374.

Singer, W., & Gray, C. M. (1995) Visual feature integration and the temporal correlation hypothesis. *Annual Review of Neuroscience, 18*, 555-586.

Steriade, M., Gloor, P., Llinas, R., Lopes Da Silva, F. H., & Mesulam, M. M., (1990). Basic mechanisms of cerebral rhythmic activities. *Electroencephalography and Clinical Neurophysiology, 76*, 481-508.

Tallon-Baudry, C., Bertrand, O., Wienbruch, C., Ross, B., & Pantev, C. (1997). Combined EEG and MEG recordings of visual 40 Hz responses to illusory triangles in human. *Neuroreport, 8*, 1103-1107.

Van Petten, C., & Luka, B. J. (in press). Neural localization of semantic context effects in electromagnetic and hemodynamic studies. *Brain and Language*.
Vandenberghe, R., Price, C., Wise, R., Josephs O., & Frackowiak, R. S. (1996). Functional anatomy of a common semantic system for words and pictures. *Nature*, *383*, 254-6.
Von der Malsburg, C. (1995). Binding in models of perception and brain function. *Current Opinion in Neurobiology*, *5*, 520-526.
Zatorre, R. J., Evans, A. C., Meyer, E., & Gjedde, A. (1992). Lateralization of phonetic and pitch discrimination in speech processing. *Science*, *256*, 846-9.
Zhuang, P., Toro, C., Grafman, J., Manganotti, P., Leocani, L., & Hallett, M. (1997). Event-related desynchronization (ERD) in the alpha frequency during development of implicit and explicit learning. *Electroencephalography and Clinical Neurophysiology*, *102*, 374-381.
Zygierewicz, J., Durka, P. J., Klekowicz, H., Franaszczuk, P. J., & Crone, N. E. (2005). Computationally efficient approaches to calculating significant ERD/ERS changes in the time–frequency plane. *Journal of Neuroscience Methods*, *145*, 267-276.

INDEX

LITERACY STUDIES

1. Brain Research in Language — 978-0-387-74979-2
   Zvia Breznitz (Ed.)